CLEAN EATS

Also by Alejandro Junger

Clean

Clean Gut

CLEAN EATS

Over 200 Delicious Recipes to Reset Your
Body's Natural Balance and Discover What It
Means to Be Truly Healthy

Alejandro Junger, M.D.

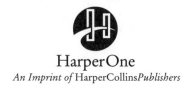

HarperOne
An Imprint of HarperCollinsPublishers

HarperOne

This book contains advice and information relating to health care. It should be used to supplement rather than replace the advice of your doctor or another trained health professional. If you know or suspect that you have a health problem, it is recommended that you seek your physician's advice before embarking on any medical program or treatment. All efforts have been made to assure the accuracy of the information contained in this book as of the date of publication. The publisher and the author disclaim liability for any medical outcomes that may occur as a result of applying the methods suggested in this book.

CLEAN EATS: *Over 200 Delicious Recipes to Reset Your Body's Natural Balance and Discover What It Means to Be Truly Healthy.* Copyright © 2014 by Alejandro Junger. All rights reserved. Printed in the United States of America. No part of this book may be used or reproduced in any manner whatsoever without written permission except in the case of brief quotations embodied in critical articles and reviews. For information, address HarperCollins Publishers, 195 Broadway, New York, NY 10007.

HarperCollins books may be purchased for educational, business, or sales promotional use. For information, please e-mail the Special Markets Department at SPsales@harpercollins.com.

HarperCollins website: http://www.harpercollins.com

HarperCollins®, ⏹®, and HarperOne™ are trademarks of HarperCollins Publishers.

FIRST EDITION

Interior Design by Laura Lind Design

Recipe photographs by Vanessa Stump

Library of Congress Cataloging-in-Publication Data.

Junger, Alejandro.
Clean eats: over 200 delicious recipes to reset your body's natural balance and discover what it means to be truly healthy / Alejandro Junger, M.D.—First edition.
    pages cm
    ISBN 978–0–06–232781–9
    ISBN 978–0–06–232783–3
    1. Detoxification (Health) I. Title.
    RA784.5.J87 2014
    641.5'63—dc23
                    2013051294

15 16 17 18   RRD(H)   10 9 8 7 6 5

Dedicated to all who teach that
food is medicine.

CONTENTS

Introduction   1

How to Use This Book   5

Creating Your Clean Kitchen   9

The Big Picture: Seven Essays on Clean Eating   23
    What Is Clean Eating?   24
    Food Is Information   26
    Cook More   28
    Master Five   30
    Money   31
    Community   33
    Live More   35

Recipes by Chef Frank Giglio   37
    Breakfast Ideas   41
    Salads, Sauces, and Dressings   63
    Sides, Starters, and Snacks   95
    Fish   133
    Poultry   155
    Meat   175
    Vegetables   191
    Soups and Stews   223
    Shakes, Elixirs, Drinks, and Tonics   245
    Desserts   267

Appendices

Our Programs   289

21-Day Clean Cleanse Meal Plan   291

21-Day Clean Gut Meal Plan   292

7-Day Clean Refresh Meal Plan   293
Contributors   295

Nutrient Analyses of Recipes   303

Acknowledgments   327

Index   329

INTRODUCTION

There is an old proverb: Give a man a fish and you will feed him for a day. Teach a man how to fish and you will feed him for a lifetime.

After many years of helping people become healthier, I know firsthand that what happens in the days and weeks following any health program can determine the long-term results. It can be the difference between looking and feeling amazing for just a few weeks and a complete health transformation that reverberates positively, affecting your family, friends, and community. That is why I am tremendously excited to share this book. These pages offer the tools, knowledge, and recipes to make eating *clean* part of your life for good.

Years ago, after moving to the United States from my native country, Uruguay, I got sick, really sick. The drastic change in lifestyle, especially in my diet, left me with severe allergies, irritable bowel syndrome, and depression. These three diagnoses led to my being prescribed seven medications indefinitely, which did not "feel right." So I started an intense search for a different, more natural solution. I tried everything I could find. My search took me around the world. I found many things that, alone or in combination, helped a great deal. But it wasn't until I stumbled upon the concepts and practices of cleansing and detoxification that I completely restored my health. Within ten days of an intense cleansing-detox program at the We Care Spa near Palm Springs, all my symptoms completely disappeared. Not only was I suddenly symptom-free, but I also felt and looked years younger.

In the days and weeks after the cleanse, everybody asked me what had changed. They wanted to do what I had done. I started guiding my family and friends through cleansing and detox programs that I designed, observed, and improved on. Soon after, my patients demanded the same. Wherever I went, I put people on cleansing programs.

After Palm Springs, I moved to Venice, California. The "cleansing wave" followed me wherever I went. I found a great property, three blocks from the beach, with three small craftsman cottages that shared a garden. I lived in one of them and my guests stayed in the other two. The cottages all had blenders, juicers, and water filters. My guests stayed for some time and followed the programs I designed for them. Soon my neighbors started stopping by. We prepared smoothies, juices, and all kinds of healthy foods. Many great chefs came by and prepared food for whoever was there at the time. And it was always packed with people. They started coming to me from all over the world.

Anyone who started a program would be glowing just a few days later, which prompted people to ask them what they had done. Next thing, their friends would show up in my Venice cottages, and then their friends. Everyone was welcome, and the results were astounding. Some had such a profound transformation that every-body noticed. Those people brought me their family and friends by the dozens. Or they went on to create their own wave of healthy living. Many of them became well known and are doing amazing work.

Day and night I discussed good nutrition, explaining the value of protein, fat, carbohydrates, fiber, minerals, and vitamins. I suggested books on nutrition and asked people to watch the many great educational movies about food from which I had learned myself. I suggested they buy a blender, a juicer, and a few other tools that I use every day. Countless times I went with patients to the supermarket to help them shop, and to the natural pharmacy to help them choose the right supplements.

No matter the specific results, as they came to the end of their programs, every single patient asked, "So, Doc, now what? How do I keep the results? What do I eat? How do I prepare healthy meals?"

Clean eating isn't just one thing. It is not a straightforward list of foods to eat and not eat. It is a way of thinking about food and how it makes us feel. Clean eating does have a foundation based on whole foods, but what makes it work is personalization. It can't be as simple as "just stay away from gluten" or "stop eating sugar forever." I'm not a fan of gluten, and I know processed sugar isn't healthy, but blanket statements like that don't give us the tools we need for our complicated lives. What we need is template recipes to get us started but also strategies to help us figure out what works for us in the long term.

So I started showing people what to eat and how to prepare it. Or I told them to come and learn from the great chefs that continually visited the cottages. This was the most effective way of helping people maintain the benefits of a cleanse, and it often went way beyond what they had already achieved. People started taking notes, and so did I. After collecting a number of recipes, I started sharing recipes by e-mail. These were passed around and soon a community grew, discussing, changing, and developing recipes.

These days my team and the community are much larger, and we are all still collecting and coming up with great recipes. My friend, the talented chef Frank Giglio, has prepared 180 recipes inspired by the Clean community. We also have many fantastic recipes contributed by our community of friends. These dishes not only taste great but also provide the nutritional punch that will help your body thrive. Whether you are using this book to help you through one of our programs or whether you are totally new to Clean, you'll find the recipes in this book simple and straightforward.

In addition to the recipes, the book offers some amazing insights from my team members Dhru Purohit and John Rosania on the key principles to better navigating the world of food, cooking, and clean eating; some invaluable tips for setting up your kitchen; and several meal plan options for anyone wanting additional guidance.

Our goal is to make this book an important tool in your journey to lifelong health. Enjoy these recipes and, like the proverb we started with, happy fishing.

HOW TO USE THIS BOOK

This book is a celebration—a celebration of great-tasting food and of the power of whole foods to heal us. This book is also a tasty guide to taking back your health. By making the incredible meals developed by chef Frank Giglio and our guest contributors, you are upgrading the quality of your food with every bite. Recent nutritional science has taught us that food is not just calories; it is information. This information is telling our bodies how to run and which genes to turn on and off. With every dish prepared, smoothie blended, or salad created from this book, you are upgrading the quality of the information you are sending your body. We've seen it happen over and over again; when people eat clean, true health becomes a possibility. Our hope is that using this book will turn that possibility into a reality.

The Recipes: Gluten- and Dairy-Free

All the recipes in this book are made from whole plants and animals. We focus on unprocessed, organic ingredients, free of chemicals and preservatives. The recipes are also gluten- and dairy-free. We have removed gluten and dairy because we have found they are the two foods that give people the most trouble with their health. Simply removing gluten and dairy for a period of time can produce impressive health benefits. Let's recap some of the reasons why taking a break from these foods is beneficial.

The Problem with Gluten and Dairy

Gluten is the protein found in wheat and other cereal grains, such as barley, rye, spelt, and kamut. The list of syndromes and diseases associated with gluten sensitivity seem to be endless. It causes irritation and direct damage to the gut, contributing to a host of problems in the body. Gluten triggers autoimmune responses and thyroid issues and creates the conditions for leaky gut. Gluten sensitivity has been associated with chronic headaches, cancer, type 1 diabetes, neuropathy, and increased mortality rates. With our clients at Clean, we see gluten contribute directly to indigestion and bloating as well as fatigue and brain fog. While some people may have a serious allergy to wheat, nearly everyone has an immune response to it. This immune response can create a cascade of negative reactions that we are only beginning to understand. As opposed to foods like fish and vegetables, gluten-containing foods, such as cakes and cookies, are also more likely to be highly processed and contain chemicals, preservatives, and sugar.

Dairy has its own problems and can cause trouble for people even if they are not lactose intolerant.* The most common symptoms associated with dairy are sinus issues, postnasal drip, skin breakouts, allergies, ear infections, digestive distress, and constipation. Each person may tolerate dairy differently. Some people have difficulty with any dairy, while others can have dairy infrequently or in small amounts. It also may be the type of dairy that matters—cow's milk is out, but goat and sheep work fine.

Whatever your relationship to dairy or gluten, we have seen incredible health results by removing them for a period of time. While it may not be necessary for you

---

*For those of you who do well with dairy, we have indicated the recipes to which some dairy—such as feta cheese or ghee—can be added.

to remove these foods completely from your diet, we think having a trove of great recipes that don't include them bypasses the potential problems these foods can cause and is a real asset to your health.

Icons Explained

Throughout this book you will see three different icons appear on the recipes. Each of these icons provides details about what is in the recipe and how it can be used.

C **Cleanse:** When you see this icon, it means the recipe is suitable for use during our twenty-one-day Clean Cleanse program. The Clean Cleanse is explained in *Clean: The Revolutionary Program to Restore the Body's Natural Ability to Heal Itself*. The program focuses on supporting the body's continuous process of cleansing and detoxification. You can find out more about this program in the appendix (see page 289).

G **Gut:** This icon means the recipe is appropriate for our twenty-one-day Clean Gut program. This program expands on the work of the cleanse and focuses on gut repair and digestive health. In my book *Clean Gut* I explain how the root of almost all chronic diseases, from heart disease to cancer to depression, can be traced back to an injured gut (see page 289 for more information).

V **Vegan:** If you see this icon, the recipe is completely free of animal products. Even if you're new to vegan cooking, don't be shy. These meals are a great way to add more tasty and nutrient-dense plant foods to your diet.

Guest Contributors

There's no one way to eat clean. That is why in addition to chef Frank Giglio's recipes we asked a few of our friends to share their favorite clean meals. These guest contributors come from all walks of life. They're mothers, fathers, coaches, actors, doctors, businesspeople, humanitarians, and more. We included them in the book not only because they're part of our community but also because their personal take on food just might inspire you to make clean eating your own.

CREATING YOUR CLEAN KITCHEN

In my parents' house in Uruguay, where I grew up, the kitchen was the heart and belly of our house. We had breakfast, lunch, and dinner in the kitchen, which had a table as big as the one in the dining room. The latter was much fancier, but we all preferred the kitchen. We also snacked there, and in my late teens, I met my two sisters there countless times at five A.M. after returning from dance parties. We would then tell each other about our night's adventures and prepare elaborate snacks.

Our appreciation of cooking, and eating together in the kitchen, came from our parents. My father especially loved making food. He also loved having people over to enjoy it. One tradition he brought to Uruguay from his hometown in Hungary was preparing goulash for the family. The goulash took three full days to prepare. By the time it was done cooking, we were so excited because we knew how delicious it was going to be. Our neighbors were excited too, and every year more and more of them would show up to feast on my father's masterpiece.

One weekend, after coming home from playing with my friends, I saw a fleet of black cars parked outside my house. A dozen men were there, all dressed in black suits with walkie-talkies in their hands. One of the men had a gun holstered on his waist. Something was obviously wrong. My heart started pounding and I ran into my house ready to fight. I heard noises in the kitchen, so I went there first. And there, sitting in my favorite spot at the kitchen table, having a plate of my dad's famous goulash, was the president of Uruguay.

Oh, if my childhood kitchen could talk . . .

Today, as a father, I have continued the tradition of keeping the kitchen as the heart and belly of our house. And as a doctor, I have taken it one step further. My kitchen is the main pharmacy in my medical practice and the most important tool in my medical toolbox. I often see patients at my home, and after their consultation I always take them to my kitchen. I show them inside my fridge and teach them the important role food plays in their health. If we have time, we even make a few simple recipes together. Right before they leave, I tell them something very important. I tell them that the path to vibrant health starts in the kitchen, and that setting up their clean kitchen is the best way to support their long-term health goals.

Clean Kitchen

A clean kitchen is the heart and soul of your clean lifestyle. It is the space in your home where you keep the ingredients and tools you will need to make clean meals that nourish you and your entire family. Keeping your kitchen well stocked with the following items is one of the most important ways to make clean eating and cooking from scratch easy and fun. Having a wide variety of ingredients and condiments around will also take the stress out of preparing recipes that satisfy whatever taste you're craving at the moment.

We have included descriptions of how to buy and use the best-quality whole foods, which tools and cooking utensils are needed, and some essential clean cooking skills. Finally, we've listed the Clean team's favorite food items for you to try out and incorporate into your life.

Clean Foods

Produce

Fresh fruits and vegetables are the foundation of clean eating. Look to purchase a wide and colorful variety of organic, chemical-free produce. Stock up on inexpensive leafy greens, such as arugula, chard, collards, and kale. Carrots, turnips, and root vegetables are great for adding density to a meal. Keep fresh onions, garlic, ginger, and herbs, such as basil, parsley, thyme, and dill, around to make it easy to add flavor to meals. Finally, keeping fresh produce on the kitchen counter or in a hanging basket will encourage you to eat it more frequently.

Meat

Purchase good-quality meat: grass-fed, organic, and pasture-raised. Chicken, turkey, beef, and lamb are easily found, but duck, goat, wild game, and rabbit can make interesting additions to your meals. Meat can be bought in bulk from farmers' markets and stored in the freezer. Animal organs are inexpensive and nutrient-dense, and they can be used in soups and turned into pâtés. Bones are great for making gut-healing bone broths and stews.

Fish

When it comes to fish, smaller cold-water fish are good options because they contain fewer heavy metals and toxins. Consider eating salmon, trout, mackerel, sardines, herring, and small halibut. Whole wild-caught fish can be expensive, so supplement with canned fish (and look for "wild-caught" on the label). Canned anchovies, sardines, and salmon are good sources of omega-3 fatty acids, vitamin D, and protein. When not doing one of the Clean programs, shellfish like shrimp, crab, clams, and oysters can also be a good source of lean protein, minerals, and iodine.

Eggs

Eggs are one of nature's most nutrient-dense foods and a relatively inexpensive source of protein. Look for organic and pasture-raised eggs. Pasture-raised varieties contain lower amounts of pro-inflammatory omega-6 fatty acids and higher amounts of omega-3, vitamins A and E, and beta-carotene.

Dairy

We haven't included any recipes in this book that include dairy because it's one of the whole foods that gives people the most trouble.* Skin and digestive issues, constipation, and excess mucus are some of the common symptoms. However, if you have tested dairy and found that it works for you, small amounts can give a meal that extra flair and flavor. There are many different kinds of dairy. We recommend organic varieties, free of added vitamins. Some people do better with raw dairy, while others have found goat and sheep (both unpasteurized and pasteurized) work best for them. Cooking with butter and ghee produced from grass-fed cows can also be a great way to add nutrient-rich fats to your diet, but only if dairy does not cause you issues.

Grains

We do not include grains that contain gluten in any of our recipes. Gluten is the protein found in grains such as wheat, rye, and barley and has been associated with an almost endless list of syndromes and diseases. However, non-gluten grains, such as quinoa, millet, amaranth, buckwheat, and rice, can be great additions to one's diet. Having these inexpensive foods around the kitchen can be very useful in making all types of gluten-free breads, pancakes, and side dishes. Soaking the grains for a few hours before cooking can make them easier to digest.

Beans and Legumes

Beans, legumes, and lentils are all useful sources of quality calories and protein. Having a variety of these ingredients in the pantry can make stews and soups more hearty and add protein to vegetarian dishes. For some people, beans and legumes can be difficult to digest and often produce gas and bloating. Soaking and thoroughly cooking them can help with these difficulties. It's a good idea to test these foods to see how much or how little makes you feel the best.

Starches

Starches, such as rice, potatoes, sweet potatoes, yams, winter squash, taro, and plantains, can make great side plates to meals. They are also helpful and nourishing during

---

*Some recipes suggest where you can add dairy if it is a food that works for you.

periods of increased exercise, when more carbohydrates can be tolerated. Sweet potatoes and rice can also be used to create delicious sugar- and gluten-free desserts.

Nuts and Seeds

Good sources of healthy fats and proteins, nuts and seeds contain a wide range of vitamins and minerals. Look for raw and toasted varieties free of preservatives, sugar, and seed oils. They make great snacks and can be used to make nondairy nut cheeses. A jar of nut or seed butter (almond, sesame, etc.) kept in the cabinet can be used to quickly create sauces and dips and thicken shakes and smoothies. However, nuts and seeds can often be difficult to digest. Soaking them for a few hours will help, or if you feel heavy after eating them, reduce the amount you include in your diet.

Oils and Fats

Our bodies need healthy fats for every system to function, especially our digestive system and brain. Look for organic expeller and cold-pressed, unrefined oils. Oils such as coconut oil, ghee, and lard are higher in saturated fats and best for medium-temperature cooking. Coconut oil is our recommendation as an all-purpose cooking oil and provides a good source of saturated fat. It is also a wonderful moisturizer and addition to shakes. Olive oil is good for medium-temperature cooking but is best used in salad dressings or as a condiment. Avocado oil has a high smoke point and is good for high-temperature cooking. Nut and seed oils, such as pumpkin and walnut, can provide essential fatty acids and nourishment but should not be used regularly for cooking because they are unstable at high temperatures and can turn rancid. Avoid oils high in polyunsaturated fats, such as soybean, peanut, corn, cottonseed, and canola.

Gluten-Free Flours

There is a whole world of gluten-free grains and flours out there. These can be used to make your own cakes, cookies, breads, and biscuits. Almond and coconut flours are higher in protein and fiber and lower in carbs. Rice, potato, and chickpea flours are other useful alternatives.

Herbs and Spices

To flavor our food, we choose herbs and spices that are organic and/or locally sourced from the huge array of plants and seeds growing on this earth. Spices do more than add to the taste and depth of our dishes. They can have medicinal and nutritional benefits too. For example, cinnamon helps slow our insulin response to sugar, while cayenne helps promote circulation. Ginger supports digestion, and turmeric is anti-inflammatory. The list goes on and on for every herb and spice you have in your pantry. Some of our other favorite medicinals are rosemary, black pepper, dill, and thyme. Herbs do lose their potency and flavor, so replace them every few months. Plus, look to supplement your dried herbs with fresh ones from time to time.

Salt
Salt is essential to the human body. We need it for adrenal function, digestion of proteins and carbohydrates, metabolism, and overall cellular function. Choose real sea salt such as Celtic or Maine (white or gray), or Himalayan (pink) salt for the highest mineral content. Avoid refined and bleached table salt with added chlorine and aluminum.

Sweeteners
We can enjoy small amounts of natural sweeteners from time to time. Our favorites are raw honey, maple syrup, coconut nectar, molasses, date sugar, stevia, xylitol, and Lakanto.

We suggest staying away from high-fructose corn syrup, agave nectar, and artificial sweeteners, which are made with chemicals.

Must-Haves for This Book

- *Almond Butter:* A wonderful and sweet peanut butter replacement, this works in smoothies, soups, sauces, cookies, or straight out of the jar.

- *Coconut Oil:* Coconut oil is an essential saturated fat that supports immune functioning, weight loss, and digestive health with additional antibacterial and antiviral properties. It's our main cooking oil.

- *Coconut Butter:* Made from the flesh of the coconut, coconut butter is thicker and creamier than coconut oil and perfect for smoothies or frostings. Or you can just eat it off the spoon for an energy boost.

- *Celtic Sea Salt or Himalayan Salt:* An essential seasoning agent, salt is present in just about every recipe, and having too much or too little can make or break a meal.

- *Coconut or Almond Milk:* A staple in clean cooking, these milks are something to always keep on hand for soups, dressings, sauces, desserts, shakes, and as thickeners. Buy them organic and unsweetened, or make your own.

- *Wheat-Free Tamari:* A gluten-free fermented soy sauce adds a wonderful salty flavor to many of our recipes.

- *Whole-Grain Mustard:* A very useful condiment, mustard can be used to create a quick, clean sauce or salad dressing. We like the varieties that are sugar-free and made with apple cider vinegar.

- *Balsamic Vinegar:* Another useful ingredient to always have on hand, this vinegar is one of our favorite all-around flavorings.

Clean Team Favorites

These are products our team loves keeping in the kitchen. They make great snacks and will enhance some of the recipes listed in this book.

- *Green Powders:* These handy powders are a useful way to add more mineral-rich food to your meals. You can add a scoop to salad dressings, smoothies, and even desserts like cookies, energy bars, or chocolate mousse.

- *Coconut Water:* An excellent source of natural electrolytes, with lots of potassium and a low natural sugar content, coconut water is nature's sports drink replacement. It's great in shakes or as a post-workout beverage.

- *Coconut Manna:* This is the flesh (and some oil) of the coconut, so you get extra fiber, protein, and saturated fat. It has a creamy and slightly sweet taste and is wonderful as a butter or frosting substitute.

- *Liquid Chlorophyll:* A natural internal cleanser and deodorizer, mint-flavored liquid chlorophyll is a tasty way to get a boost of nutrition into your shakes. Add it to a chocolate-flavored one and you'll make it taste like a mint chocolate milk shake.

- *Maca Powder:* This is a South American root ground into a powder and used for its health properties. Full of B vitamins, enzymes, and amino acids, it boosts stamina and libido, balances hormones, and has a great malty flavor that's wonderful in nut milk shakes or smoothies.

- *Yerba Maté:* This is an adaptogenic South American herb that's a great pick-me-up and a nervous-system support, leaving you energized but without the crash and acidity of coffee. We like to have it around for anyone who is removing coffee from his or her diet during one of our programs.

- *Kombucha:* Made from fermented mushrooms, kombucha adds healthy flora to your system and aids digestion. It's easy to make yourself but also easy to find at most supermarkets. It's deliciously sparkling and can even take the place of alcohol in festive drinks and cocktails.

- *Xylitol Chewing Gum:* This sugar-free gum supports dental health. Chewing gum after a meal encourages good digestion.

My Favorite Salad Toppings

When I make a salad, it's not just some lettuce and a few lonely vegetables. I fill it with loads of ingredients and toppings that add flavor and make each salad unique. Here are some of my favorite salad toppings.

- *Spirulina:* This blue-green algae is rich in protein and minerals and contains all essential amino acids.

- *Nutritional Yeast:* This deactivated yeast is rich in B vitamins and protein. It has a cheesy and nutty flavor.

- *Sea Salt:* There are a wide variety of flavored sea salts available, from smoked to rosemary to ginger.

- *Bragg Liquid Aminos:* This certified non-GMO protein concentrate is made from soybeans. It's gluten-free and has a salty flavor.

- *Apple Cider Vinegar:* Often considered the healthiest vinegar, unpasteurized apple cider vinegar is loaded with enzymes and aids digestion. You can also add a tablespoon to water with a dash of honey or stevia for a refreshing drink.

- *Olive Oil:* Look for organic, extra-virgin olive oil in dark glass bottles.

- *Seaweed:* Mineral-rich sea vegetables like dulse, kelp, or nori can be bought in strips, sheets, or powdered.

- *Dr. Schulze's SuperFood:* My favorite and best-tasting superfood powder, this product is full of organic vegetables, minerals, and nutrients.

- *Lucuma Powder:* This is a dried version of the lucuma fruit from Peru. It has a sweet maple-like taste.

- *Sesame Seeds:* These seeds make any salad more beautiful to look at, and they add a boost of calcium.

- *Freshly Squeezed Lemon Juice:* A classic in any salad, lemon juice adds just enough acidity to give it some kick.

Kitchen Tools

- *High-Speed Blender:* This is an essential tool for making smoothies, soups, sauces, dressings, desserts, and purées. There are many great ones on the market, but if you want the top of the line, something that can blend absolutely anything, go for a Vitamix or a Blendtec.

- *Food Processor:* Another kitchen tool for blending, this serves a different function than a blender. A food processor chops and mixes, but it's not meant for a lot of liquid. It's best for drier ingredients, such as crumbles or thicker sauces, pestos, and dressings.

- *Slow Cooker:* This cooking device is invaluable for busy families. It cooks or warms meals without you having to stand over the stove or keep the oven on. Safe to leave on overnight or while you're not home, a slow cooker is an incredibly convenient way to have warm meals ready when you're finished working, playing, or adventuring.

- *Large, Ovenproof Sauté Pan:* This is a tool no kitchen should be without. You can use this pan to make just about any meal on the stovetop or in the oven. Choose cast iron or stainless steel, and avoid Teflon or other nonstick surfaces. This pan and a good knife are the two most versatile and essential kitchen tools.

Utensils Under Twenty Dollars

- *Garlic Press:* The garlic press is one of those simple tools that makes life so much easier in the kitchen. Pop a clove in, squish, and out comes mashed garlic. No fine chopping needed. Use it for ginger too.

- *Microplane:* Every kitchen must have a microplane. Whether zesting citrus fruits or freshly grating nutmeg or cinnamon over a smoothie, the flavor created from this tool is priceless.

- *Vegetable Peeler:* We love the Kuhn Rikon Swiss peeler for its lightweight, ergonomic shape and long-lasting, sharp blade. The best part: it costs under five dollars. Pick up a few different colors and enjoy peeling with ease.

- *Strainer:* You will see fine-mesh strainers called for throughout this book. They come in various dimensions; we suggest you pick up both a small and a large one. These tools are very handy and really get those small bits out of your puréed soups, sauces, and smoothies.

- *Cutting Board:* Besides having a solid chopping block, a few smaller boards will always have a use in your clean kitchen.

- *Mini Offset Spatula:* These inexpensive spatulas are perfect for decorating cakes, portioning out cookie dough, or scraping batter from the sides of a bowl. A mini one is great, but you can use one of any size for smoothing the tops of dips, pâtés, or chocolates when you pour them into molds.

- *Stainless-Steel Ice Cream Scoops:* You will also see these called "portioning" scoops. They come in various sizes and are labeled with a number. Besides being used for ice cream, these are great whenever you need exact amounts. I use this tool to portion out cookie dough, fudge, and savory items like falafel batter and pesto.

Some Basic Skills

Soaking

Grains, beans, legumes, nuts, and seeds all contain anti-nutrients in the form of phytates and enzyme inhibitors. Consuming these foods in excess without properly preparing them can cause bloating and digestive issues. Soaking these foods deactivates the enzyme inhibitors and creates an easy-to-digest and nutrient-rich food. Although there are different soaking times for each type of ingredient, just remember that the smaller or less dense the item, the less soaking time required. The opposite is true for dense beans and nuts. They require more soaking time. Using warm water and an acidic medium is also beneficial. Add a splash of lemon juice or unpasteurized apple cider vinegar to your liquid.

Small seeds (sesame, sunflower, pumpkin seeds, etc.) should soak 1 to 2 hours. Dense beans and legumes (almonds, dry beans, rice, chickpeas, etc.) should soak 8 to 12 hours. Once your items are soaked, use them right away or drain well and store in the fridge for up to three days. It may be helpful to rinse them each day while they are stored.

> *TIP: Do your soaking before bed. Gather your ingredients and place them in glass bowls or jars. Cover them with water, by at least 1 inch or more as they will absorb a lot of liquid, and soak overnight. When you're ready in the morning, drain and rinse them, then refill with water if your ingredient requires more soaking time.*

Dry Roasting

Dry roasting (or toasting) nuts, seeds, and spices helps to release naturally present oils and bring out more flavor. You can roast them in an oven (350°F) or in a dry sauté pan. Without overcrowding them, place the seeds, whole spices, or nuts into a sauté pan over medium heat or on a baking sheet in the oven. Once the pan warms up, shake it continuously until everything turns golden brown. This happens quickly, so keep an eye on the pan to make sure they don't burn. If you're roasting them in the oven, keep a close watch and stir them frequently, again making sure they don't burn.

Infusions vs. Decoctions

Making a daily herbal tea is a simple way to take in the health benefits of herbs. There are two ways to draw out the medicinal qualities from your herbs: infusions and decoctions.

An infusion is the process of extracting chemical compounds from plant material via water, oil, or alcohol. For a daily tea, we use water. Boil 1 quart of water and pour it into a glass jar that contains 2 tablespoons of dried herbs (4 tablespoons fresh). Cover it with a tight-fitting lid, then allow it to steep for 10 minutes to 8 hours. The longer you steep your herbs, the more medicinal properties will be extracted. Infusions are ideal for making tea from the leaves of a plant that contains volatile compounds. Short brewing times allow for these compounds to be retained. For general purposes, a 15-minute steep before consuming is great, but if you become a regular tea drinker, you can plan ahead and do your infusions overnight. This will allow enough time to fully extract your herbs. Your infusion can then be strained and reheated as needed.

A decoction is another method of extraction used for the roots, stems, barks, and rhizomes of a plant. This term can also refer to cooking methods. When you make a chicken stock, you are essentially making a decoction from the bones and aromatics in the water. Before decocting, the plant material is often mashed to provide more surface area and to release more of the volatile compounds. A proper decoction is boiled for about 1 hour using a 2-tablespoons-dried-herb to 1-quart-water ratio. Because of the long cooking process, we recommend using a high-quality pot. Heavy-bottom stainless-steel pots are ideal, since the materials in the pan will not leach into your simmering liquid. A slow cooker is a very simple and inexpensive alternative. Try to find a brand that does not use lead in its glaze.

Elixirs

In the "Shakes, Elixirs, Drinks, and Tonics" section (page 245) you will see that elixirs use the technique of smoothie making and combine with herbal infusions to create a warm medicinal beverage. Add a base of warm or cold herbal tea to your blender along with some flavorings and spices, a fat, and finally a sweetener. Once you get comfortable with the formula, you can start making drinks using herbs designed for your specific needs and health issues.

Here are a few examples of elixir ingredients.

- *Base:* mushroom tea, nettle infusion, peppermint, hibiscus, dandelion, horsetail

- *Flavorings:* chocolate powder, cinnamon, nutmeg, allspice, vanilla, mesquite meal, lucuma powder

- *Fats:* coconut oil, coconut cream, hemp seeds, cashews, almonds, brazil nuts, cacao butter

- *Sweeteners:* stevia, coconut nectar, maple syrup, honey

THE BIG PICTURE: SEVEN ESSAYS ON CLEAN EATING

Dhru Purohit and John Rosania

Today, we have more access to health information than ever before. These essays will give you direction to help cut through the noise and learn how to make clean eating your own.

What Is Clean Eating?

Clean eating isn't a list of foods to eat and not to eat. It isn't a stringent approach to what's on your plate. And it certainly isn't a diet. Clean eating is a perspective, a way to help you make better decisions about which foods you consume each day.

For some of us, we labeled ourselves as "vegetarian" or "paleo" for a period of time, tried a few weeks as a macrobiotic, or took a shot at Atkins. Others of us have never tried to describe how we eat; we just want to know how to eat "healthily." The problem with strict diets is they rarely give us broad enough tools to account for the real diversity of how we eat throughout the year. And the problem with just eating "healthily" is this word has been so overused by food companies that it lacks any useful meaning.

When we look at what is happening around us, we see that people are less attached to diets and diet definitions. They're realizing that the "perfect" or "optimal" diets doctors and health gurus are selling are overhyped and often fail. More and more, people use terms like "clean" and "whole foods" to describe how they eat. Then they mention a few foods they try to stay away from or that don't work well for them.

This changing way we talk about healthy diets can be used to help define what it means to eat clean.

Clean eating begins with the simple idea of eating whole foods as the primary foods in your diet. This idea is something that all doctors and health gurus can agree upon. They may not agree on which foods or how much, but across the board, they agree that whole, unprocessed plants and animals are an essential element for health.

So let's get clear about what we mean by "whole foods." They're foods found in nature and made of one ingredient. You find them at your local farmers' market or on the outer edges of the supermarket. Fruits, vegetables, leafy greens, meat, fish, nuts, and seeds are some examples.

Whole foods are the foundation of clean eating. They're your home base, the foods to focus on daily and to return to when you're not feeling your best. There are no magic bullets or perfect diets needed—just simple, clean, whole foods. The idea isn't the sexiest. But maybe our search for the next sexy diet is one of the reasons why we've become so confused about how to eat. Sexy may sell, but clean eating works.

When we eat primarily whole foods, we've automatically removed most of the junk foods, sodas, preservatives, and chemicals that are flooding our food supply. This alone is a huge step in the right direction and might by itself, over time, clear up our health issues.

But there's still one caveat. This is the second part of what clean eating means: some whole foods can cause us trouble. Remember, we're not talking about junk foods or the processed foods we know don't help our health. We're talking about the *whole foods* that may not make us feel our best. When we start getting into the whole foods that might create challenges for us, we start to see why there are so many different diets. Each person is a little bit different, and each person develops his or her own approach. In our opinion, though, the fundamentals seem to stay the same for everyone: eat whole foods, but what the foods are, and how much, will differ from person to person.

We call the whole foods that give us problems "toxic triggers." These foods can cause indigestion, bloating, inflammation, skin issues, fatigue, and a whole host of health challenges. The more we continue to eat them, the more we may experience health issues, even if we're primarily eating a diet of whole foods.

While not everyone has the same toxic triggers, we do see patterns. Within the whole foods context, gluten and dairy rank among the most problematic for the most people. After that, toxic triggers are manifested on a person-by-person basis. Whatever the whole food is, for one person it's God's gift, while for another person it's a stomachache. We'd love to be able to tell you which foods to avoid, but the reality is that getting clear on your toxic triggers requires some personal testing. There's no one diet that will solve it for you. You'll need to experiment and play around to see which whole foods help you feel the best. This is a process that takes time and helps to explain why a diet may work incredibly well for some people and not at all for others. The interplay between toxic triggers and our bodies just makes some diets and ways of eating not work for us, regardless of what we've been told.

So let's recap. Clean eating means two things: eating whole foods and staying away from your toxic triggers. Once you've consistently put these ideas into practice and found the foods that work for you, you're in a great place. Your food choices, tastes, and preferences will most likely change over time, but the foundation of clean eating stays the same. It's something you can depend on and use to make real food choices in the world. "Is it a whole food?" "Is it one of my toxic triggers?" No longer do we have to stick to one rigid diet or try to make choices based on some vague notion of "healthy" or "natural."

Clean eating is an idea whose time has come, an idea that guides us toward a life of great meals and great health.

Food Is Information

Food is more than just calories; it's information. And that information plays a much greater role than just providing us fuel for energy. Every bite we eat contains information that tells our genes how to express themselves. Food literally has the ability to turn our "good" genes on and our "bad" genes off. This is called "gene expression" and the study of it is known as epigenetics.

Think of your genes as the hardware and the food you eat as the software. Even if your hardware is great, downloading crappy software will slow your system down. It could even cause your system to crash. That's exactly what is happening today. Eating low-quality and toxic food is not just making people gain weight; it's also causing increased rates of autoimmune issues, infertility, heart disease, autism, and diabetes.[1]

It's amazing to think that even today, we still have doctors telling their patients that cancer has nothing to do with what they eat and nutritionists telling their clients that there is no difference between the calories from a bagel and the calories from a salad. It's no wonder that so many people think food is just a collection of proteins, fats, and carbohydrates. And that the definition of health is simply a slim waistline, regardless of how you feel. And that the best form of cancer prevention is being born with better genes or waiting for some miracle pill.

The role food plays in telling our bodies how to "show up" is deep. Every year, through new research, we're learning that the relationship is even deeper than we could have ever imagined.

Let's take phytonutrients, for example. They are found in nature's most colorful foods, such as blueberries and dark, leafy greens. They are natural chemicals that protect plants from bad bacteria and bugs. Many studies have found that phytonutrients provide our bodies with the beneficial information needed to reduce inflammation, increase immune function, and even improve memory.[2] When phytonutrients are missing from our diets, it's no different from when a computer is running an outdated operating system—things break and the operating system becomes weak.

On the flip side, vegetable oils, which are high in omega-6 polyunsaturated fatty acids (PUFAs), are examples of foods that can contain harmful information. These oils are often seen as healthy because they are called "vegetable" oils, but this couldn't be further from the truth. The reality is that oils like corn oil, canola oil, soybean oil, sunflower oil, and safflower oil are highly fragile and produce toxic compounds in the body. These compounds, like free radicals, have been associated with a range of health problems, such as cancer and heart disease. When we cook with these oils, instead of stable oils like coconut oil, we're sending our bodies tiny bits of information that move us further away from health.

Phytonutrients send one type of information, unstable vegetable oils send another, and everything we eat is telling our genes how to express themselves. When we see food as a delivery mechanism for information, and not just as a fuel source, we begin to make better food choices. Our awareness opens up and we start asking ourselves, "What information am I providing my body?"

1. Loren Cordain, S. Boyd Eaton, Anthony Sebastian, Neil Mann, Staffan Lindeberg, Bruce A. Watkins, James H. O'Keefe, and Janette Brand-Miller, "Origins and Evolution of the Western Diet: Health Implications for the 21st Century," http://ajcn.nutrition.org/content/81/2/341.abstract.

2. Jessica Maki, Brigham and Women's Hospital Communications, Harvard Medical School, "Berries Keep Your Brain Sharp," http://news.harvard.edu/gazette/story/2012/04/berries-keep-your-brain-sharp/.

Cook More

We're working more and cooking less. Since the 1960s, Americans have put in an extra 150 hours per year at work. At the same time we've reduced our hours in the kitchen by 40 percent.[1] What are the health effects of these broad cultural changes? By cooking less, we end up buying more prepared, processed, and increasingly cheaper packaged foods to make up the difference. Or we're eating out or on the run. Either way we look at it, cooking less means we're outsourcing our health to food companies, restaurants owners, fast-food joints, and delis. In fact, dietary data indicates that each meal away from home adds over 130 calories and lowers diet quality.[2] It also increases our intake of fat and sugar and decreases the amount of vegetables and whole grains.[3]

So what happens when we flip our priorities and place our attention back on making our own food? Cooking more clean food for ourselves takes back control of *what* we eat and *how* it's prepared. By purchasing whole, organic foods, we limit our exposure to chemicals and preservatives used to keep packaged items shelf-stable. And by cooking more meals at home, we reduce our exposure to restaurants using poor-quality ingredients and cooking with poor-quality oils. Over time, the simple act of cooking more can become one of our most powerful health strategies. No complicated protocols or supplements, no doctors' waiting rooms or expensive tests this time. Just a few clean recipes and your motivation to put them to use.

Now, you might be saying, "How am I supposed to do that when I'm already so busy?" The thing is, we're not saying that it's necessary to cook every meal at home. In fact, studies have shown that it takes just an extra hour a week of cooking or replacing two away meals with home-cooked meals to shed weight and increase the quality of your diet.[4] It's these small changes that, over time, produce huge benefits. A few meals a week turns into hundreds of meals a year and thousands of meals over a lifetime, not to mention all of the unhealthy meals you haven't consumed. When looked at from this perspective, cooking your own clean food is quite possibly the most important strategy you have to reduce health issues and continue to build robust health into the future.

Cooking more also does something else. It brings more attention to the food we're eating. When we cook clean foods at home, we take a moment to slow down and focus on the simple task of creating a nourishing meal. Think about how good it feels to cook a meal that tastes great *and* is nourishing. Or think about a time when someone prepared you a healthy meal that also excited your taste buds. The flavors and experience of the food are heightened, all from giving the meal a little bit of attention. This attention can very quickly turn into a joy of cooking. For some people, this joy springs from the creative component of taste, touch, and smell, the blending of flavors and spices. For others, it's the knowledge that a meal was prepared with love for family and friends. Centenarians advise us to "find the joy in cooking," since one of the most common traits of people living past one hundred is their love of cooking.[5] Whatever the reason—whatever *your* reason—finding the joy of cooking is how clean eating becomes a sustainable and lifelong practice.

It doesn't have to happen overnight or all at once. Step by step, prepare a few more breakfasts here, a few more dinners there, substituting some homemade snacks for the cakes left at work. And before you know it, "cook more" becomes a habit, a compass to guide you in the minefield of junk food that surrounds us all. It is both a way out and a way in, into a life of more health, of more control over what you eat and how you eat it.

1. Michael Pollan, "Out of the Kitchen, Onto the Couch," *New York Times Magazine,* August 2, 2009, http://www.nytimes.com/2009/08/02/magazine/02cooking-t.html?pagewanted=all&_r=0.

2. Lisa Mancino and Christian A. Gregory, "Does More Cooking Mean Better Eating? Estimating the Relationship Between Time Spent in Food Preparation and Diet Quality," presented August 12–14, 2012, Annual Meeting, Agricultural and Applied Economics Association, Seattle, Washington, http://agecon search.umn.edu/bitstream/124025/2/Mancino%20Gregory--AAEA%202012.pdf.

3. Jessica E. Todd, Lisa Mancino, and Biing-Hwan Lin, "The Impact of Food Away from Home on Adult Diet Quality," Economic Research Report No. ERR-90, Economic Research Service, U.S. Department of Agriculture, February 2010, http://www.ers.usda.gov/Publications/ERR90/.

4. Mancino and Gregory, "Does More Cooking Mean Better Eating?"

5. Paul Jaminet and Shou-Ching Jaminet, *Perfect Health Diet* (New York: Scribner, 2012).

Master Five

Eating clean can seem confusing. According to one study, half of all Americans polled think it's easier to do their taxes than to eat healthfully.[1] If a food is unfamiliar to us or the preparation new, it can quickly push us outside our comfort zone. Even the initial enthusiasm to clean up our diet, to *live* healthily, can easily peter out when faced with a week of meals to prepare.

But the reality of clean eating is not so complicated. For most people, the bulk of their diets are made up of around five basic meals rotated seasonally. Think of soup and salad, chicken and rice, fish and veggies, even a burger and fries. They're the same meals made over and over again. The spices, sauces, and combinations may change, but the basic meal remains the same. It's exactly the same with clean eating.

Instead of worrying about complex recipes or eating clean forever, *just focus on mastering five healthy meals* to start. These five meals will make up the base of your diet, what you eat most of the time. You can change them around, add a new sauce or a different vegetable, but the structure of the meals will stay the same. In time, these five meals will become your creative templates, inspiration to invent a lifetime of your own clean recipes. They'll also become your health allies, friends you can turn to when you don't know what to eat or you feel you've fallen off track with your health. You can always build on your five core meals, but starting with just five ensures that you don't get overwhelmed or make learning clean recipes a bigger deal than it needs to be.

The final result is that your five meals will help you eat cleaner and more consistently. With more clean food in your diet, the long-term effect will be fuller and robust health.

Keep it simple. Master five.

1. http://www.foodinsight.org/Content/5519/IFICF_2012_FoodHealthSurvey.pdf

Money

One of the biggest criticisms of eating clean is the idea that clean food is expensive and unaffordable. In a time where expenses are going up and more families are struggling with their monthly budget, is it really fair to expect people to spend more money on clean eating?

The challenge with a lot of the criticism is that it is often misguided. Sure, if we compare the immediate cost of eating clean to the immediate cost of eating crap, eating crap will almost always be cheaper, there's no doubt about it. But that's only part of the story. When it comes to calculating the price of food there are two things to consider. First, what's the immediate cost, the price tag, on the item? And second, what's the true cost, the long-term impact of our food choices? Let's explore them both.

Getting Sick Is Expensive

We've all heard about the mortgage crisis, but have you heard of the medical bill crisis? Unpaid medical bills are the number one cause of bankruptcy today. In 2013 over 20 percent of Americans reported significant challenges paying their medical bills and more than 1.7 million of them filed for bankruptcy.[1] And while universal insurance will help, it isn't expected to fix the problem. Medical costs are rising so quickly that even those with insurance are finding it hard to keep up. Considering that most chronic diseases are preventable by better food and lifestyle choices, it's safe to say that getting sick is much more expensive than eating clean.

Whole Foods, Not Packaged Foods

A few years ago Whole Foods Market, the natural foods grocery chain, was given an unflattering nickname, a name that has stuck even today. The nickname "Whole Paycheck" came from the sticker shock many people experienced at the checkout register. But if you hang out at the register at most natural food stores across America, including Whole Foods, you'll notice something interesting. The majority of foods that drive up the checkout total aren't whole fruits, vegetables, and meats. The foods that cost the most are processed or boutique health foods like organic kettle cooked chips, strawberry-melon kombucha, gluten-free oatmeal cookies, and raw food maca bars. Don't get us wrong, these foods taste great, but a diet of packaged natural foods isn't what clean eating is all about. Clean eating is about focusing on a solid foundation of fruits, veggies, natural meats, and other whole foods. When we spend our hard-earned money on these items, instead of on packaged health foods, we'll see an immediate drop in our grocery bills.

Eat In

Here's an easy way to cut your food expenses: eat in. Today it is estimated that over 40 percent of our food budget is spent eating outside the home.[2] Restaurants, regardless of whether they are healthy, are expensive. Depending on restaurants, even clean ones, to make almost half of our meals is one of the easiest ways to ensure that we'll break the monthly food budget. When we're not reliant on restaurants and the prepared food buffet at our local natural food store, clean eating becomes extremely affordable.

Understanding Why

Type the phrase "eating healthy on a budget" into Google and you'll find thousands of articles, tips, and tricks that will show you, in detail, how to eat clean in an affordable way. Some of these tips include joining a community-supported agriculture club, avoiding expensive out-of-season produce, starting a small container garden, and preparing weekly meals in bulk. All these tips are great, and there are a thousand more online just like them. What we've found, however, is that if we don't understand why clean eating matters, we'll never make it a priority and we won't put these tips to work. When we get educated about health and wellness, and the true costs of our food choices, we'll be more inspired to make clean eating a reality and see it as one of the best investments we can make in our long-term health.

1. NerdWallet Health finds medical bankruptcy accounts for majority of personal bankruptcies: http://www.nerdwallet.com/blog/health/2013/06/19/nerdwallet-health-study-estimates-56-million-americans-65-struggle-medical-bills-2013/.

2. Over 40 percent of the typical American food budget is spent on eating out, with family meals often being relegated to holidays and special occasions: http://www.sciencedaily.com/releases/2012/04/120423184157.htm.

Community

The communities we grow up in teach us how to live and what to eat. We learn about food from those around us and eat whatever they eat. In the past, we lived in tribes and small groups and our lifestyle and food choices were also governed by these groups. We would gather and hunt together, and cook and eat the same foods together.

Today, we still eat mostly whatever our community eats. But instead of eating the food of medieval farmers, or our hunter-gatherer ancestors, we're eating the processed food of our twenty-first-century default culture. And this is producing some serious health consequences for us.

We are living with more health problems and chronic diseases than ever before. From heart disease to autoimmune conditions to diabetes, these issues are a direct consequence of lifestyle choices of our community. Processed food, chemical-laden products, sedentary living, lack of sleep, and chronic stress are the currency our default community trades, and we are all the poorer for it.

But there is a way out of this situation. There are communities that serve our needs better. The way out is to go beyond our default community and consciously join up with people who share our interest in health and wellness. When we actively engage in a community of people who value wellness, we gain the support we need to get out of the health rut our default culture has fallen into.

What is it about community that makes it such a powerful tool for our health? A community gives us a forum to explore and learn about best practices. It's a place to share stories, recipes, and information, and learn the skills to live a clean lifestyle. It's also a place where we can find accountability. We can ask our community to help us stay on track with whatever health practice we are working on. In our experience, people who are supported by a purposeful community find it easier to make significant and lasting changes to their health.

Most of all, though, community provides us with connection and a sense of belonging. Who hasn't had the experience of sharing a new health practice with family or friends only to be ridiculed? When this happens, we can feel like an outsider and can quickly lose the enthusiasm and motivation to take care of ourselves. It's then easier to outsource our health to someone else, to food companies and organizations who often care more about their bottom line than our well-being. But a consciously chosen community can turn this loss of enthusiasm around and give us the energy and inspiration to continually recommit to living clean each day.

Feel free to start small. Join a clean eating community online. Share some clean recipes with a friend. Make a plan to eat one lunch or dinner together each week. Then expand and try hosting a meet-up or potluck. Invite other people in your area who are interested in clean eating. Just one potluck here and there is enough to make you feel rejuvenated and connected for weeks to come. Technology has created more possibilities than ever before to connect and engage with people of similar interests. Use these to improve your health and expand your community.

So whether it's a virtual or physical community, an email list or a potluck, begin to actively cultivate your community now. In the end, we may have been part of a default community, but we're not stuck there. We can actively choose to create a newer and cleaner one where we can grow year after year.

Live More

When food starts working for us, instead of against us, our entire life changes. Not only do we feel better meal to meal and day to day, but we also have the lasting energy and health we need to show up strong for the areas of life that we care about most.

Clean eating is a vehicle, an approach, that helps make food work for us. But it is also much bigger than that. It is a way of thinking that helps us move away from the fear around aging and getting ill, and moves us toward the strength of knowing that we can take control of our health.

Even the Centers for Disease Control and Prevention's very conservative estimates tell us that more than 60 percent of the leading causes of death are preventable. Heart disease, stroke, most cancers, and diabetes are all examples of leading killers that are preventable through lifestyle changes. Clean eating alone isn't the answer, but it is a major part of the solution to preventing chronic disease and feeling better day to day. Without a doubt, clean eating helps us live more.

Living more means that we have the ability to give love and attention to the priorities in our life. When we're feeling unhealthy, sick, or tired, it's hard to show up fully for ourselves and others. But when we feel grounded in our health, we have the energy to stay active, explore new hobbies, work on new projects, or volunteer our time to our favorite nonprofit.

Clean eating is not just about upgrading our food. Clean eating is about upgrading our entire life. Clean eating is about living more.

RECIPES BY CHEF FRANK GIGLIO

Ever since I was a young boy, cooking has been of interest to me. I can still taste the aroma of tomato sauce that filled my home as it simmered for hours. Watching my Italian grandparents cook instilled a passion that would demand I go deeper. Culinary school was a natural choice for me, and after graduation, I took the opportunity to travel the United States, learning from great chefs along the way. As a chef, I was always taught to make food taste good, without ever paying attention to how it made us feel. Somewhere along the line I stopped seeing my health as a priority until I hit a personal rock bottom. I was sluggish, overweight, and lacking a true connection to my career.

After this heavy moment, I embarked on a personal journey toward health and vitality. I began experimenting with diets, went to nutrition school, and learned what worked and didn't work for me. Each health program had its pros and cons, but I took the best parts and incorporated them into my life.

Ultimately, I landed on the important idea that it was the farm-fresh whole foods that helped me thrive, not the restrictive diets. Pairing these with daily exercise, positive relationships, and clean water, I developed a recipe for success.

Today I live off the grid with my wife and son in central Maine, where we share clean eating with our surrounding community. For me, clean eating is less about what you can't eat and more about all the foods you can eat. It has become about building a community around you and, most important, as Dr. Junger teaches, that food is our medicine.

With Dr. Junger's inspiration and my twenty years of culinary experience, we've put together a collection of recipes that are delicious, fun to prepare, and good for you. My goal is to inspire a culinary revolution within you, to inspire you to craft the foods that will bring forth a vigorous and harmonious lifestyle.

Think like a Chef

Before we get started, here are five skills to bring out your inner chef:

Plan

If there is one thing I learned in culinary school, it is the power of planning. There are two lists I use that will help you save time and money. The first is your weekly meal planner. Spend a few minutes planning what you are going to eat for the week. This may include simply having a few breakfast options stocked in the pantry and then planning out your dinners, or putting together a full three-meal seven-day calendar. Then, prepare a grocery list *before* you head to the farmers' market or grocery store. This will keep you from stumbling around the aisles and wasting time. Both of these planning techniques are simple but essential to making clean food more often.

Prep

There's nothing that helps to create a smooth cooking experience more than prepping your ingredients before you start. Doing this helps to ensure you don't get halfway through your recipe before realizing you are missing an ingredient. I notice that when everything is prepped and ready to go, a calm is created in the kitchen that allows me to savor and enjoy what I'm doing. Prepping and organizing are also easy ways to include children in the process and teach them the basics of clean cooking.

Taste

It's amazing to think that many people don't taste their food throughout the cooking process. I can't imagine anything more satisfying. This simple idea could easily save more than a few recipes from the trash can. By frequently tasting the food and sauces you are preparing, you learn how flavors develop and how to balance the basic tastes. Sweet, sour, salty, bitter, and umami all have specific characteristics that can be neutralized, balanced, or accented based on your personal preference. But you won't learn to recognize this if you don't give a taste to everything you make.

Improvise

It is easy to get attached to following recipe instructions or using the exact ingredients. At first, this works great as you hone your skills and discover which foods you like best. But over time, letting your intuition guide you in the kitchen can lift your recipes to a whole new level. The more you cook with whole foods, the more you can improvise and let the recipes serve as guides rather than hard-and-fast rules. Improvising based on your taste and what's fresh and available at your market will go a long way in developing your own inner chef and unique clean cooking style.

Experiment

In my opinion, cooking is an art form. And like any good art form, it develops and progresses by practicing *and* experimenting. When you take a chance and experiment with a new ingredient or spice, you open up new possibilities. Taking chances is an important skill as you develop as a clean chef. Once you've gotten through the first four skills, challenge yourself in the kitchen by trying a new flavor or dish each week. This will not only help you develop your own unique cooking style but also help you discover your favorite dish to make and your favorite dishes to eat.

BREAKFAST IDEAS

How you feel during the day has a lot to do with what you eat for breakfast. It's similar to how putting on certain clothing can change how you feel about yourself. When you start the morning with a clean breakfast, you're setting yourself up for better eating habits throughout the day. It might seem strange at first to make breakfast without gluten and dairy, but we promise you that these protein-packed, clean versions of classic breakfast dishes will satisfy and energize you.

BUCKWHEAT GRANOLA

C Cleanse

V Vegan

Makes: ½ gallon

Prep time: overnight

Cooking time: 4 to 6 hours if cooking, up to 24 hours if dehydrating

This recipe takes some time to make, but it's well worth it. Crunchy and full of flavor, this gluten-free granola will keep the whole family energized and ready to enjoy whatever the day holds. This is a nice break from traditional granola made with oats and also gives smoothies or coconut yogurt a delicious added crunch. Also perfect for grain- and dairy-free parfaits.

3 cups buckwheat groats, soaked for 2 hours, then rinsed in a strainer until the water runs clear
1½ cups raw pumpkin seeds, soaked overnight, drained, and rinsed
1½ cups raw sunflower seeds, soaked overnight, drained, and rinsed
1½ cups raw almonds, soaked overnight, drained, and rinsed
3 crisp apples
¼ cup mesquite meal
¼ cup ground cinnamon
¾ cup shredded unsweetened coconut
1½ cups coconut nectar
2 teaspoons sea salt

Soak the groats, seeds, and nuts the night before you wish to prepare the recipe. Once they are drained and rinsed, process them in several batches, if necessary, in a food processor. Roughly pulse them to break them up, but stop before they are completely blended. You don't want them puréed; just roughly chopped. Repeat until all the groats, seeds, and nuts are processed, then place them in a large bowl and set aside.

Wash and grate the apples, adding them to the groat, seed, and nut mixture. Stir to combine, then add the mesquite meal, cinnamon, coconut, coconut nectar, and salt. Combine thoroughly.

If you have a dehydrator, you can spread the mixture in a thin layer over the screens and dehydrate it at 200°F for 6 to 8 hours, or until crisp.

If you do not have a dehydrator, preheat the oven to 275°F.

Spread the mixture onto a parchment-lined baking sheet or baking dish and bake it for 4 to 6 hours, or until crisp. Once crisp, store the granola in an airtight container. It will keep for several weeks.

QUINOA AND SUGAR PUMPKIN PORRIDGE

C Cleanse

V Vegan

Serves: 2

Prep time: overnight

Cooking time: 30 minutes

A seasonal twist and nutritional upgrade to traditional oatmeal, this porridge is warm and comforting, making it perfect for a chilly morning. Pumpkin is a complex carbohydrate and quinoa is a great protein source, so this meal is also a stellar post-workout recovery meal.

½ cup quinoa
½ teaspoon lemon juice
1 cup unsweetened coconut milk
¾ cup pumpkin purée (canned will work, freshly cooked is ideal)
1 tablespoon mesquite meal
½ teaspoon ground cinnamon
¼ teaspoon ground ginger
¼ teaspoon vanilla bean powder or ½ teaspoon vanilla extract
Pinch of sea salt
2 tablespoons coconut nectar or maple syrup

Garnish
Chopped pecans
Toasted unsweetened coconut flakes
Freshly grated nutmeg
¼ cup fresh blueberries

Before you make this dish, soak the quinoa in 2 cups of water with a ½ teaspoon of lemon juice. Allow the quinoa to soak for a minimum of 8 hours (overnight works well). Strain, rinse well, and set aside.

In a heavy-bottomed sauce pot set over medium heat, combine the quinoa, coconut milk, pumpkin purée, mesquite meal, cinnamon, ginger, vanilla bean powder or extract, and salt. Simmer the mixture for about 20 minutes, or until the quinoa is tender and the coconut milk thickens, stirring often to prevent sticking and burning.

Once fully cooked, stir in the coconut nectar or maple syrup. Pour the porridge into a bowl, garnish it with the pecans, coconut flakes, nutmeg, and blueberries, and serve.

Variations: Feel free to replace the quinoa with millet, amaranth, or rice.

BLUEBERRY QUINOA CEREAL

Lina Fedirko, Clean community member

Ⓒ Cleanse

Ⓖ Gut*

Ⓥ Vegan

Serves: 4

I love this recipe for its convenience. After doing the Clean Cleanse program, it's very easy to slip into old habits and not find time to prepare meals. I make sure to make my breakfast quinoa on Monday so I can eat it for the next few days. It helps me keep my breakfast clean and healthy.

1 cup quinoa, rinsed well
1 cup unsweetened almond milk
1¼ cups unsweetened coconut milk
⅔ cup fresh blueberries
Coconut yogurt or coconut milk cream to taste
Sweetener of your choice to taste

In a saucepan, combine the quinoa, almond milk, coconut milk, and blueberries. Bring the mixture to a boil, then lower the heat and simmer it for 30 minutes, or until it is very tender. Serve the cereal warm with coconut yogurt or coconut milk cream and a drizzle of sweetener. Enjoy!

Variations: This cereal is great with banana, if you are not doing the cleanse.

*For sweetener, use stevia, xylitol, or Lakarto

EXPERIENCE: The Clean program changed my life in such a positive way that I will always be in deep gratitude to Dr. Junger and the Clean team. I completed my first Clean Cleanse program last October and then completed the Clean Gut program in April. I went from getting sick three to four times a year and taking antibiotics each time, having constant eczema episodes all over my hands, never cooking and always eating out, and having constant indigestion issues to rarely getting sick, cooking all my beautifully healthy meals, and having no signs of eczema (didn't think that was possible!) or stomach issues. Clean really taught me how to be kind to my stomach and how to take care of my body.

CASHEW YOGURT

C Cleanse

G Gut

V Vegan

Makes: 1 pint

Prep time: 15 minutes

Fermentation time: 8 to 24 hours

A delicious replacement for dairy-based yogurt, this cashew version is easy to digest and works with a variety of sweet and savory recipes. For a breakfast treat, top yogurt with a sprinkle of granola and fresh berries.

1½ cups raw cashews
¾ to 1¼ cups water

In a blender, purée the cashews with ¾ cup of the water, adding more water as needed to achieve a thick but spreadable consistency. Scoop the mixture into a glass mason jar, then cover it with cheesecloth and allow to sit in a warm place for 8 or more hours. The yogurt is finished once you see tiny air pockets spread throughout the mixture. Eat immediately, or store it in a jar in the fridge for three to four days.

Pairings: Serve with Buckwheat Granola (page 42), Blackberry Cobbler (page 268), or crumbles, or use it in smoothies.

BLUEBERRY PANCAKES

Vegetarian*

Serves: 4

Prep time: 10 minutes

Cooking time: 10 minutes

Whether eaten for breakfast or warmed up in a toaster oven as a snack, these pancakes are sure to bring smiles to every face around the table.

1¾ cups brown rice flour
¼ cup buckwheat flour
¼ cup almond flour
¼ cup tapioca starch
1 tablespoon coconut flour
1 teaspoon ground cinnamon
¼ cup coconut palm sugar
1½ teaspoons baking powder
½ teaspoon sea salt
2 large pasture-raised eggs
½ cup frozen or fresh blueberries
1 cup unsweetened almond milk
1 cup water
¼ cup coconut oil, melted, plus more for the skillet
1 teaspoon vanilla extract
Coconut nectar or maple syrup to taste

In a large bowl, stir together the brown rice flour, buckwheat flour, almond flour, tapioca starch, coconut flour, cinnamon, coconut palm sugar, baking powder, and salt. In a separate bowl, whisk the eggs, then stir in the blueberries, almond milk, water, coconut oil, and vanilla. Pour the wet ingredients over the dry ingredients, and stir until the mixture is just incorporated.

Heat a large skillet over medium heat. Melt a few tablespoons of coconut oil, then spoon ¼-cup portions of the batter into the pan, cooking each pancake for 2 to 3 minutes before flipping and cooking for an additional 1 to 2 minutes. You want each side to be golden brown. Serve warm, topped with a drizzle of coconut nectar or maple syrup.

*Contains eggs

Chef Frank on Gluten-Free Flours

While I generally see baked goods and refined-flour products as something to use only as an occasional treat, there are ways to make them healthier. My favorite flours to use are coconut and almond, because they are high in protein and fiber and lower in carbohydrates. Coconut flour is very absorbent, so make sure to adjust and add more liquid when using it. There are also lots of other gluten-free flours you can try, such as teff, brown rice, chestnut, sorghum, and millet. Each has its own quality and will slightly change the texture of a recipe. Many gluten-free flour mixes have corn and potato, which are fine in small amounts as long as you're not on the Clean Cleanse or Clean Gut programs.

FRENCH TOAST WITH VANILLA CREAM

Vegetarian*

Serves: 2

Prep time: 10 minutes

Cooking time: 5 minutes

For breakfast or brunch, this French toast is insanely good. You can make large batches to keep in the freezer and warm up as the best toast ever. This treat makes the ordinary extraordinary.

For the French Toast
4 pasture-raised eggs
½ cup unsweetened coconut milk
2 teaspoons ground cinnamon
½ teaspoon ground allspice
¼ teaspoon ground clove
½ teaspoon freshly ground nutmeg
Up to ¼ cup coconut oil
2 to 3 slices gluten-free bread per person (Sami's Bakery millet bread is our favorite
      clean brand)

For the Vanilla Cream
3 ounces unsweetened coconut milk
1 teaspoon vanilla extract
½ cup coconut cream (in a can)
1 to 2 tablespoons coconut nectar
Pinch of sea salt

First, make the vanilla cream. Slowly warm the coconut milk, vanilla, coconut cream, coconut nectar, and salt until the coconut cream melts and the sauce thickens. Keep this mixture warm while prepping the rest.

Whisk together the eggs, coconut milk, and spices in a large shallow dish.

Heat a large skillet or griddle over medium heat and melt a few tablespoons of coconut oil in it. While the skillet warms, transfer four slices of bread into the egg mixture (if your dish allows it; if not, do however many you can at a time) and allow both sides to absorb a lot of the moisture. Carefully transfer the bread slices onto the skillet and cook until golden brown (you can check the bottoms by lifting with a spatula) before flipping and cooking the other side for an additional few minutes.

Once cooked through, cut each slice of bread in half, top with fresh berries, and drizzle with the vanilla cream.

*Contains eggs

Chef Frank on Saturated Fats

You'll notice we use saturated fats for most of our cooked recipes rather than vegetable oils. It's because fat from pasture-raised animals such as lard and duck fat, along with avocado and coconut oil, stay stable at medium-high temperatures, reducing free radicals in the body. These fats are the healthiest cooking choices and provide usable energy. They also boost immunity, aid digestion, and help brain function. Save olive and other vegetable oils for low-temperature cooking, use in vinaigrettes, or drizzle them over your meal after it's been cooked.

BANANA BREAD

Jenny Nelson, Clean wellness coach, chef, and photographer

Vegetarian*

Makes: 1 full-size loaf or 2 small loaves

Prep time: 8 minutes

Cooking time: 40 to 50 minutes

It's wonderful to be able to share kitchen time with your family, especially giving kids a chance to help make (and then eat!) a refined-sugar-free version of a sweet treat. There's no need to sacrifice taste when you're eating healthy food, so enjoy sharing this delicious bread with the people you love.

4 tablespoons softened coconut oil
4 medium-large spotted, mushy bananas
2 pasture-raised eggs
½ cup coconut nectar
1 cup gluten-free flour of your choice (Bob's Red Mill brand or Trader Joe's gluten-free baking mix are great)
1 cup almond meal/flour
1 teaspoon sea salt
½ teaspoon baking soda
¼ teaspoon baking powder
1 teaspoon ground cinnamon
½ teaspoon ground nutmeg
½ teaspoon ground cardamom (optional)
¾ cup nuts (pecan, walnut, almond pieces, etc.), shredded coconut, or chocolate chips

Preheat the oven to 350°F.

Grease 1 full-size loaf pan, or 2 small loaf pans, with the coconut oil.

In a large bowl, combine the bananas, eggs, and coconut nectar using a fork or potato masher until the mixture is soft. It's fine if small chunks of banana are left in the batter. It doesn't have to be perfectly smooth.

In another bowl, stir together the flours, salt, baking soda, baking powder, cinnamon, nutmeg, and cardamom, then add the wet ingredients to the dry ingredients and combine well. Add any nuts, coconut flakes, or chocolate chips you like, then pour the dough into the prepared pan(s).

Bake the bread until the top is golden brown and a toothpick comes out clean, roughly 40 to 50 minutes, depending on the loaf size. (Smaller pans will cook faster, and large ones will take longer.) Let the bread cool for 8 minutes, then remove it from the pan, slice it, and serve. The bread will keep for several days at room temperature, or you can freeze it and toast slices as needed.

*Contains eggs

CHAI-SPICED CHIA PORRIDGE

C Cleanse

V Vegan

Serves: 2

Prep time: 15 minutes plus 20 minutes to let stand

Chia seeds are an ancient endurance food. They're a complete protein, they're hydrating, and they contain valuable essential fatty acids. Chai spice adds warmth and aids digestion. The ground sesame seeds balance the dish by helping to regulate blood sugar.

1 quart water
4 chai tea bags or ¼ cup loose chai tea
1 cup hulled raw sesame seeds or 6 tablespoons tahini
6 tablespoons chia seeds
4 Medjool dates, pitted and roughly chopped
1 to 2 tablespoons coconut nectar or a few drops of stevia to taste

Garnish
¼ cup shredded unsweetened coconut
1 cup fresh berries (blue, black, or raspberries)

Bring the water to a boil with the tea bags or loose chai tea, then turn off the heat and let the brew steep for 5 to 10 minutes (the longer it steeps, the stronger it will be), allowing it to cool slightly. Strain (if using loose tea) or remove the tea bags.

In a blender, blend the warm chai tea with the sesame seeds or tahini for 45 seconds on a high setting, then strain the "milk" into a 1-quart mason jar. Stir in the chia seeds and chopped dates. Screw on a lid and shake to mix the seeds with the milk.

Let the mixture stand for 20 minutes before sweetening to taste with the coconut nectar or stevia and topping with the coconut and fresh berries. It should be nice and thick for serving.

SALMON SCRAMBLE WITH CAULIFLOWER AND DILL PURÉE

Orlando Bloom, actor and UNICEF Goodwill Ambassador

Ⓖ Gut

Serves: 1 to 2

Prep time: 20 to 30 minutes

A warm and tasty meal perfect for all seasons. This is a fantastic breakfast or brunch option.

6- to 8-ounce fillet wild-caught salmon, with or without skin (king salmon is great)
½ cup (2 to 3 ounces) chopped cauliflower
2 large pasture-raised eggs
2 tablespoons coconut oil or ghee / clarified butter
Handful of fresh dill
Sea salt and freshly ground black pepper to taste
½ small ripe avocado, pitted and left in its peel
Apple cider vinegar, lemon juice, or olive oil for the avocado

In a saucepan, bring 1 inch of water to a boil. Poach the salmon on both sides, cooking it only halfway. It will finish cooking when you add it to the eggs.

While the salmon is cooking, add the cauliflower to a steamer. Steam it until you can pierce it easily with a sharp knife.

In a bowl, whisk the eggs. Warm 1 tablespoon of the coconut oil or ghee in a nonstick skillet set over low heat, and add the eggs. Be sure to keep the eggs moving in the pan as you cook them, which will ensure they will be creamy and not dry.

While the eggs are still cooking and the salmon is waiting, add the cauliflower, 1 tablespoon of the coconut oil or ghee, and the dill to a blender. Add salt and pepper to taste. Purée the mixture, adding some of the salmon's poaching water little by little, if necessary, to help the ingredients combine smoothly. When it is the right consistency, leave the lid on the blender so it stays hot until you're ready to serve.

Shred the poached salmon. Add it to the cooking eggs when two-thirds of the eggs are solid. Keep the mixture all moving together in the skillet until the eggs are fully cooked, but still not dry. Remove the skillet from the heat, and spoon the eggs and salmon onto a serving plate. Add the cauliflower to the plate too.

In the avocado half, pour apple cider vinegar, lemon juice, and/or olive oil into the small "bowl" where the pit used to be and sprinkle it with salt and pepper. Include it on the serving plate and enjoy. (By leaving the avocado in its peel, you stop the juices from running all over the plate.)

This dish is also very yummy with a couple of strips of bacon!

SUNKEN EGGS

Ⓖ Gut

Vegetarian*

Serves: 2

Prep time: 5 minutes

Cooking time: 15 minutes

This Italian-themed egg dish is perfect for Sunday brunch or if you're cooking for a crowd. The bright yellow of the eggs set inside the deep red tomatoes is gorgeous, and looks amazing in the center of the table.

3 cups organic tomato sauce (preferably homemade)
3 tablespoons chopped fresh herbs, such as basil, parsley, thyme, oregano, rosemary, and/or scallions
4 pasture-raised eggs
Sea salt to taste
Kale, chard, or spinach, sautéed (optional)

Preheat the oven to 350°F.

Heat the tomato sauce in a small saucepan. When warm, transfer it to a baking dish and stir in the fresh herbs. Create four indentations in the sauce, and carefully crack an egg into each one. Bake the mixture for 10 to 12 minutes, depending on how you like your egg yolks cooked. Remove the pan from the oven and sprinkle everything with a dash of sea salt.

Divide the sunken eggs between two plates and serve with a side of sautéed greens, if you like.

*Contains eggs

ROASTED ASPARAGUS WITH POACHED EGGS

G Gut

Vegetarian*

Serves: 2

Prep time: 5 minutes

Cooking time: 15 minutes

Asparagus is loaded with antioxidants and nutrients, and helps rid the body of excess salt and fluid in the tissues. Combined with protein-packed eggs, this is truly the breakfast of champions.

1 bunch (about 12 ounces) asparagus, woody bottom stalks removed
2 tablespoons extra-virgin olive oil
Sprinkle of sea salt
¼ teaspoon freshly ground black pepper
4 cups water
2 tablespoons apple cider vinegar
2 to 4 medium-large pasture-raised eggs (1 to 2 per person)

Preheat the oven to 400°F.

Arrange the asparagus in a baking dish. Drizzle them with the olive oil, sprinkle them with salt and pepper, then roast them until they are fork-tender, about 10 minutes.

While the asparagus are roasting, bring the water to a simmer in a small pot. Add the apple cider vinegar.

In a small bowl, crack 1 egg. Gently whisk the simmering water and vinegar mixture to create a whirlpool, then carefully drop the egg into the middle. Simmer the egg for 2 to 3 minutes, being mindful not to fully cook the yolk. Use a slotted spoon to remove it from the water, drain well, and sprinkle the egg with salt. Repeat with all the eggs.

Divide the roasted asparagus between two serving plates and top each with 1 or 2 poached eggs, depending on how many you have for each person. Cut open the egg and allow the runny yolk to become a flavorful sauce for the asparagus.

*Contains eggs

SCRAMBLED EGGS WITH SMOKED SALMON

G Gut

Serves: 1

Prep and cook time: 5 minutes

A protein-packed meal that works for breakfast, brunch, lunch, or dinner. Kids love scrambled eggs as a meal or as a snack anytime of the day. Eggs also provide vitamins, minerals, choline and cholesterol, all necessary for growing bodies. Serve over mixed greens or plenty of sautéed kale for a heartier dish.

1½ tablespoons avocado oil
4 large pasture-raised eggs
¼ cup unsweetened coconut milk
Pinch of sea salt
Freshly ground black pepper to taste
2 ounces smoked salmon
1 tablespoon chopped fresh chives

Heat a heavy-bottom saucepan over medium-high heat. Add the oil and let the pan get very hot.

While the pan is heating, whisk together the eggs and coconut milk in a small bowl, and season the mixture with salt and pepper.

When you start to see wisps of smoke in the saucepan, add the eggs and stir them vigorously, using a wooden spoon. When they are cooked halfway through, toss in the salmon and chives. Continue stirring until the eggs are just cooked. Transfer the eggs to a plate and serve.

VEGETABLE FRITTATA

G Gut

Vegetarian*

Serves: 2

Prep time: 10 minutes

Cooking time: 15 to 25 minutes

The frittata is a wonderful go-to meal when you're short on time or have a lot of extra produce kicking around. This also travels well, since it holds together. As a bonus, it doesn't have to be warmed up to taste good, so it's perfect for a meal at the office or school. In terms of combining foods, proteins go well with greens so try pairing this with a salad.

2 tablespoons coconut oil
3 to 4 cups seasonal vegetables, such as summer squash, zucchini, kale, spinach, and/or broccoli
1 medium yellow onion, thinly sliced
2 garlic cloves, minced
6 pasture-raised eggs
½ cup unsweetened coconut milk
¼ cup chopped fresh herbs, such as chives, basil, and/or parsley
1 to 2 teaspoons sea salt

Preheat the oven to 350°F.

Heat a large ovenproof sauté pan, preferably cast iron, over medium-high heat. Melt the coconut oil, then add the vegetables and onion. Cook them, stirring occasionally until everything is soft. Add the garlic and continue stirring occasionally until the mixture is aromatic.

While the vegetables are cooking, in a medium bowl whisk together the eggs, milk, herbs, and salt.

Pour the egg mixture into the pan with the vegetables, then transfer the pan to the preheated oven. Bake for about 15 to 25 minutes (the size of the pan will determine how long it takes in the oven). Once the center is firm or "set," remove the pan from the oven and serve the frittata either warm or at room temperature.

*Contains eggs

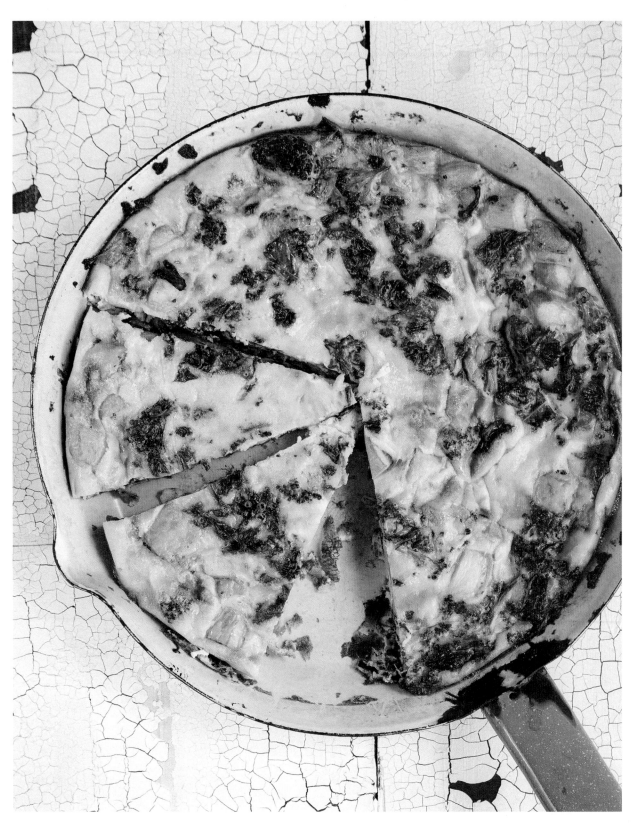

Vegetable Frittata, page 56

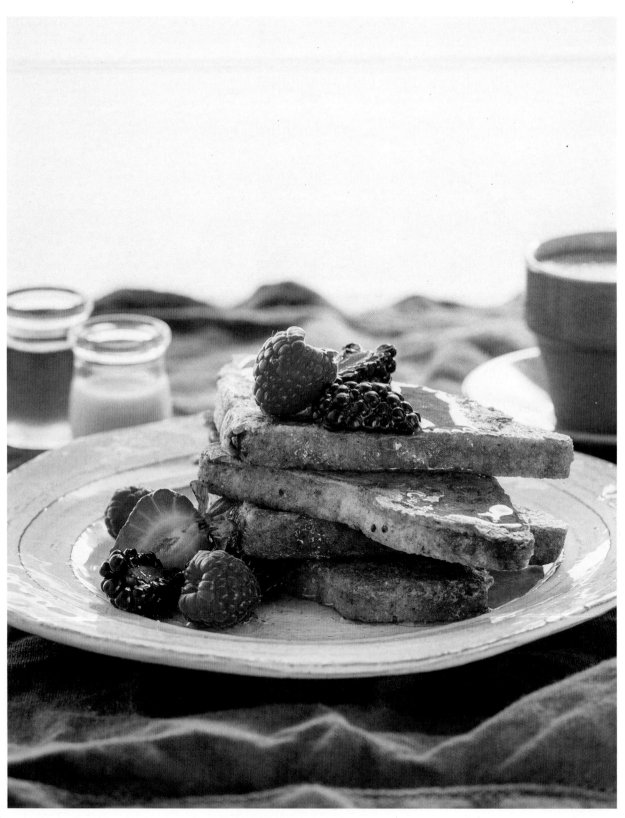

French Toast with Vanilla Cream, page 48

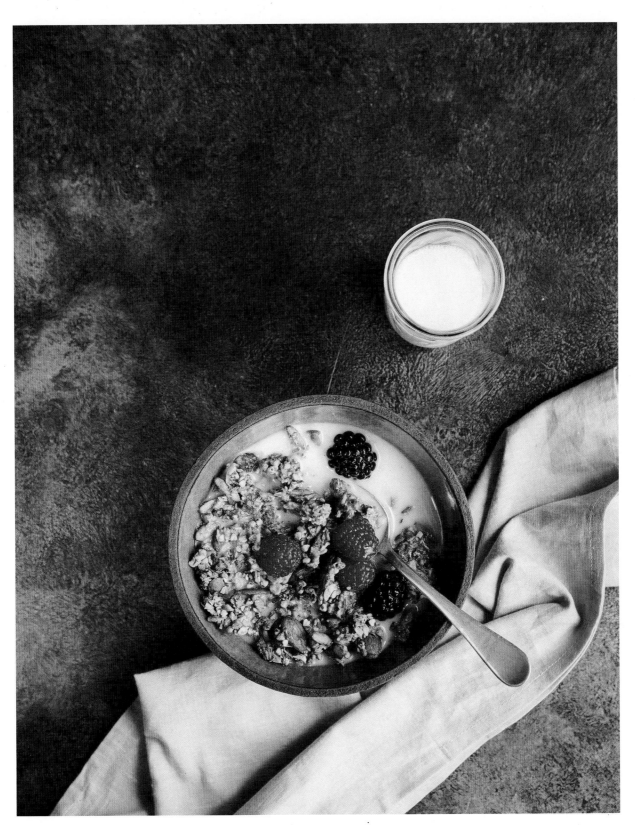

Buckwheat Granola, page 42

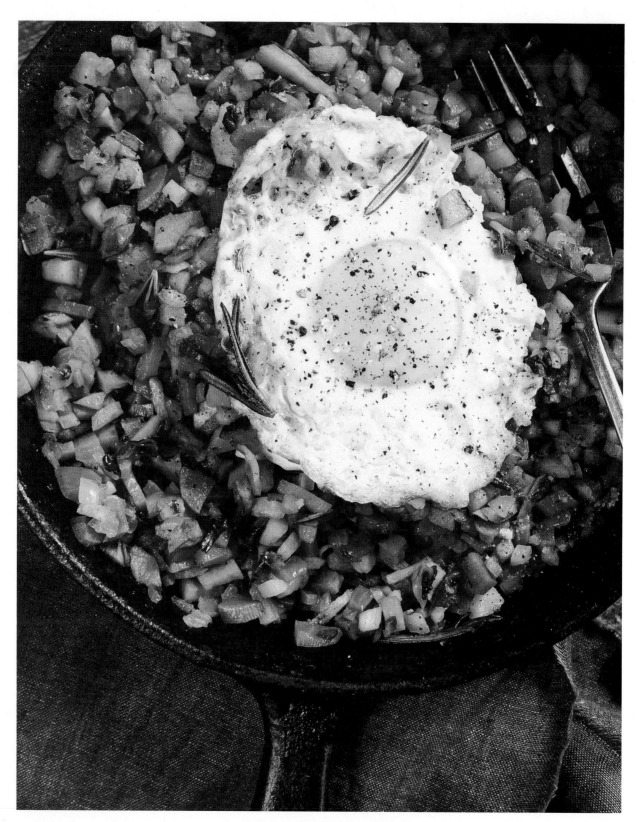

Root Vegetable Hash, page 60

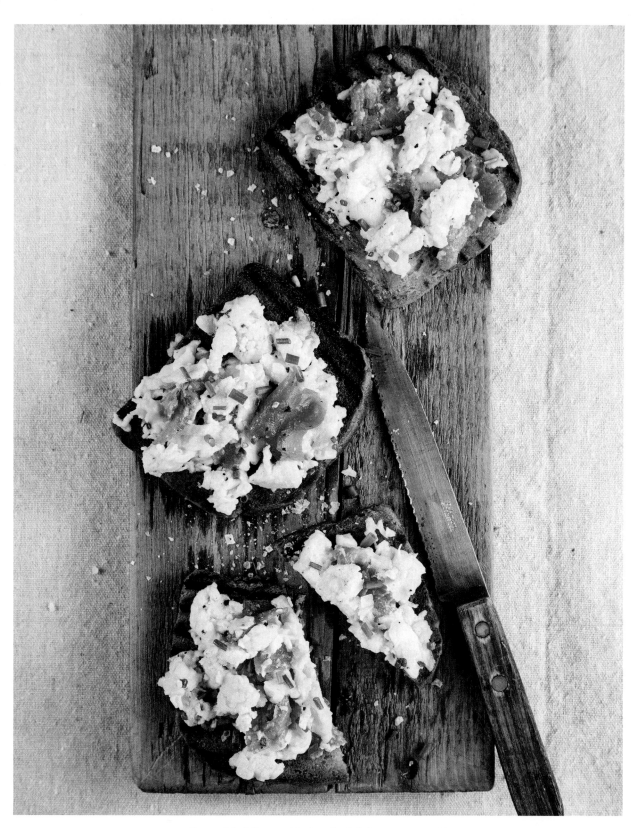

Scrambled Eggs with Smoked Salmon, page 55

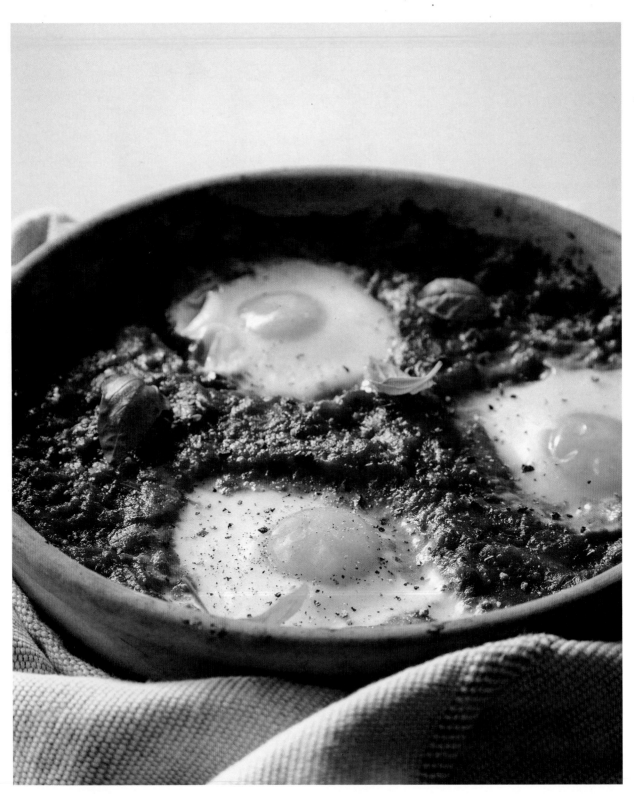

Sunken Eggs, page 53

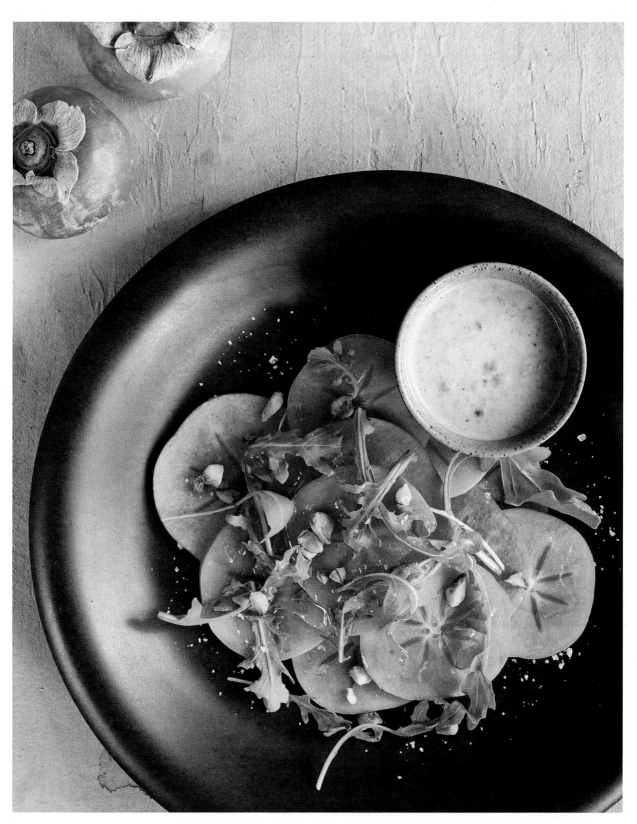

Arugula and Persimmon Salad with Pistachio Vinaigrette, page 68

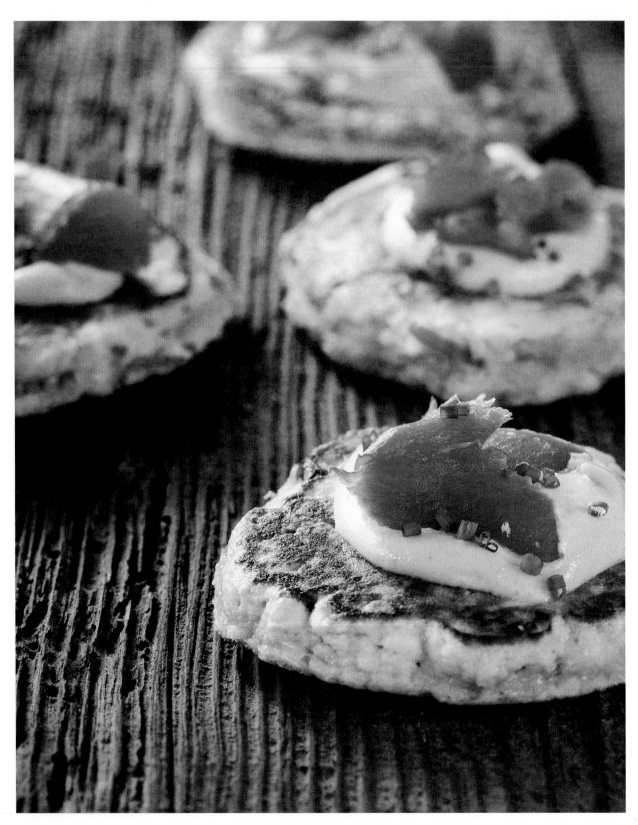

Scallion Pancakes, page 57

SCALLION PANCAKES

G Gut

Vegetarian*

Makes: 8 to 16 pancakes

Prep time: 5 minutes

Cooking time: 5 minutes

These are uniquely tasty. The sweet spice of scallions, cooked in healthy coconut oil, make for a wonderful crunchy meal, snack, or side anytime of the day. You can add a variety of toppings, such as Apple Onion Chutney (page 126), Tomato Salsa (page 124), Sour Cream (page 98), or Cashew Cheese (page 97).

6 pasture-raised eggs
3 scallions, thinly sliced
¼ cup coconut flour
½ teaspoon baking powder
1 teaspoon sea salt
¼ cup water
Coconut oil for cooking

In a large bowl, whisk the eggs. Then add the scallions, coconut flour, baking powder, salt, and water. You may need to switch to a wooden spoon or spatula to fully incorporate everything.

Heat a large skillet, preferably cast iron, over medium heat. Coat the pan with coconut oil, then add ⅛- to ¼-cup portions of the batter. Lightly brown each pancake on one side, about 2 minutes, then flip and finish cooking.

Pairings: Serve the pancakes as a side or as a brunch item with sour cream and smoked salmon.

*Contains eggs

LACY POTATO CAKES

Vegetarian*

Makes: 8 cakes

Prep time: 5 minutes

Cooking time: 10 minutes

This is a twist on traditional latkes. We use coconut oil to fry them, which promotes gut health, immunity, and metabolism function. You could also use lard or pasture-raised animal fat, if you can get it from local farmers. These potato cakes are wonderful alone or with Apple Onion Chutney (page 126).

1½ pounds Yukon Gold potatoes
1 large pasture-raised egg, lightly beaten with a fork or whisk
¼ cup minced onion
2 tablespoons tapioca starch
2 teaspoons sea salt
2 tablespoons coconut oil

Wash and peel the potatoes, then grate them into a large bowl. Squeeze the grated potatoes in your hands to get rid of any excess liquid. Once they are dry, combine them with the eggs, onion, tapioca starch, and salt.

Heat a heavy-bottom skillet over medium-high heat. Melt the coconut oil in the pan and, when the oil is hot, drop in ⅓-cup portions of the potato mixture, shaping them into small cakes. Fry them for 4 to 5 minutes on each side, until they are crisp, golden brown, and warmed all the way through.

Pairings: Serve with pasture-raised eggs cooked to your preference, salads, Hanukkah meals, The Most Perfect Chicken Breast (page 163), or for a delicious mix of textures, the Everything Kale Salad (page 69).

Variations: For Sunday brunch, serve them with smoked salmon and Sour Cream (page 98).

*Contains eggs

EGG-STUFFED SWEET POTATOES WITH SPINACH PURÉE

Vegetarian*

Serves: 2

Prep time: 1 hour

Cooking time: 10 to 12 minutes

This is an easy meal for two, or you can halve the recipe to serve one. Jammed with nutrients, protein, complex carbs, and starch, it makes a great post-workout dish. Similar to a toad-in-the-hole, but without the bread. This tends to be popular with kids; since it's soft, it's great for little ones learning to feed themselves.

2 large sweet potatoes
2 scallions, both greens and whites thinly sliced
Sea salt to taste
¼ teaspoon freshly ground black pepper
4 pasture-raised eggs

For the Spinach Purée
¼ pound (about 4 cups) baby spinach
1 garlic clove, minced
Juice and zest of 1 lemon
½ cup extra-virgin olive oil
Pinch of sea salt

Preheat the oven to 350°F.

In a baking dish, bake the sweet potatoes for 45 minutes to 1 hour until tender. Remove them from the oven and set them aside until they are completely cooled.

While the sweet potatoes bake, in a blender purée the spinach, garlic, lemon juice and zest, olive oil, and salt until the mixture is smooth. Store the purée in an airtight container for up to three days in the fridge until you're ready to use it.

When the sweet potatoes have cooled, cut them each in half lengthwise, then scoop out the center, trying to leave about ½ inch of potato attached to the skin. Fill each sweet potato halfway with scallions and season with salt and pepper, then carefully crack an egg into each. Return the stuffed potatoes to the baking dish and bake for an additional 10 to 12 minutes. Try to bake them just until the egg whites have cooked through but the yolks remain a bit runny.

Swirl a generous amount of spinach purée on each serving plate before topping with the sweet potatoes. Serve warm.

*Contains eggs

ROOT VEGETABLE HASH

C Cleanse
G Gut*
V Vegan

Serves: 2

Prep time: 15 minutes

Cooking time: 20 minutes

This is one of the easiest and tastiest recipes for fall vegetables. It can be a main course or a side dish; it pairs easily with anything; and leftovers can be mixed with a salad or baked in a frittata for lunch the next day. You can even purée it and make an amazing soup. Feel free to vary the vegetables with whatever you have on hand or find at your local farmers' market.

2 tablespoons coconut oil
6 cups small-diced root vegetables, such as beets, carrots, turnips, rutabagas, and/or parsnips
1 medium onion, diced small
2 teaspoons chopped fresh rosemary
Sea salt to taste

Heat the coconut oil in a large, heavy-bottom skillet over medium-high heat. When the oil is hot, add the root vegetables. Sauté, stirring occasionally to prevent sticking, for about 10 minutes. Next, add the onion, and continue sautéing until the vegetables are tender and have started to meld together. Sprinkle in the rosemary and salt to taste. Serve warm.

Pairings: Serve with eggs, fish, chicken, burgers, or salads, or use this as a taco or quesadilla filling.

*Omit beets

Chef Frank on Local and Seasonal Foods

I encourage sourcing as much of your food locally as possible. This is one of the best ways to make sure you're getting the freshest and most nutrient-rich food. Buying from small and local farms enables you to learn about their farming practices and makes it easier to avoid chemicals and inhumane animal practices. By talking with your local farmers, you may find that many of their farms are chemical-free but do not have the money to get organic certification. Buying most of your food locally also means you're eating seasonally and therefore gaining the health benefits that come from eating a wide range of foods throughout the year. It's good for our bodies and our minds to switch things up once in a while. Finally, when we support small, local farmers (or grow food ourselves), we also help the planet by reducing the resources needed to ship food around the globe.

SALADS, SAUCES, AND DRESSINGS

Salads have been given a bad rap. Many of us are used to plates of iceberg lettuce, carrots, and a lonely tomato. But salads can be incredible, *if* they're made well. When a salad is created with layers of tasty ingredients, it can be quickly transformed into a full meal. Fresh to the taste buds and simple to prepare, a well-made salad leaves you satiated without feeling sluggish and gives you a simple way to add more nutrient-rich plant food to your diet.

ROMAINE AND SEA VEGETABLE SALAD WITH CREAMY DILL DRESSING

C Cleanse

G Gut

V Vegan

Serves: 2

Prep time: 10 minutes

Mineral-rich and delectably creamy, this salad is a must-try. It's like a super healthy Caesar salad, elegant and hearty.

For the Salad
1 head romaine lettuce, leaves washed, spun dry, and cut into bite-size pieces
1 strip kelp (they normally come in a bag of roughly 6 to 8 strips), soaked for
    20 minutes, drained, and snipped into small pieces
1 small handful dulse, torn into bite-size pieces
1 medium carrot, peeled and grated

For the Dressing
1 cup raw sunflower seeds
½ cup raw hemp seeds
2 garlic cloves
1 tablespoon miso (South River brand is our personal favorite)
½ teaspoon kelp powder
1 teaspoon sea salt
1 cup water
¼ cup chopped fresh dill

First, make the dressing. In a blender, purée the sunflower seeds, hemp seeds, garlic, miso, kelp powder, salt, and water until smooth and creamy. Taste the mixture and adjust the seasonings to your liking, then blend in the dill just until incorporated.

In a large bowl, toss together the romaine, kelp, dulse, and carrot. Stir in enough dressing to evenly coat the greens, and serve.

ROASTED BEET SALAD WITH MISO DRESSING

C Cleanse

V Vegan

Serves: 2

Prep time: 10 to 15 minutes

Cooking time: 30 to 45 minutes

Miso is a wonderful enzyme-rich addition to a meal. Remember to add the miso at the end, as it should never be heated to high temperatures, which would destroy its wonderful health benefits.

6 to 8 medium red beets
1 head broccoli (about 4 cups), cut into small florets
2 tablespoons miso (South River brand is our personal favorite)
Juice of 1 lemon
¼ cup extra-virgin olive oil
2 teaspoons wheat-free tamari
¼ cup raw pumpkin seeds
¼ cup chopped fresh chives

Preheat the oven to 350°F.

Place the beets in a baking dish and cover them with tinfoil or an ovenproof lid. Roast the beets in the preheated oven for 30 to 45 minutes or until tender. Remove them from the oven, let them cool, then peel them and chop them into large chunks.

While the beets are roasting, in a pot bring 8 cups of salted water to just below a boil. Submerge the broccoli florets in the water and boil them until they are just fork-tender and bright green. Strain them and run them under cold water to stop the cooking process. Set them aside.

To make the dressing, in a small bowl whisk together the miso, lemon juice, olive oil, and tamari.

In a large serving bowl, toss together the beets, broccoli, pumpkin seeds, and chives. Pour the dressing over the mixture and stir to evenly coat everything. Allow the vegetables to mingle with and soak up the dressing for 10 to 15 minutes before serving.

CHICKEN PAILLARD WITH BUTTERNUT SQUASH AND MUSTARD VINAIGRETTE

Ⓒ Cleanse
Ⓖ Gut

Serves: 2

Prep time: 15 minutes

Cooking time: around 30 minutes

This dish is perfectly spiced and incredibly delicious. In culinary terms, "paillard" means "to flatten," so the chicken is pounded until it is thin. Then it is seared, so it cooks very quickly and retains a wonderful flavor. The mustard provides a warming kick and clears out your sinuses.

2 pasture-raised boneless, skinless chicken breasts
1 teaspoon freshly ground fennel seeds
Sea salt to taste
Freshly ground black pepper to taste
Coconut oil for coating and cooking
½ pound baby spinach

For the Squash
1¼ pounds butternut squash, peeled and diced (4 to 5 cups)
1½ tablespoons extra-virgin olive oil
1 teaspoon sea salt
½ teaspoon ground cinnamon
¼ teaspoon chipotle chili powder

For the Mustard Vinaigrette
2 tablespoons minced shallots
1 tablespoon whole-grain mustard
1 tablespoon apple cider vinegar
2 tablespoons extra-virgin olive oil
Pinch of sea salt

Preheat the oven to 375°F.

First, prepare the squash. In a large bowl, toss the squash with the olive oil, salt, cinnamon, and chipotle chili powder. Spread the mixture evenly in a baking dish and roast the squash until the pieces are tender, about 20 to 30 minutes.

While the squash is roasting, in a small bowl whisk together all the vinaigrette ingredients until well combined. Set it aside.

To prepare the chicken, season each breast well with the fennel, salt, and pepper. Lay them flat on a piece of parchment paper that has been lightly spread with olive oil, then drizzle the breasts with a touch of coconut oil and cover them with an additional piece of parchment. Use a mallet or an empty wine bottle to pound out the breasts until each is evenly about ½-inch thick throughout.

Heat a large skillet over medium-high heat. Add a touch of coconut oil. When the oil is hot, carefully place both breasts in the pan. Cook for just a few minutes, then flip them and cook on the other side for a few more minutes. Remove the breasts from the pan and let them rest for 2 to 3 minutes before slicing the chicken into thin strips against the grain.

In a large bowl, gently toss together the chicken, the cooked squash, and the fresh spinach, allowing the warm squash to lightly wilt the spinach. Pour in the vinaigrette and toss again to evenly coat everything. Divide the mixture between two plates and serve.

Chef Frank on Wild Foods

Wild foods are foods that aren't grown by humans. Found wild in nature, they are usually richer in minerals and nutrients and lower in sugar. I encourage you to add wild foods to your diet whenever you can. In the spring, try fiddlehead ferns and stinging nettle. Choose tiny wild blueberries rather than the larger hybrid ones. Sea vegetables, Brazil nuts, mesquite powder, and wild rice are other great examples available in most markets around the United States.

ARUGULA AND PERSIMMON SALAD WITH PISTACHIO VINAIGRETTE

C Cleanse   **Serves:** 2

V Vegan   **Prep time:** 15 minutes

For this gorgeous salad, choose persimmons that are super soft. The riper the fruit, the sweeter the flavor. High in fiber, B and C vitamins, and plenty of antioxidants, the sweet persimmons pair perfectly with the arugula's snap and the complexity of the pistachio dressing.

½ pound arugula, washed and spun dry
2 Fuyu persimmons, stemmed and sliced into thin rounds

For the Pistachio Vinaigrette
1 tablespoon lemon juice
2 tablespoons extra-virgin olive oil
⅛ cup water
¼ cup pistachios
½ teaspoon sea salt

In a blender, purée all the vinaigrette ingredients until the mixture is smooth and well incorporated.

Toss the arugula in a large bowl with the vinaigrette until the leaves are well coated.

Arrange the persimmon slices on two serving plates, then top them with the dressed greens and serve.

EVERYTHING KALE SALAD

Cameron Diaz, actress

Ⓖ Gut

Serves: 1

Prep time: less than 10 minutes if the chicken and grains are precooked and the quinoa is made

I eat this every day. I use it in the middle of the day because it's packed with everything I need: protein, fats, and carbs, and the microgreens and sprouts are very nutrient dense. It's balanced to keep me going while still feeling clean in my system. Plus, you can play around with the grains, proteins, greens, and seeds you prefer or have in your fridge!

6 large leaves of Tuscan (aka Dinosaur or Lacinato) kale, stems sliced out of the center of each leaf and the leaves julienned into ½-inch-wide strips
⅛ cup assorted sprouts, such as clover, alfalfa, lentil, garbanzo, and/or any kind you like
⅛ cup microkale and/or microgreens, again your choice
5 to 8 cherry or grape tomatoes, halved
2 tablespoons raw pumpkin seeds
1 tablespoon raw sunflower seeds
Flesh of ½ ripe avocado, diced
1 small piece (4 to 6 ounces) cooked pasture-raised chicken, diced or shredded
½ cup cooked quinoa
Juice of ⅓ lemon
1 tablespoon extra-virgin olive oil
1 teaspoon apple cider vinegar or other vinegar of your choice
Sprinkle of nutritional or brewer's yeast
Pinch of Maldon sea salt

In a large bowl, toss all the ingredients together in any order until everything is evenly coated, and enjoy!

BITTER GREENS AND HERB SALAD

C Cleanse

G Gut*

V Vegan

Serves: 4

Prep time: 15 minutes

Although consumed less and less these days, bitter foods play a crucial role in our diets. Bitter greens are much more nutritious than non-bitter greens. They are incredibly detoxifying and act as a wonderfully stimulating digestive tonic.

1 head radicchio
1 head endive
1 large handful frisée or watercress
1 bunch dandelion greens
1 medium fennel bulb, shaved into thin strips
1 Asian pear or any variety of crisp apple, cored and julienned
½ cup flat-leaf parsley leaves
2 tablespoons minced fresh dill
1 tablespoon fresh tarragon leaves
2 to 3 fresh mint leaves, torn into smaller pieces
½ cup raw hemp seeds
2 to 3 tablespoons extra-virgin olive oil
Juice of 1 lemon
Pinch of sea salt

Chop the radicchio, endive, frisée or watercress, and dandelion greens into bite-size pieces, then wash and spin dry them.

In a large bowl, toss all the greens with the fennel strips and the julienned pear or apple. Add the parsley, dill, tarragon, and mint. Stir in the hemp seeds followed by the olive oil, lemon juice, and salt. Toss the mixture well, then divide the salad between four serving plates.

*Omit pear and apple

SESAME BOK CHOY SALAD

C Cleanse

G Gut

V Vegan

Serves: 2, as a side

Prep time: 10 minutes

Marinating time: 10 to 12 minutes

This salad is easy to make and really delicious—perfect in the warm summer months when you don't want to cook. Bok choy is packed with antioxidants, vitamin C, folic acid, and potassium.

1 pound bok choy
1 medium carrot, julienned
½ cup dulse, torn into smaller pieces
2 tablespoons raw sesame seeds (hulled or unhulled, black or white)
1 tablespoon unrefined sesame oil
2 teaspoons toasted sesame oil
2 teaspoons brown rice vinegar
1 tablespoon wheat-free tamari

Roughly chop the bok choy, then wash and drain it or dry it in a salad spinner.

In a large bowl, toss together the bok choy, carrot, dulse, sesame seeds, sesame oils, vinegar, and tamari. Let the mixture marinate for 10 to 12 minutes before serving.

Chef Frank on Bitter Greens

Bitter greens are loaded with nutrition. The bitter taste helps digestion by stimulating gastric acid in the stomach and by assisting in overall nutrient absorption. The greens also balance out the taste buds and can help relieve sugar cravings. Unfortunately, the bitter component has been mostly eliminated from the food we eat today. If you're new to eating bitter foods, start by mixing them with light-tasting, tender greens and sauté them in some balsamic vinegar or add some sweet nuts like pistachios or pecans to the mix. For example, mix kale, endive, dandelion greens, or radicchio with romaine lettuce, Swiss chard, or spinach.

PAPA D'S FRESH FALL SALAD

Dhru Purohit, Clean CEO

V Vegan

Serves: 4 to 6

Prep time: 15 to 20 minutes

This recipe is my go-to dinner party salad. What I love about it is all the layers and textures.

2 medium sweet potatoes, cut into 1-inch cubes (about 2 cups)
3 tablespoons coconut oil
Salt
Pepper
Dash of cinnamon
3 ounces scallion
2 bunches Dinosaur kale (Lacinato kale), approximately 14 to 16 medium leaves
2 pinches of sea salt
2 heads butter leaf lettuce
Juice of ¼ lemon
3 tablespoons nutritional yeast
¼ cup diced almonds
¼ cup pomegranate kernels
½ avocado, cubed

For the Dressing
½ cup olive oil
1 tablespoon tahini butter
2 teaspoons stone-ground mustard
1 teaspoon raw honey
Juice of ¼ lemon
2 pinches of sea salt
½ teaspoon dill spice

Bring about 5 cups of water to simmer in a pot. Place the sweet potato cubes into the simmering water and cover. Cook the sweet potatoes for 12 to 14 minutes, or until tender enough to eat. Once ready, place the sweet potato cubes into a small bowl and add 1 tablespoon of the coconut oil, some salt, pepper, and a dash of cinnamon to taste.

Dice the scallions and place them into a cup. De-stem the kale and chop it into ½-inch chunks. Place the kale and scallions into a pot. Drizzle 2 tablespoons of the coconut oil into the pot. Cook the scallions and kale on low-medium heat until the kale starts to wilt, and then sprinkle 2 small pinches of sea salt on it and give it a stir in the pot. Remove the kale from the stove and place it into a large salad bowl.

Take the two heads of butter lettuce and chop or rip them into large bite-size chunks. Toss the lettuce into the salad bowl that contains the kale and scallions. Squeeze the lemon juice over the contents. Sprinkle 3 tablespoons of nutritional yeast over the salad and add in the diced almonds, pomegranate kernels, avocado, and sweet potatoes from earlier.

Mix all the contents together. At this point, even without dressing, the salad should taste fantastic on its own. If needed, add salt or pepper to taste.

Add all of the dressing ingredients to a blender. Blend all the ingredients together and pour over the salad. Mix together and serve.

ARUGULA AND PEAR SALAD WITH WALNUT VINAIGRETTE

C Cleanse

V Vegan

Serves: 2

Prep time: 20 minutes

This is a simple and lovely salad, delicately flavored. The mild sweetness of pears and the slightly fiery kick of arugula are a perfect combination. The walnuts provide omega-3s, which are anti-inflammatory.

2 large handfuls arugula
1 small head Belgium endive, roughly chopped
1 ripe pear, cored, thinly sliced
Pinch of sea salt

For the Walnut Vinaigrette
1 cup (about 4 ounces) walnuts
2 tablespoons minced shallots
2 teaspoons sea salt
½ cup water
¼ cup sherry vinegar
½ cup extra-virgin olive oil

Preheat the oven to 350°F.

First, make the vinaigrette. In a blender, purée ¾ cup of the walnuts with the shallots, salt, water, vinegar, and olive oil until everything is well incorporated. Refrigerate the vinaigrette until you're ready to serve.

Place the remaining ¼ cup walnuts on a baking sheet and toast in the oven, stirring occasionally, until they are golden brown, about 8 to 12 minutes. Set them aside to cool completely.

In a large bowl, toss together the arugula, endive, pear slices, and salt. Pour in enough vinaigrette to evenly coat the greens. Divide the salad between two serving plates and sprinkle the toasted walnuts over the top.

HEIRLOOM TOMATO, FENNEL, AND AVOCADO PRESSED SALAD

Sarma Melngailis, founder of One Lucky Duck

G Gut

V Vegan

Serves: 6

This has been on our menu at Pure Food and Wine during the summer when heirloom tomatoes are in season. We call it a "pressed salad" since we use a ring mold and press it down to compact the flavors and create a nice presentation. But if you're making it at home and don't have a ring mold, it tastes just as good served in a big messy pile. We serve it with our caper dressing.

2 fennel bulbs, cored and thinly sliced
6 large heirloom tomatoes, roughly chopped into 1-inch pieces
Flesh of 2 ripe avocados, diced into ½-inch cubes
2 shallots, minced
¼ cup raw pistachio nuts, roughly chopped
1 large handful fresh mint leaves, finely chopped
1 large handful fresh basil leaves, finely chopped
Freshly squeezed juice of 1 lemon
3 tablespoons pistachio nut oil (or substitute extra-virgin olive oil or macadamia nut oil)
Sea salt to taste
Freshly ground black pepper to taste
Chopped fresh chives or additional mint or basil leaves for garnish

Caper Dressing
½ cup capers, mashed
Zest of 1 lemon
2 tablespoons minced fresh chives
5 turns of coarse black pepper
1 cup extra-virgin olive oil

First, make the dressing. In a medium bowl, combine the capers, lemon zest, chives, and pepper. Add the olive oil slowly while mixing everything with a spoon.

To make the salad, in a large bowl very gently toss the fennel, tomatoes, avocado, shallots, pistachios, mint, basil, lemon juice, pistachio oil, salt, and pepper. Keep in mind the caper emulsion will round out the flavors, so only a small amount of seasoning is needed.

Place a wide ring mold in the center of each serving plate and fill it with the salad. Gently press down the mixture to compact it. Remove the ring and drizzle the caper dressing over and around the salad. Garnish with the chives, mint, or basil. (At the restaurant, we serve each salad with two long whole chives crossed over each other, leaning on the salad.)

Note: This recipe was taken from *Living Raw Food* (HarperCollins, 2009) by Sarma Melngailis.

SPIRULINA SPROUT SALAD

C Cleanse

G Gut

V Vegan

Serves: 2

Prep time: 10 minutes

Spirulina packs a mighty protein punch in each tiny amount. Kids tend to gobble spirulina up, which is great since it's a powerhouse of nutrition. Be aware that it tends to turn teeth green, but honestly, kids love that too!

4 to 6 ounces mixed greens
1 large handful sunflower sprouts
1 cup roughly peeled and chopped cucumber
¼ cup raw hemp seeds
Pinch of sea salt

For the Spirulina Dressing
Flesh of 1 large ripe avocado
1 garlic clove
¼ cup extra-virgin olive oil
¾ cup water
1 teaspoon sea salt
1 tablespoon lemon juice
1 teaspoon spirulina powder

First, make the dressing. In a blender, purée all the dressing ingredients until smooth, then set it aside.

In a large bowl, toss together the greens, sprouts, and cucumber, and the drizzle the mixture with enough dressing to evenly coat everything. Sprinkle in the hemp seeds and salt, toss to combine, and serve.

EGG SALAD

Ⓖ Gut

Vegetarian*

Serves: 2

Prep time: 30 minutes

This dish is the perfect picnic food, salad topping, or protein- and-choline-packed snack that kids love. Many people believe that lack of choline can contribute to fatty liver disease so it's important to include some in your diet. Pasture-raised egg yolks are a wonderfully nutritious food, especially for growing bodies and brains.

6 pasture-raised eggs
¼ cup minced shallots
1 medium dill pickle, minced
1 celery stalk, minced
2 tablespoons chopped fresh parsley
2 tablespoons extra-virgin olive oil
1 tablespoon sherry wine vinegar
2 teaspoons whole-grain mustard
1 to 2 teaspoons sea salt

Place the eggs in a pot of cold water and bring it to a boil. Turn off the heat, cover the pot, and let it stand for 5 minutes. Then run the eggs continuously under cold water until they have cooled.

Peel the eggs and place them in a large bowl. Use your hands or a fork to mash them up as much as you like. Stir in the shallots, pickle, celery, parsley, olive oil, vinegar, and mustard. Sprinkle the mixture with sea salt, stir to combine, and taste and adjust the seasonings.

Variations:

Replace the sherry vinegar and mustard with 2 teaspoons curry powder and 1 tablespoon lemon juice.

Try fresh dill instead of the parsley.

*Contains eggs

CHUNKY AVOCADO SALAD

Josh Radnor, actor and director

C Cleanse*

G Gut

V Vegan

This is a simple salad that's quick to prepare and uses some interesting ingredients like hearts of palm and dill. Add in the spirulina and nutritional yeast for a boost of protein, nutrition, and flavor.

Flesh of 2 ripe avocados, cut into large chunks
1 large tomato, cored and cut into chunks
1 medium cucumber, peeled and cut into ¼-inch-thick rounds
1 can (14 ounces) hearts of palm, drained and cut into ½-inch-thick rounds
¼ cup toasted sunflower seeds or walnuts
Juice of 1 lemon
¼ cup extra-virgin olive oil
¼ cup roughly chopped fresh dill
2 tablespoons nutritional yeast
Pinch of sea salt
1 to 2 tablespoons spirulina (optional)

In a large bowl, toss all the ingredients together and let the mixture sit for 5 to 10 minutes before serving, to allow the flavors to combine.

*Omit tomato

THE CLEAN NIÇOISE

Serves: 2

Prep time: 30 minutes

A lovely take on the French classic, this salad has every flavor and texture you could want: salty, mild, creamy, and crunchy. It takes some time to prepare, but it's well worth it.

½ pound red potatoes, scrubbed but not peeled, and cut into chunks
4 cups water
2 teaspoons sea salt, plus a pinch for the asparagus
1 bunch (12 ounces) asparagus, woody ends removed
2 teaspoons olive oil
1 head (3 to 4 ounces) romaine lettuce, chopped, washed, and spun dry
4 hard-boiled eggs, peeled and each egg cut in half
1 3- to 6-ounce can sardines, kippers, or wild-caught salmon
Approximately 20 Kalamata olives, pitted
¼ cup thinly sliced red onions
1 large scoop (about 4 ounces) sauerkraut

For the Lemon Herb Vinaigrette
¼ cup lemon juice
½ cup extra-virgin olive oil
2 tablespoons water
1 tablespoon whole-grain mustard
½ teaspoon sea salt
¼ teaspoon freshly ground black pepper
2 tablespoons chopped fresh herbs, such as tarragon, thyme, oregano, parsley,
    and/or marjoram

Place the potato chunks in a pot with the water and 2 teaspoons of the salt. Bring them to a boil, then lower the heat and gently simmer them until they are fork-tender. Drain, and run cold water over them until they have cooled.

While the potatoes cook, prepare the asparagus. Place them in a baking dish or cast-iron pan and coat them with the olive oil and the pinch of salt. Set them in a broiler for 5 to 8 minutes, until they are lightly brown and tender. Remove them and let them cool.

Arrange the romaine leaves on a large serving platter. Top the leaves with the egg halves, fish, olives, red onions, sauerkraut, potatoes, and asparagus.

Place all the ingredients for the vinaigrette into a pint-size jar. Secure the jar's lid and shake the mixture until it's evenly combined. Drizzle the vinaigrette over the salad, and enjoy!

FARMERS' MARKET SALAD

Ⓥ Vegan

Serves: 2

Prep time: 10 minutes

This salad celebrates the bounty of fresh produce that comes from our local farmers, true community heroes who supply the nourishing food for our families every day all around the world. People are growing their own food everywhere, in the smallest of lots, in the cities or just outside, so make a point to find out where the family-owned farms are near you and support them however you can.

4 ounces mixed greens
1 carrot, cut into thin half-moons
1 ripe tomato, roughly chopped
1 medium beet, peeled and grated
1 cucumber, peeled, thinly sliced
¼ cup shaved fennel bulb
¼ cup raw pumpkin seeds
Salad dressing of your choice

Wash and spin-dry the greens, then toss them in a large bowl with the carrot, tomato, beet, cucumber, fennel, and pumpkin seeds. Drizzle with your favorite salad dressing and serve.

Dr. Junger on Farmers' Markets

When I was growing up in Uruguay, everything was farm-fresh and organic. We didn't think of it as "special" or "clean" food; to us it was just food. It wasn't until I came to the United States that I realized how amazing the food I ate growing up was. That's why I love farmers' markets. The food the farmers have there reminds me of what I ate when I was young. If you have one near you, it's really the simplest way to get the freshest and tastiest clean food into your diet.

FOREVER-GREEN SOUP AND SALAD

Donna Karan, designer and founder of the Urban Zen Initiative

Ⓒ Cleanse

Ⓖ Gut*

Ⓥ Vegan

A simple and elegant soup and salad combo where the creaminess of the Cashew Basil Dressing balances perfectly with the saltiness of the soup's white miso.

For the Salad
1 bunch kale
1 bunch baby arugula
1 bunch baby spinach
1 green apple (shaved or diced)
2 tablespoons sprouted pumpkin seeds
2 tablespoons lemon juice

For the Cashew Basil Dressing
Handful of basil leaves
1 garlic clove
1 tablespoon grated ginger
½ cup olive oil
2 tablespoons raw cashew butter
Juice of 1 whole lemon
½ teaspoon Celtic sea salt

For the Soup
2 cups organic spinach
2 stalks celery, chopped
½ fennel bulb, chopped
1 medium-size zucchini, chopped
1 tablespoon white miso
1 tablespoon raw tahini
1 teaspoon Celtic sea salt
4 cups filtered water
½ cup sprouted sunflower seeds (garnish)

Remove ribs from kale and tear leaves into small pieces. Combine all greens in a salad bowl. Toss greens with apple, pumpkin seeds, and lemon juice. For the Cashew Basil Dressing, add all ingredients into a blender and blend for 1 minute.

Place all soup ingredients (except sunflower seeds) in a Vitamix and blend on high until warm (approximately 5 minutes). Garnish with sprouted sunflower seeds and serve with love.

*Omit apple

SMOKED SALMON AND FENNEL SALAD

C Cleanse

G Gut

Serves: 2

Prep time: 10 minutes

This perfect combination of melt-in-your-mouth smoked salmon and crisp fennel is entirely satisfying. It's wonderful with any meal or, as a large portion, it's a filling entrée—a tasty way to get heart-healthy omega-3s.

1 large fennel bulb plus a clump of fennel fronds
1 small dill pickle or 1 tablespoon capers
Juice of 1 lemon
2 tablespoons olive oil
Pinch of sea salt
Freshly ground black pepper to taste
4 ounces smoked wild-caught salmon

Trim the top of the fennel, then using a sharp knife or mandoline, slice the bulb paper-thin. Place the fennel slices in a large bowl along with some roughly chopped fennel fronds. Mince the pickle or roughly chop the capers and add them to the fennel. Add the lemon juice and drizzle in the olive oil. Season the salad with salt and pepper to taste, and toss everything well.

Divide the smoked salmon between two serving plates. Top with portions of the fennel salad.

MEXICAN BLACK BEAN SALAD

C Cleanse*

V Vegan

Serves: 2

Prep time: overnight

Cooking time: overnight plus 15 minutes

Protein rich, this simple salad is full of flavor. Serve it on its own as a meal or as a side dish with any Southwestern-themed entrée.

1 cup dried black beans
2 quarts water
1 tablespoon apple cider vinegar
1 small red onion, diced small
1 jalapeño pepper, minced
12 cherry tomatoes, halved, or 1 medium tomato, roughly chopped
Flesh of 1 ripe avocado
2 garlic cloves, minced
¼ cup roughly chopped cilantro
1 heaping tablespoon Mexican seasoning
2 teaspoons sea salt
Juice of 1 lime
¼ cup extra-virgin olive oil

The night before you make this dish, soak the black beans in 1 quart of the water with the apple cider vinegar for a minimum of 8 hours.

Strain and rinse the black beans, then add them to a large pot with the remaining quart of water. Bring the pot to a boil, then lower the heat and simmer until the beans are tender, about 20 minutes. Strain the black beans again and rinse them. Allow them to cool to room temperature.

In a large bowl, stir together the cooled beans, red onion, jalapeño, tomatoes, avocado, garlic, cilantro, Mexican seasoning, salt, lime juice, and olive oil. Adjust the seasonings to taste, then serve.

*Omit tomatoes

CHINESE CHICKEN SALAD

Ⓒ Cleanse

Ⓖ Gut*

Serves: 2

Prep time: 20 minutes

Cooking time: 10 minutes

Well spiced and versatile, this salad can be used in a variety of ways: over mixed greens, in a wrap, or on its own. It will bring a unique flavor to your next gathering or picnic.

1 pound pastured boneless, skinless chicken breasts or leftover cooked chicken
2 cups thinly shaved napa cabbage
1 large carrot, julienned
¼ cups roughly chopped fresh cilantro
¼ cup raw cashews
2 tablespoons raw sesame seeds

For the Dressing
¼ cup brown rice vinegar
¼ cup extra-virgin olive oil
2 tablespoons toasted sesame oil
1 to 2 tablespoons coconut nectar
1 tablespoon wheat-free tamari
1 tablespoon freshly grated ginger
1 bunch (about 3 ounces) scallions, thinly sliced

Place the chicken in a small pot with 1 cup of water. Cover and cook the chicken over medium heat until it's cooked through, about 10 minutes. Let the chicken cool, then use your hands to shred the meat or use a knife to thinly slice it.

In a large bowl, toss the chicken with the cabbage, carrot, cilantro, cashews, and sesame seeds. Set aside.

In a separate bowl, whisk together all the ingredients for the dressing. Pour enough dressing over the chicken mixture to evenly coat everything, then serve.

*Omit coconut nectar

ZESTY ROASTED CHICKEN SALAD

Michelle Hartgrove, Clean community member

Ⓒ Cleanse

Ⓖ Gut

Serves: 4

This dish takes salad to the next level. Juicy lemon- and garlic-roasted chicken is perfect on top of a super fresh salad bursting with flavor. This recipe lasts me for several lunches during the week and has even encouraged colleagues to skip dining out and join me. It leaves you feeling satisfied and happy.

1 lemon, peeled and cut into quarters
3 garlic cloves
1 whole (4 to 5 pounds) pasture-raised chicken
Lemon-flavored olive oil, for the chicken, plus more for the salad
1 large pinch fresh rosemary
2 generous pinches sea salt
2 generous pinches freshly ground black pepper
Salad greens of your choice (I use lamb's lettuce or rocket), roughly 1 to 2 handfuls
    per person
1 cup quinoa, cooked and cooled
1 medium cucumber, peeled and diced
Flesh of 1 ripe avocado, sliced
1 cup chopped mushrooms
2 carrots, grated
Balsamic vinegar

Preheat the oven to 350°F.

Stuff the lemon quarters and the whole peeled garlic cloves inside the chicken. Drizzle olive oil over the chicken, then season it with generous pinches of rosemary, salt, and pepper. Roast the chicken in a baking dish for 1 hour and 30 minutes, until it's tender and golden brown on top, then set it aside while you prepare the salad.

In a large bowl, toss together the greens, quinoa, cucumber, avocado, mushrooms, and carrots, then drizzle all with lemon-flavored olive oil and balsamic vinegar to taste, coating the salad evenly. Divide the salad between four serving plates. Carve up the chicken and add however much you like to each salad, then serve.

ROASTED SWEET POTATO AND SPINACH SALAD

(V) Vegan*

Serves: 4

Prep time: 10 minutes

Cooking time: 30 minutes

If you can tolerate dairy, try some crumbled goat or feta cheese with this salad, and it'll be even more fantastic. Either way, it's stunning as a holiday centerpiece with the bright red, green, and orange medley.

3 pounds sweet potatoes, peeled and chopped into ½-inch dice
3 tablespoons extra-virgin olive oil
2 teaspoons coriander seeds
1 teaspoon fennel seeds
¾ teaspoon ground cinnamon
1½ teaspoons sea salt, plus more for final seasoning
½ pound fresh spinach, roughly chopped
1 cup raw or toasted walnuts
½ cup dried cranberries, goji berries, or dried cherries
Goat or feta cheese to taste (optional)

Preheat the oven to 350°F.

In a large bowl, toss the chopped sweet potatoes with the olive oil, coriander seeds, fennel seeds, cinnamon, and 1½ teaspoons of the salt, coating the chunks evenly. Spread the potatoes in a baking dish and roast them until they are fork-tender, about 25 to 30 minutes. Remove them from the oven.

In a large serving bowl, toss the still-warm sweet potatoes with the chopped spinach, using the heat of the sweet potatoes to lightly wilt the spinach. Once the potatoes cool, stir in the walnuts and dried fruit along with a sprinkle of salt and goat or feta cheese, if you're using it, then serve.

*Omit cheese

BASIL VINAIGRETTE

C Cleanse

G Gut

V Vegan

Makes: about ⅔ cup

Prep time: 10 minutes

When it's summer and the gardens are exploding with flavor and variety, we love adding basil to as many of our recipes as possible. This vibrantly green vinaigrette will enhance your salads or pairs perfectly with grilled chicken or roasted vegetables.

2 cups loosely packed fresh basil leaves
1 large garlic clove, minced
2 tablespoons slivered raw almonds or 4 whole raw almonds
½ cup plus 1 tablespoon extra-virgin olive oil
3 tablespoons white wine vinegar
1 teaspoon sea salt
¼ teaspoon freshly ground black pepper

Purée all the ingredients together in a blender for about 30 seconds, or until the mixture is smooth.

Store the vinaigrette in a container in the refrigerator for up to five days.

Chef Frank on Dairy

Even if you haven't had great luck with dairy, there are some different types you may want to try. Many people who have a problem with cow's milk products can tolerate goat's or sheep's milk, or fermented dairy products like yogurt, kefir, or aged cheese. You may also find that unpasteurized (raw) dairy of any kind works for you where pasteurized dairy doesn't. Organic, whole-fat dairy from pastured animals is higher in all nutrients, including choline, healthy cholesterol, vitamin E, vitamin D, and calcium. For a nutrient-rich fat that stays stable at medium- to high-temperature cooking, try butter from grass-fed cows. Even for people who may be sensitive to dairy or are lactose intolerant, butter from grass-fed cows is often handled well.

GREEN GODDESS DRESSING

Ⓒ Cleanse

Ⓖ Gut

Ⓥ Vegan

Makes: just over 1 pint

Prep time: 10 minutes

This is one of the yummiest and most versatile dressings. We suggest keeping a jar of it in the fridge at all times! Apple cider vinegar and miso aids digestion while the olive oil and tahini provide essential fats and protein to any salad.

½ cup tahini
½ cup extra-virgin olive oil
3 tablespoons apple cider vinegar
2 tablespoons lemon juice
2 garlic cloves, minced
¼ cup miso
¼ cup fresh parsley leaves
¼ cup fresh cilantro leaves
¼ cup fresh basil leaves
1 scallion, roughly chopped
½ teaspoon sea salt

In a blender, purée together the tahini, olive oil, vinegar, lemon juice, garlic, and miso until the mixture is smooth and creamy. Add the parsley, cilantro, basil, scallion, and salt, and blend again, but only until the dressing is just incorporated.

Store dressing in the fridge, in a container, for up to one week.

THAI DIPPING SAUCE

C Cleanse

Makes: about 1 pint

Prep time: 10 minutes

Who doesn't love Thai food? Unfortunately, the ingredients in Thai dishes and sauces are rarely clean, so we've made our own and it's delicious; it's perfect for any and all sweet and spicy comfort-food cravings.

½ cup fish sauce (Red Boat is a Clean-approved brand)
1 cup lime juice
2 tablespoons chopped fresh cilantro
1 tablespoon chopped fresh mint
1 tablespoon freshly grated ginger
¼ cup extra-virgin olive oil
2 tablespoons coconut nectar

Place all the ingredients in a jar, secure a lid, and shake the mixture vigorously for 10 seconds, until the mixture is well incorporated.

Store the dressing in a container, refrigerated, for up to one week.

TERIYAKI SAUCE

Lara Whitley, Clean community member

V Vegan   **Makes:** sauce for 4 portions of protein (chicken, fish, etc.)
                      or a green salad

This was one of the first recipes with which I figured out how to both please my family and honor my clean eating in one dish. We eat it frequently with broiled protein (chicken thighs and wild-caught salmon are favorites), though it would work well with vegetables too. The secret is to slather it on during the final minutes of cooking. My favorite sides are sesame noodles and sunomono (Japanese cucumber) salad.

¼ cup wheat-free tamari
¼ cup coconut nectar
¼ cup sake
¼ cup mirin

Combine all the ingredients in a small saucepan. Bring everything to a boil and simmer the mixture, uncovered, until it reaches a desired thickness.

Use this dressing on a large green salad, or broil your favorite protein, such as chicken or fish, and generously cover the protein with the sauce during the final 5 or so minutes of cooking, until the sauce thickens and just begins to bubble. Serve immediately.

EXPERIENCE: Remarkable. Eye-opening. Educational. Transformative. After three weeks of the Clean program, I spent another four weeks food testing. I learned more about my nutrition and my body in seven weeks than in the previous forty-six years. And with this knowledge I have made lasting changes to my diet and my living and I hope to my future!

THOUSAND ISLAND DRESSING

Ⓖ Gut

Ⓥ Vegan

Makes: 1 pint

Prep time: 5 minutes

This is a multipurpose dressing that's so much better than the store-bought kind. Use it with a variety of meals in this book, including Lemon Herb Chicken Burgers (page 156) or any salad.

1½ cups (about 4) quartered plum tomatoes
½ cup raw macadamia nuts or cashews
⅛ cup lemon juice
⅛ cup extra-virgin olive oil
2 garlic cloves
1 teaspoon sea salt
1 dill pickle, minced

In a blender, purée the tomatoes, nuts, lemon juice, olive oil, garlic, and salt for 45 seconds, until the mixture is thick and creamy. Transfer the contents to a bowl and fold in the minced pickle.

Store the dressing in a container, in the fridge, for up to three days.

MAYONNAISE

G Gut

Vegetarian*

Makes: 1 pint

Prep time: 10 minutes

A standard condiment, real homemade mayonnaise is packed with good fats and energizing protein. When you find out how easy it is to make, and how much better it tastes, you'll never want store-bought mayo again!

2 pasture-raised egg yolks
1 tablespoon whole-grain mustard
2 tablespoons lemon juice
Sea salt to taste
Up to 2 cups extra-virgin olive oil, avocado oil, or grapeseed oil

In a food processor or blender, combine the egg yolks, mustard, lemon juice, and salt. Very slowly, drop by drop, add the olive, avocado, or grapeseed oil. The mixture will slowly begin to emulsify. When the mayonnaise starts to emulsify, you may add the olive oil in a faster stream, but be mindful that if the oil is added too quickly, or too much is added at one time, the emulsification can break and you'll have to start over again. Once you have slowly poured in 1½ cups of the oil, you can additionally season the mayonnaise to taste. Stored in the fridge, it keeps for a week or more.

*Contains eggs

AIOLI (GARLIC MAYONNAISE)

G Gut

Vegetarian*

Makes: 1 pint

Prep time: 10 minutes

This is the same as mayonnaise, but with a garlic kick!

2 pasture-raised egg yolks
2 garlic cloves
1 tablespoon whole-grain mustard
2 tablespoons lemon juice
Sea salt to taste
Up to 2 cups extra-virgin olive oil, avocado oil, or grapeseed oil

In a food processor or blender, combine the egg yolks, garlic, mustard, lemon juice, and salt. Very, very slowly add the oil. The mixture will slowly begin to emulsify. When the aioli starts to emulsify, you may add the olive oil in a faster stream, but be mindful that if the oil is added too quickly, or too much is added at one time, the emulsification can break and you'll have to start over again. Once you have slowly poured in 1½ cups of the oil, you can further season the aioli to taste. Stored in the fridge, it keeps for a week or more.

*Contains eggs

SPICY CASHEW DIP

Meghan Markle, actress

Ⓒ Cleanse

Ⓖ Gut

Ⓥ Vegan

This is a simple dip with tons of flavor that takes no time to make. I love using it with crudités or on salad greens.

½ cup raw cashews
Juice of 1 lime
Juice of 1 small lemon
1 to 2 handfuls fresh cilantro leaves (I like more cilantro flavor, so I use 2 handfuls from the garden)
1 garlic clove
About ⅓ cup water
Half of a fresh jalapeño (keep the seeds in for more spice)

In a blender, purée all the ingredients for exactly 15 seconds so the mixture stays a little chunky. I promise—it's a winner.

ROSEMARY MUSTARD MARINADE

C Cleanse   **Makes:** 1 cup

G Gut   **Prep time:** 5 minutes

V Vegan

This versatile marinade works on everything from eggplant to chicken breasts. Vary ingredients with the seasons, changing up the herbs as you see fit. Basil, thyme, oregano, and tarragon will all work perfectly here.

½ cup extra-virgin olive oil
2 tablespoons balsamic vinegar
2 tablespoons lemon juice
2 tablespoons wheat-free tamari
1 teaspoon chopped fresh rosemary
2 teaspoons whole-grain mustard
1 large garlic clove, minced

Whisk together all the ingredients in a bowl, or blend them in a blender, until the mixture is well combined.

Refrigerate the marinade in a container for up to one week.

SIDES, STARTERS, AND SNACKS

Unhealthy snacks are everywhere. That's why knowing how to make some great clean snacks and starters can be a major way to maintain your health. From the Avocumber Rolls to the Vegetable Pakoras, these recipes can provide quick energy throughout the day, delight guests at a dinner party, or add that final touch to a great entrée.

THE PERFECT HARD-BOILED EGG

G Gut

Vegetarian*

Prep time: 10 minutes

Cooking time: 1 minute

Once you perfect this recipe, deviled eggs, egg salad, and many other dishes become a joy to cook and super simple. A great source of necessary choline and protein, this egg comes wrapped in its own little package and is fun to peel, which both kids and adults love.

Pasture-raised eggs (the number is up to you)
Water

Place the eggs in a pot and cover them with 1 inch of cold water. Bring the water to a boil, and cook the eggs for 1 minute. Cover the pot, remove it from the heat, and let it stand for 5 minutes.

Run the eggs under cold water for a few minutes to stop the cooking.

Keep them in the fridge, in their shells, until you are ready to eat them.

*Contains eggs

CASHEW CHEESE

C Cleanse

G Gut

V Vegan

Makes: 1 pint

Prep time: 10 minutes

Fermentation time: overnight (optional)

Nut "cheeses" have quickly become a staple in the diets of those avoiding dairy or dealing with allergies. Fatty nuts like cashews, pine nuts, and macadamias can be blended and aged to provide a tangy cheese-like flavor and texture. Once you've got this recipe dialed in, you can alternate the nuts and flavorings used in each batch.

2 cups raw cashews
1 tablespoon lemon juice
1 teaspoon sea salt
¼ cup or more water, for thinning
¼ teaspoon probiotic powder (optional)
2 tablespoons chopped fresh herbs, such as parsley, chives, rosemary, and/or dill (optional)
1 tablespoon nutritional yeast (optional)

Place the cashews, lemon juice, and salt into a blender and process the mixture until it's smooth but thick, using water as needed to help thin out the paste. Once a consistency similar to soft goat cheese (chèvre) is achieved, use a rubber spatula to transfer the mixture to a large bowl.

At this point you can choose to ferment the cheese overnight. This will give it more of a tangy, cheesy flavor. If you decide to ferment it, fold in the probiotic powder and either keep the mixture in the bowl or transfer it to kitchen molds or cheesecloth. Cover it or wrap it snugly in the cheesecloth and allow it to sit in a warm area (about 70°F) for 8 to 12 hours. You should start seeing small air pockets forming throughout the paste.

If you choose to serve the cashew cheese freshly blended, you can immediately season it with the optional fresh herbs, nutritional yeast, or any spices you like.

Store refrigerated in a container for up to one week.

SOUR CREAM

Ⓒ Cleanse

Ⓖ Gut

Ⓥ Vegan

Makes: ¾ cup

Prep time: 10 minutes

Sour cream is the hidden ingredient in many dishes, both sweet and savory, that makes it moist and absolutely delicious. Here's an easy recipe to make your own dairy-free version.

1 cup raw pine nuts
1 tablespoon plus 1 teaspoon lemon juice
½ teaspoon sea salt
¼ cup water

In a blender, purée all the ingredients until the mixture is smooth, thick, and creamy.

Store the sour cream in a container in the refrigerator for up to four days.

ASIAN-INSPIRED CHICKPEAS

Ⓒ Cleanse

Ⓥ Vegan

Serves: 4 to 6

Prep time: overnight soaking (8 to 12 hours)

Cooking time: 20 minutes plus 10 minutes to marinate

This is a simple recipe that gives a boost of protein. Fresh chickpeas taste better than canned, so leave time to soak them overnight and cook them the next day.

4 cups of cooked chickpeas
½ cup minced red onion
2 scallions, sliced thin
1 tablespoon sesame seeds
2 tablespoons toasted sesame oil
2 tablespoons rice wine vinegar
1 teaspoon balsamic vinegar
3 to 4 tablespoons wheat-free tamari

Soak chickpeas overnight for 8 to 12 hours then strain and rinse well. Cook the chickpeas in 2 quarts of water for 15 to 20 minutes, or until tender. Stirs all the ingredients together and let marinate for 10 minutes. Taste, adjust seasonings as needed and serve.

Pairings: Serve with Herbed Buffalo Burgers (page 187), the Most Perfect Chicken Breast (page 163), or Marinated Carrot Ribbons (page 101).

ROASTED CAULIFLOWER WITH A MIDDLE EASTERN TWIST

Lisa and Mehmet Oz, founders of HealthCorps

Ⓒ Cleanse*

Ⓥ Vegan

1 head cauliflower, broken into bite-size florets
1 cup canned garbanzo beans, rinsed and drained (or dry beans soaked overnight, rinsed, and drained)
2 tablespoons extra-virgin olive oil
2 garlic cloves, minced
1 tablespoon whole cumin seeds
1 tablespoon nigella seeds (also known as kalonji seeds or black onion seeds)
2 shallots, minced
1 teaspoon red pepper flakes (optional)
½ cup golden raisins (unsulfered)
Juice of ½ lemon
Sea salt to taste

Preheat the oven to 400°F.

Mix all the ingredients together in a large bowl, then spread the mixture into a baking dish and roast it in the oven for about 40 minutes. Toss the mixture once or twice while it cooks to roast it evenly. The cauliflower should brown a bit and the top should get a little crispy.

*Omit raisins

PICKLED RADISHES

C Cleanse

G Gut

V Vegan

Makes: 1 pint

Prep time: 10 minutes

Fermentation time: 3 to 5 days

This basic fermentation yields a salty and tangy product that not only boosts good bacteria in the gut but also works perfectly in salads, sushi, or just out of the jar as a yummy snack. You'll need a ½-gallon mason or similar glass jar for this recipe.

1 quart water

2 tablespoons unpasteurized apple cider vinegar

3 tablespoons sea salt

1 pound daikon, watermelon, or common red radishes, sliced into thin rounds or julienned ⅛-inch thick

Pour the water, vinegar, and salt into the ½-gallon mason jar. Stir until the salt is dissolved, then add the radishes to the brine and loosely cover the jar with its lid. Place the jar in a warm, dark space for three to four days, being mindful to open and close the jar one to two times per day. Doing this releases gasses and helps prevent the jar or bottle from potentially exploding.

After four days, store the jar in the fridge. The radishes will keep up to one month.

Chef Frank on Fermented Foods

I love fermented foods, not just because of their health benefits but for the flavors they add to dishes. Miso, sauerkraut, or other fermented foods like kimchi or pickled vegetables can be added to spreads, dips, and dressings for a tangy element. Fermented foods are used daily in most traditional cultures, and when eating grains and animal proteins, I always try to incorporate a scoop of fermented foods to aid in digestion and add beneficial gut flora.

MARINATED CARROT RIBBONS

Ⓒ Cleanse

Ⓖ Gut

Ⓥ Vegan

Serves: 2

Prep time: 10 minutes

Marinating time: 15 to 20 minutes

In a tasty marinade, these carrots become gently "cooked," perfect for summer meals or as sides. The olives and lemon create a simple yet incredible flavor profile, and the pine nuts round it out with richness and protein.

1 pound carrots, peeled
½ cup sliced green olives
¼ cup sliced shallots or red onion
¼ cup toasted pine nuts
2 teaspoons chopped fresh thyme
1 tablespoon freshly squeezed lemon juice
2 tablespoons extra-virgin olive oil
2 pinches sea salt

Using a vegetable peeler or mandoline, slice the carrots lengthwise to create long, noodle-like pieces. In a large bowl, combine the carrot "noodles," olives, shallots or onion, pine nuts, thyme, lemon juice, olive oil, and salt. Use a pair of tongs to gently toss it all together. Allow the carrots to marinate and soften for 15 to 20 minutes before serving.

GRACY'S AVOCUMBER ROLLS

Ⓒ Cleanse

Ⓖ Gut

Ⓥ Vegan

Serves: 2

Prep time: 10 minutes

Dr. Junger and his daughter Grace created this simple and delicious snack, which is both satiating and hydrating. Cut the rolls like sushi and add any of Dr. Junger's favorite salad toppings (pages 16–17).

2 large cucumbers
Flesh of 2 ripe avocados
Sea salt to taste
Lemon juice to taste
Bragg Liquid Aminos to taste

Peel the cucumbers, cut off the ends, and cut them in half widthwise. With a knife, cut out the center flesh and seeds of each piece, creating a tubelike hole through the cucumbers (you should be able to see through them like a telescope). Stuff the avocado flesh into the open tubes of the cucumbers.

Set the filled cucumbers on their sides and slice them like sushi, making 4 to 5 rolls total. Season the rolls with sea salt, lemon juice, and a dash of liquid aminos. Serve and eat immediately.

ASPARAGUS, SORREL, AND CHESTNUT PURÉE

Ⓒ Cleanse

Ⓖ Gut

Ⓥ Vegan

Serves: 2 to 4

Prep time: 20 minutes

This dish is an elegant side dish to any meal (vegetables, fish, chicken, or wild game) and also a wonderfully healthy baby food! The chestnuts provide protein and healthy fat, while the taste is sweet and simple.

1 bunch asparagus (12 ounces), woody portions removed and each stalk cut into thirds
1 cup (5 to 6 ounces) raw, peeled chestnuts, plus 4 for garnish
½ cup raw pine nuts
1 bulb Slow-Roasted Garlic (page 113)
½ cup water
1 tablespoon lemon juice
1 to 2 teaspoons sea salt, or to taste
1 handful fresh sorrel or baby spinach
¼ teaspoon freshly ground black pepper

Bring 4 cups of salted water to a boil. Blanch the asparagus for just 2 to 3 minutes, then remove the asparagus with a slotted spoon and immediately submerge them in a bowl of ice water to stop the cooking process. Cut and set aside half the cooked asparagus tops for use as a garnish later.

In a blender, purée the blanched asparagus, chestnuts, pine nuts, garlic, and the ½ cup water until the mixture is smooth, about 45 seconds. Add the lemon juice, salt, and greens, blending until the mixture is well combined. Sprinkle in the black pepper. Serve garnished with the reserved asparagus tops.

GINGERED CARROT PURÉE

C Cleanse
G Gut
V Vegan*

Makes: 2 cups

Prep time: 10 minutes

Cooking time: 15 to 20 minutes

This simple but vibrantly colored purée pairs well with baked fish, grilled lamb, or roasted vegetables. Like the Asparagus, Sorrel, and Chestnut Purée (page 103), it also makes yummy baby food for lucky little ones!

1 pound carrots (about 4 cups), peeled and evenly chopped
1 garlic clove
2 tablespoons apple cider vinegar
1 cup water, vegetable stock, or chicken stock
1 tablespoon freshly grated ginger
1½ tablespoons coconut butter/manna (the oil and flesh together, not just the oil)
Sea salt to taste

In a small saucepan, combine the carrots, garlic, vinegar, and water or stock. Cover and bring the mixture to a boil, then lower the heat and simmer until the carrots are tender.

Transfer the mixture to a blender and purée until it's smooth and creamy.

Return the purée to the saucepan and reheat it over medium heat, stirring in the ginger and coconut butter/manna until they are well incorporated. Add a pinch or two of salt to taste. Keep the purée warm until you're ready to serve it.

*If using water or vegetable stock

ZA'ATAR-ROASTED CARROTS

Ⓒ Cleanse

Ⓖ Gut

Ⓥ Vegan

Serves: 4, as a side

Prep time: 5 minutes

Cooking time: 30 to 40 minutes

This is one of my favorite ways to enjoy carrots. Za'atar is a Middle Eastern condiment and provides a complex earthy balance to the sweetness of the roasted carrots.

2 pounds medium carrots
2 to 4 tablespoons extra-virgin olive oil
1 heaping tablespoon za'atar spice
2 teaspoons sea salt

Preheat the oven to 375°F.

Place the whole carrots in a baking dish. Drizzle them with olive oil, then sprinkle in the za'atar spice and salt. Bake them for about 30 minutes, stirring occasionally, until the carrots are fork-tender.

MINTY RICE DOLMAS WITH GARLIC DIPPING SAUCE

C Cleanse

V Vegan

Makes: 10 to 12 dolmas

Prep time: 20 minutes

Dolmas, a Middle Eastern staple, are easy to prepare and a perfect way to use up leftover rice or even quinoa. They make perfect passing appetizers or starters for any occasion.

¼ cup extra-virgin olive oil
¼ cup finely chopped raw walnuts
2 cups cooked brown rice
Zest of 1 lemon
Juice of ½ lemon
½ cup roughly chopped fresh parsley
2 tablespoons roughly chopped fresh mint
1 teaspoon ground coriander
1 teaspoon sea salt
12 large pickled grape leaves

For the Garlic Dipping Sauce
1 cup raw sesame seeds
4 garlic cloves
2 tablespoons lemon juice
¼ cup extra-virgin olive oil
1 teaspoon sea salt
½ cup plus 2 tablespoons water, or just enough for the correct consistency

Heat the olive oil in a small skillet over medium heat. Add the walnuts and slowly roast them, stirring occasionally, until they are lightly browned.

In a medium bowl, toss together the walnuts, rice, lemon zest, lemon juice, parsley, mint, coriander, and salt until the mixture is well combined.

Spread the grape leaves on a cutting board. If they are attached, remove their stems, then depending on the size of the leaves, add 1½ to 2 tablespoons of the rice mixture. Fold in the sides to meet in the middle then roll each one away from you until the rice is securely wrapped. Continue until all the seasoned rice is used up.

To make the dipping sauce, in a blender purée the sesame seeds, garlic, lemon juice, olive oil, and salt, adding enough of the water to create a yogurt-like consistency.

CRISPY POTATO WEDGES WITH ROASTED RED PEPPER AND CASHEW MAYO

V Vegan

Serves: 4

Prep time: 10 minutes

Cooking time: 30 minutes

Classically comforting and beyond tasty, this is a healthier method of fried potatoes. Everyone will love these, and a homemade dipping sauce is always the best.

3 pounds potatoes (we recommend Yukon Golds)
2 to 3 tablespoons extra-virgin olive oil
1 to 2 teaspoons sea salt, plus a bit extra
½ teaspoon freshly ground black pepper
2 tablespoons freshly chopped herbs (parsley, rosemary, thyme, oregano)

For the Mayo
1 cup raw cashews
2 roasted red bell peppers, seeded and peeled
2 garlic cloves
½ teaspoon chipotle chili powder
Juice of 1 lemon
½ cup extra-virgin olive oil
½ cup water, or more if needed

Preheat the oven to 375°F.

Give the potatoes a rinse and peel them only if desired. Cut each potato in half lengthwise, then cut each half into 3 or 4 wedges. Place all the cut potatoes into a large bowl and toss them with the olive oil, salt, and pepper.

Spread the seasoned potatoes evenly in a baking dish, skin (rounded) side down. Roast them in the oven until they are tender, about 30 minutes.

While the potatoes are roasting, prepare the mayo. In a blender or food processor, purée all the mayo ingredients until the mixture is smooth and spreadable. Use more water if you need to thin the consistency.

After removing the potatoes from the oven, toss them in a large bowl with the chopped herbs and an extra sprinkle of sea salt. Serve them warm with a side of the mayo.

VEGETABLE PAKORAS

C Cleanse

V Vegan

Serves: 4

Prep time: 15 minutes

Cooking time: 15 minutes

Crisp little bites with just the right amount of spice, these fritters are perfect alongside any Indian dish or on their own as a snack. It's important to choose a high-quality fat to fry these in. We recommend coconut oil, lard, or another wild or pasture-raised animal fat that will remain stable at high temperatures.

1 cup garbanzo bean flour
¼ cup brown rice flour
¼ cup roughly chopped fresh cilantro
1 jalapeño, roughly chopped (optional)
1 teaspoon ground turmeric
1 teaspoon cumin seeds
2 teaspoons roughly ground coriander seeds
½ to 1¾ cups water
About 1 cup coconut oil
1 zucchini, sliced lengthwise, then sliced into ¼-inch-thick half-moons
½ head (about 2 cups) broccoli, cut into small florets
½ head (about 2 cups) cauliflower, cut into small florets
Sea salt to taste

In a large bowl, combine well the garbanzo bean and brown rice flours, cilantro, optional jalapeño, turmeric, cumin seeds, and coriander seeds. Stir in just enough water to create a thick consistency, so that when the vegetables are dunked in the mixture they will be well coated but the batter will not run off.

Melt the coconut oil in a 2-quart pot set over medium-high heat. If you have a thermometer, heat the oil to 325°F. Test the oil by adding a drop of the batter. If it's hot enough, the batter should create bubbles and rise in the oil.

Dip the zucchini, broccoli, and cauliflower pieces one by one into the batter, coating each well, then drop each into the hot oil. Fry them for about 2 to 3 minutes each, until they are golden brown and crispy. Drain them on a paper towel and sprinkle each piece with sea salt before serving.

SARDINES ON ENDIVES

Sarah Marchand, Clean community member

C Cleanse

G Gut

Serves: 2

Prep time: 10 minutes

To me, living a clean lifestyle means using fresh, wholesome ingredients to make often simple but delicious meals and being thoughtful about everything we eat. Serve this dish, rich in omega-3s, calcium, and protein, as an appetizer for guests or pair it with a fresh green salad for a clean and easy evening meal. The sharpness of the lemon and the crisp endives are a perfect complement to the rich-tasting sardines.

1 4- to 5-ounce can sardines packed in olive oil
1 tablespoon capers
1 tablespoon lemon juice
1 tablespoon fresh thyme
Dash of cayenne
Sea salt and freshly ground black pepper to taste
1 to 2 heads (about ½ to ¾ pound) endives

In a medium bowl, mash the sardines with the oil from the can, the capers, and the lemon juice. Stir in the thyme and cayenne, and season with salt and pepper.

Wash and separate the heads of endives into single leaves. Fill each leaf with the sardine mash and arrange the leaves on two serving plates. Makes about 8 to 10 endive leaves.

BRAZIL NUT PÂTÉ

C Cleanse*

G Gut

V Vegan

Makes: 1 pint

Prep time: overnight plus 5 to 10 minutes

This is a tasty and versatile pâté you'll want to keep on hand for many occasions. The miso adds extra enzymes and good gut flora, and the Brazil nuts contain selenium and healthy fats as well as protein. Thin the pâté with olive oil to use it as a salad dressing.

2 cups raw Brazil nuts, soaked overnight in 4 cups of water with 1 teaspoon apple cider vinegar
2 tablespoons miso (preferably soy-free South River brand)
2 garlic cloves
2 tablespoons tomato powder or ¼ cup sun-dried tomatoes in olive oil
½ cup chopped fresh parsley
Leaves from 3 to 4 sprigs fresh thyme
2 tablespoons lemon juice
¼ cup or more extra-virgin olive oil

Drain the soaked Brazil nuts, then pulse them in a food processor until they are coarsely chopped.

Add the miso, garlic, tomato powder or sun-dried tomatoes, parsley, and thyme, and purée the mixture until it's smooth. While the machine is running, slowly drizzle in the lemon juice and olive oil. I prefer a thicker consistency, but use more oil if you like it a thin consistency. Store in the fridge for three to four days.

*Omit tomatoes

STUFFED MUSHROOMS

C Cleanse*
G Gut
V Vegan

Serves: 4
Prep time: 20 minutes
Cooking time: 30 minutes

One of the quintessential potluck or holiday party dishes, this easily becomes a hearty family meal (perfect for Meatless Mondays) by using large portobello caps. But the stuffing works for any mushroom, so make them both ways!

5 large portobello mushroom caps
Extra-virgin olive oil, for liberal drizzling
2 tablespoons minced fresh rosemary leaves
Sea salt and freshly ground black pepper to taste
2 tablespoons avocado oil
2 celery stalks, diced small
1 medium carrot, diced small
½ small onion, chopped
2 teaspoons dried sage
1 teaspoon dried thyme
½ cup roughly chopped fresh parsley
1 cup cubed gluten-free bread
2 plum tomatoes, chopped
Juice of 1 lemon

Preheat the oven to 350°F.

In a baking dish, place 4 of the mushrooms and drizzle them with a few tablespoons of olive oil, then season them with rosemary, salt, and pepper. Allow them to marinate for 15 to 20 minutes.

While those mushrooms rest, chop the remaining mushroom into small pieces. Heat the avocado oil in a pan and lightly sauté the chopped mushroom with the celery, carrot, and onion until the vegetables are soft. Remove them from heat and allow them to cool.

In a medium bowl, stir together the cooked vegetables, sage, thyme, parsley, bread cubes, tomatoes, and lemon juice. If the stuffing seems too thick, add a bit of water to moisten it. Season the mixture to taste, then distribute it between the four marinating mushrooms.

Bake the stuffed caps for 20 to 30 minutes or until the mushrooms are tender and the stuffing begins to crisp. Serve warm.

*Omit tomatoes

ASIAN LETTUCE WRAPS

Brent Kronk, Clean community member

C Cleanse

G Gut*

Serves: 4

16 Boston or butter lettuce leaves
1 pound ground pasture-raised chicken or turkey
2 tablespoons extra-virgin olive oil
1 medium red onion
1 garlic clove, minced
1 tablespoon wheat-free tamari
1 teaspoon freshly grated ginger
1 tablespoon rice wine vinegar
½ cup teriyaki sauce (recipe included below)
1 8-ounce can water chestnuts, drained and finely chopped
1 bunch scallions, chopped
2 teaspoons toasted sesame oil

For the Teriyaki Sauce
⅓ cup balsamic vinegar
⅓ cup coconut nectar
1 teaspoon freshly grated ginger
¼ teaspoon freshly ground black pepper
1 teaspoon brown rice miso
1 tablespoon water

First, make the sauce. In a small saucepan, combine the balsamic vinegar, coconut nectar, ginger, and pepper. Bring the mixture to a boil, then lower the heat and simmer for 10 minutes. Remove it from heat and let it cool before stirring in the miso and water. Set aside.

Rinse the whole lettuce leaves and pat them dry, being careful not to tear them. Set them aside.

In a medium skillet, brown the chicken or turkey in 1 tablespoon of the olive oil, stirring often. Reduce the heat if the meat starts to brown too fast and turn too dark. When it is cooked through, set it aside to cool.

In another skillet, heat the other tablespoon of olive oil and sauté the onion, garlic, tamari, ginger, and vinegar, and add ½ cup of the teriyaki sauce. Stir until everything is well mixed and turning tender and slightly browned. Add the water chestnuts, scallions, sesame oil, and browned chicken or turkey. Continue cooking for about 2 minutes.

Arrange the lettuce leaves around the outer edges of a large serving platter, and pile the filling mixture in the center of the plate. Serve, allowing each person to spoon a portion of the filling into a lettuce leaf and wrap the leaf around the filling like a burrito. Dip burrito in leftover teriyaki sauce.

*Omit coconut nectar

SLOW-ROASTED GARLIC

C Cleanse

G Gut

V Vegan

Makes: ½ cup

Prep time: 5 minutes

Cooking time: 30 to 40 minutes

Roasting garlic aids in mellowing out the intensity of raw garlic and, in return, delivers a soft and sweet bulb of nutrition. To maximize the best-tasting garlic, be sure to choose fresh garlic that is firm in texture.

4 whole garlic bulbs
2 tablespoons extra-virgin olive oil
Sea salt to taste
¼ teaspoon freshly ground black pepper

Preheat the oven to 300°F.

Carefully, make a horizontal cut across the top of the garlic bulbs to expose the garlic flesh. Place the bulbs in a baking dish, drizzle them with olive oil, and add a dash of salt and the pepper. Bake the bulbs for 30 minutes, or until the garlic is lightly browned on the outside and soft on the inside. You can poke down into the bulbs and see it.

Remove the bulbs from the oven and allow them to cool slightly before removing the soft garlic from the skins or squeezing it out like you would with a pastry bag of frosting.

Variations: Shallots, onions, or bell peppers can be roasted in this same fashion, though you may need to increase the cooking time.

EXPERIENCE: I enjoy exploring the ingredients I found in the recipes in the original *Clean* book. They were not always the ingredients I was accustomed to using in my pre-clean life! How wonderful it is to be able to eat healthily but also have amazing taste at the same time. Who knew? Thank you, Clean community, for helping me stay clean.

GARLICKY GREENS

C Cleanse

G Gut

V Vegan

Serves: 2

Prep time: 10 minutes

Cooking time: 10 minutes

This recipe is a great way to get dark, leafy greens into your family's diet, building your immune systems and getting a dose of iron and magnesium, plus plenty of antioxidants. We love our greens!

2 tablespoons avocado oil
1 tablespoon olive oil
3 to 5 garlic cloves, or more if you prefer, thinly sliced
6 cups chopped greens, such as kale, Swiss chard, and/or spinach
Lemon juice to taste
Sea salt and freshly ground black pepper to taste

In a large sauté pan, heat the avocado and olive oils, then add the garlic and sauté it until it is lightly toasted. Add the greens, using a pair of tongs to quickly toss them in the pan. Then add a few tablespoons of water, cover the pan, and allow the greens to steam for a few minutes. Once the greens have wilted, add a splash of lemon juice and salt and pepper to taste. Serve warm.

BUTTERNUT SQUASH RAGOUT

C Cleanse

G Gut

V Vegan*

Serves: 2 to 4

Prep time: 10 minutes

Cooking time: 30 minutes

This delicious, creamy side dish will quickly become an autumn staple. It pairs perfectly with wild mushrooms, green beans, lamb, or poultry.

2 tablespoons coconut oil
½ cup minced shallots
4 cups peeled and diced butternut squash
1½ cups chicken or vegetable stock
2 to 3 teaspoons sea salt
Freshly ground black pepper to taste
1 tablespoon chopped fresh sage
2 tablespoons coconut butter

Warm the coconut oil in a 2-quart saucepan set over medium-high heat. Add the shallots and lightly sauté them until they are translucent, about 2 to 3 minutes. Stir in the squash and sauté for another minute or 2. Add 6 ounces of the stock and stir, allowing the squash to absorb all the liquid before adding more. Continue to cook, stirring often to create a creamy, risotto-like consistency. Add more stock as needed, but not so much that it turns the squash into soup.

When the squash is cooked through, add the salt, pepper, and sage. Stir in the coconut butter and allow it to melt into the squash mixture. Serve warm.

*If using vegetable stock

SWEET AND SPICY SQUASH AND APPLE PURÉE

C Cleanse

V Vegan

Makes: 1 9-inch pie, 4 to 6 servings

Prep time: 15 minutes

Cooking time: 20 minutes

A side to a savory meal? A savory snack? A dessert? All of the above. This is an amazing flavor blend and an autumn food at its most comforting. Remove the cayenne and pecans when serving this to little ones.

1 3- to 5-pound butternut squash, peeled, seeded, and cut into 1-inch chunks
2 crisp apples, cored and cut into 1-inch chunks
3 tablespoons coconut oil, melted
Sprinkle of cinnamon
Pinch of cayenne
2 sprinkles sea salt
2 tablespoons coconut nectar
½ cup pecans, toasted, roughly chopped

Preheat the oven to 350°F.

Spread the squash and apples evenly in a casserole dish. Stir in the coconut oil, cinnamon, cayenne, and salt until everything is evenly incorporated. Bake the mixture for about 20 minutes, until the squash is tender when pierced with a fork.

Remove the mixture from the oven, then purée it in a food processor with the coconut nectar until it is smooth and silky. Fold in the toasted pecans and serve.

ROASTED PEARS AND PARSNIPS

C Cleanse

V Vegan

Serves: 4

Prep time: 10 minutes

Cooking time: 30 minutes

This is a wonderful snack food that's both sweet and savory. The pears and parsnips are lovely and yummy. Kids adore them!

4 large parsnips (about 2 pounds)
2 medium Bosc or Anjou pears
1 to 2 tablespoons extra-virgin olive oil
1 teaspoon chopped fresh thyme
1 teaspoon sea salt
¼ teaspoon freshly ground black pepper

Preheat the oven to 400°F.

Peel the parsnips, then cut them in half lengthwise, then into 2-inch-thick pieces. Cut the pears in half, remove the cores, then cut them into wedges about the same thickness as the parsnips. Toss the parsnips and pears together in a large bowl with the olive oil, thyme, salt, and pepper.

Scatter the seasoned parsnips and pears in a baking dish. Roast them for 25 to 30 minutes, until they are golden brown, but halfway through the roasting be sure to flip the pears and parsnips so they brown on both sides.

SLOW-ROASTED TOMATOES

G Gut

V Vegan

Makes: 2 quarts

Prep time: 15 minutes

Cooking time: 3 hours

When tomatoes are past their peak, this is a great recipe to make. When they're dehydrated or roasted for a long time at a low temperature, their flavors concentrate, which yields a sweeter and more intense-tasting tomato. This is a great way to enjoy the taste of tomatoes year-round, in salads, over noodles, or as a pizza topping.

3 to 5 pounds Roma tomatoes, halved
Extra-virgin olive oil
Sea salt
Freshly ground black pepper
A few 3-finger pinches (thumb, pointer, and middle fingers pinched together) dried thyme
A few 3-finger pinches dried oregano

Preheat the oven to 325°F.

In a large bowl, drizzle the tomatoes with enough olive oil to evenly coat them. Sprinkle them with some salt, pepper, thyme, and oregano, and toss so the tomatoes are evenly coated.

Place the tomatoes, skin side down, on a large baking sheet. Roast them for about 2 to 3 hours, or until the tomatoes are shrunken, generally half their original size or less. Remove them from the oven and leave them to cool.

Store them for three to four days in an airtight container, refrigerated.

Pairings: Include the tomatoes on gluten-free pizza, in tarts, in salad toppings, with pasta, or in egg dishes.

SPINACH PECAN PESTO

C Cleanse

G Gut

V Vegan

Makes: about 2 cups

Prep time: 10 minutes

Pesto is one of those versatile and always-usable food items, and there are many unique variations on the basic basil recipe. We love this one. Use it with salads, as a dip, on roasted vegetables, or with noodles.

1 cup raw pecans
2 garlic cloves
4 to 5 cups (6 to 8 ounces) baby spinach
2 teaspoons chopped fresh rosemary
Zest of 1 lemon
Sea salt to taste
1 teaspoon freshly ground black pepper
½ cup extra-virgin olive oil

Pulse the pecans and garlic in a food processor until they are coarsely chopped. Add the spinach and rosemary and continue to process. Add the lemon zest, salt, and pepper, and drizzle in the olive oil as the processor is running until the pesto reaches a smooth, creamy consistency. Store in a container, refrigerated, for up to a week. A little olive oil drizzled over the top will act as a barrier and keep from oxidizing.

BLACK OLIVE TAPENADE

C Cleanse

G Gut

V Vegan

Makes: about 1½ cups

Prep time: 10 minutes

Olive tapenade is simple to make and can be made with any type of olive. This versatile spread can be used on crackers or cucumbers, or as a crust on roasted fish, lamb, chicken, or even roasted vegetables.

2 cups Kalamata olives, pitted
2 garlic cloves
Zest of 1 orange
1 teaspoon minced fresh thyme
2 teaspoons minced fresh oregano
¼ cup chopped fresh parsley
¼ cup extra-virgin olive oil

Pulse the olives and garlic in a food processor until they are coarsely chopped. Add the orange zest, thyme, oregano, parsley, and olive oil, and continue to process the mixture until it is well puréed.

Store the tapenade in a container, in the fridge, for up to one week.

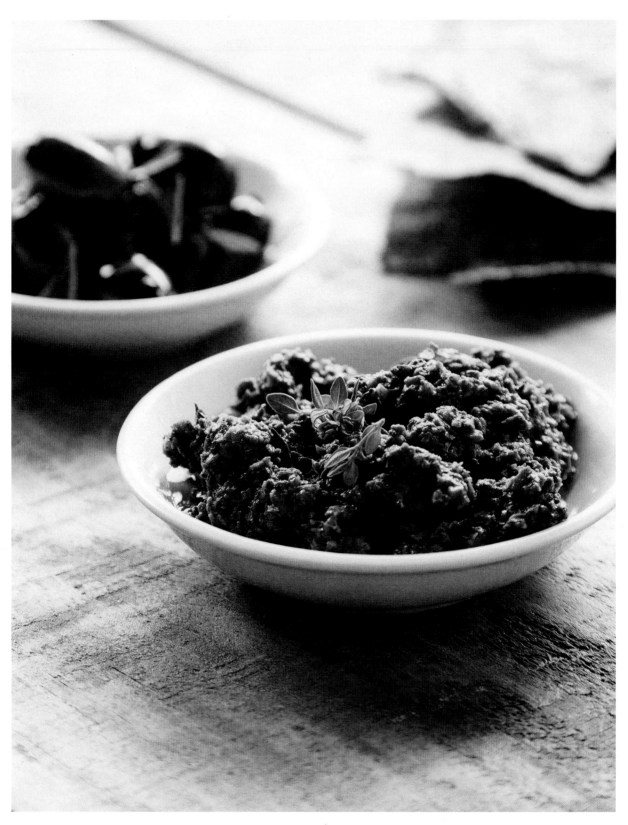

Black Olive Tapenade and Almond Poppy Seed Crackers, pages 120 and 128

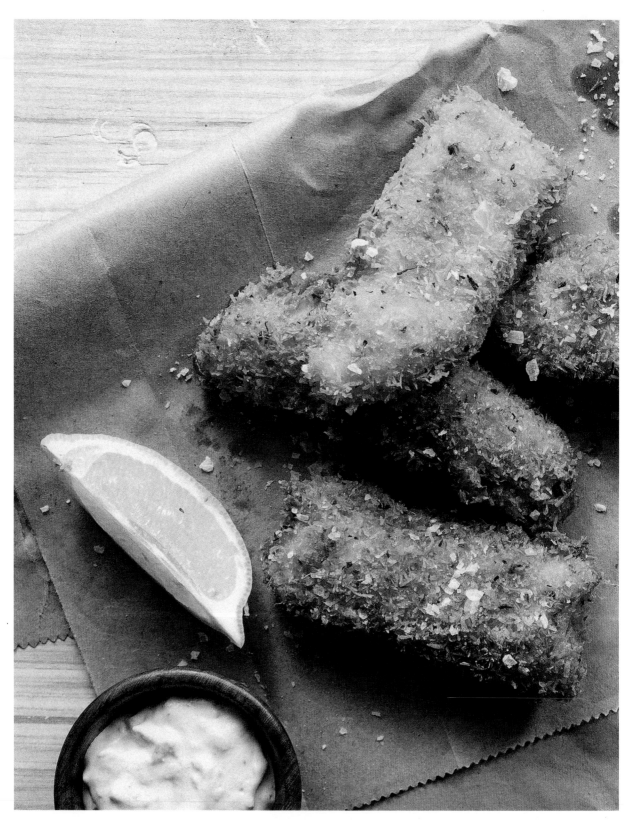

Fish Sticks with Tartar Sauce, page 142.

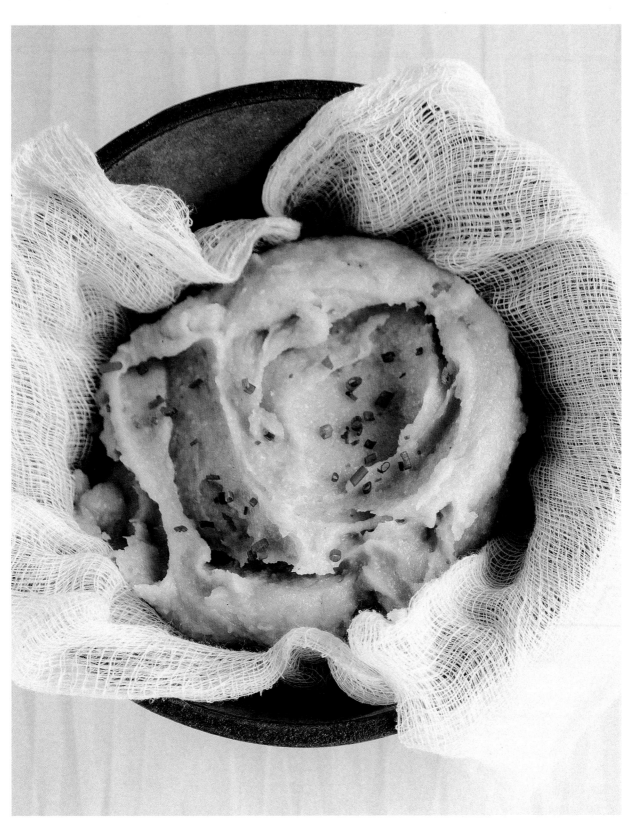

Cashew Cheese, page 97

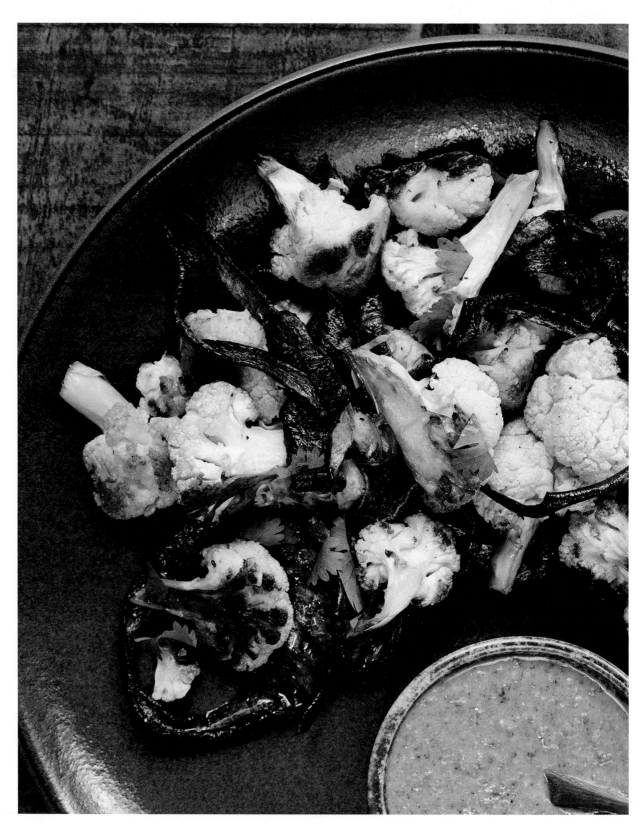

Roasted Cauliflower with Pistachio Dressing, page 203

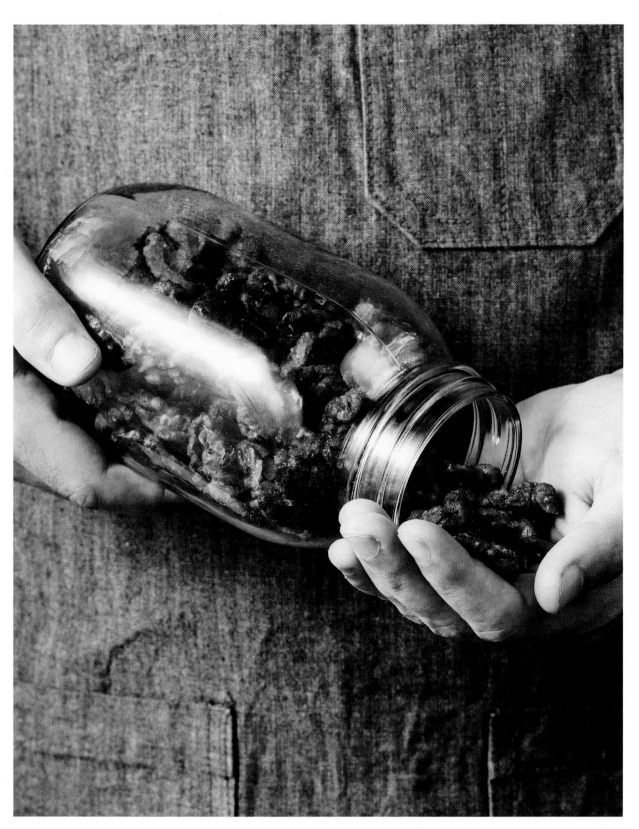

Crunchy Maple Mesquite Walnuts, page 132

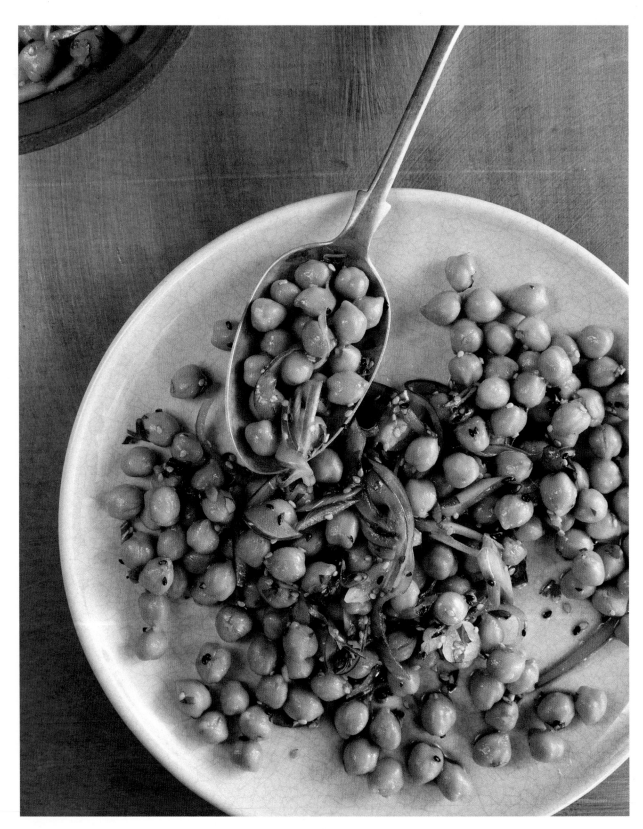

Asian-Inspired Chickpeas, page 98

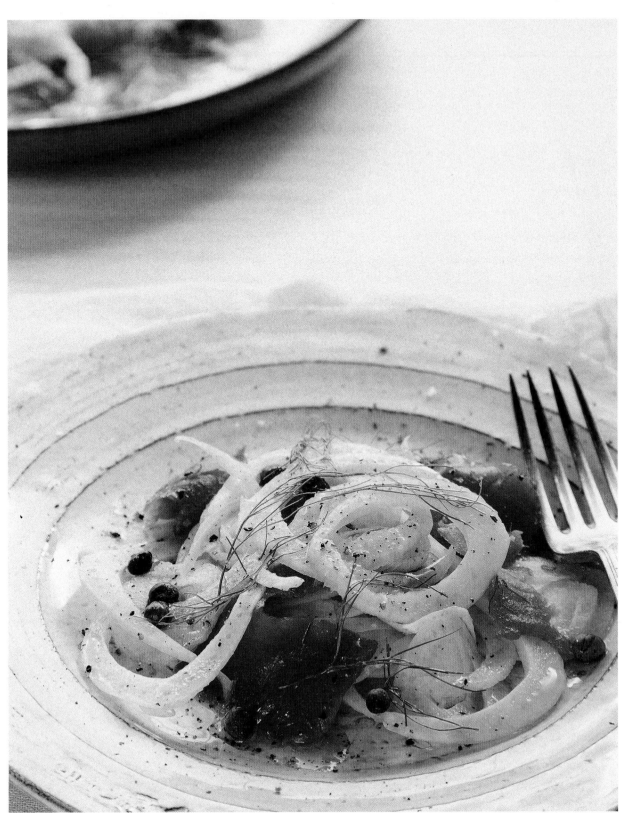

Smoked Salmon and Fennel Salad, page 81

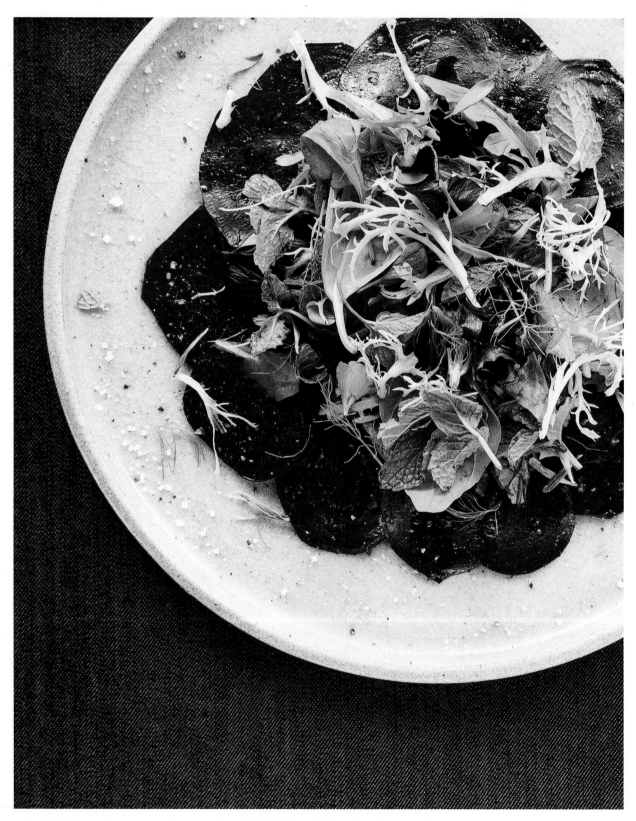

Roasted Beet Carpaccio, page 121

ROASTED BEET CARPACCIO

C Cleanse

V Vegan

Serves: 2 to 3

Prep time: 10 minutes

Cooking time: 45 minutes

This is a favorite for dinner parties or special occasions where you want a gorgeous starter or passed appetizer. Typically carpaccio is beef or seafood sliced thinly, so this is a vegetarian take on it, yet it's still as mouthwateringly delicious and elegant.

4 large beets, peeled
2 handfuls frisée, spinach, or arugula
1 small handful herbs, such as mint, dill, parsley, and/or cilantro, plus edible flowers
Juice of 1 lemon
About ¼ cup extra-virgin olive oil, plus more for the beets
Sea salt and freshly ground black pepper to taste

Preheat the oven to 350°F.

Put the beets in a baking dish, pour in about ½ inch of water, then cover the dish with tinfoil. Roast them for about 45 minutes or until the beets are tender. Remove them from the oven, drain them, and allow them to cool.

Once the beets have cooled, use a mandoline or a sharp knife to slice them into very thin rounds.

Arrange the thinly sliced beets over two or three serving plates, covering the entire surface of each plate. Drizzle the beets with a little olive oil and a sprinkle of sea salt.

In a medium bowl, toss the greens, herbs, and flowers with lemon juice, olive oil, and salt and pepper to taste. Place a small bundle of greens in the center of each plate, on top of the beets, and serve.

ROSEMARY GARLIC WHITE BEAN DIP

Ⓒ Cleanse

Ⓥ Vegan

Makes: 1½ cups

Prep time: 10 minutes

This goes perfectly with so many meals and snacks, it's another one you'll want to make often and keep on hand. Perfect with Snappy Crackers (page 127) or vegetables.

2 cups cooked white beans
1 batch Slow-Roasted Garlic (page 113)
Juice of 1 lemon
¼ cup extra-virgin olive oil
1 large sprig fresh rosemary (about 2 teaspoons chopped)
Sea salt to taste
¼ teaspoon freshly ground black pepper

Purée the cooked white beans in a food processor or blender with the roasted garlic, lemon juice, and olive oil. Add as much water as needed for your desired consistency, then add the rosemary, salt, and pepper, blending until the mixture is smooth.

Store the dip in a container, refrigerated, for four to five days.

CLEAN AND GREEN GUACAMOLE

Todd Lepine M.D., Integrative Functional Medicine expert

C Cleanse*

G Gut

V Vegan

Makes: ½ pint

Prep time: 15 minutes

Make your own whenever you can. Fresh and organic ingredients are best. Guacamole goes great with fish tacos or nachos, on salads, or as a dip for sprouted corn chips, gluten-free crackers, or vegetables. Enjoy!

2 medium-size ripe avocados
Fresh juice from 1 lemon
2 to 3 tablespoons cumin
Salt and pepper to taste
½ sweet onion (Vidalia onion is the best!)
1 big ripe tomato
Handful of cilantro (coriander)
3 cloves garlic (more or less to taste, depending on how much you like garlic)

In a large bowl, combine the avocado with the lemon juice, cumin, salt, and pepper. Use a fork to mash the mixture, then fold in the onion, tomato, cilantro, and garlic. You can make the guacamole as chunky or smooth as you like it. Allow the guacamole to sit for a while at room temperature to allow the flavors to meld before serving.

Variations: For a bulky guacamole version, add a few tablespoons of raw hemp seeds and minced carrot.

*Omit tomato

TOMATO SALSA

Ⓖ Gut

Ⓥ Vegan

Makes: about 1 quart

Prep time: 15 minutes

What are tacos and nachos without salsa? This fresh and yummy salsa is the perfect accompaniment to Fish Tacos (page 148) and goes great with guacamole. For the best flavor, use the freshest ingredients possible and use tomatoes that are at the height of their ripeness.

3 cups roughly chopped tomatoes
1 cup minced red onion
1 jalapeño or other fresh chili pepper
1 tablespoon minced garlic
½ cup roughly chopped fresh cilantro
¼ cup extra-virgin olive oil
Juice of 1 lime
1½ teaspoons ground cumin
1 tablespoon sea salt
¼ teaspoon freshly ground black pepper

In a large bowl, stir together all the ingredients, then let the mixture stand for 1 hour to allow the flavors to develop.

BEST DIP / SAUCE / SALAD DRESSING EVER

Belinda Rachman, Esq., Clean community member

C Cleanse

G Gut

V Vegan

Makes: 2 cups

Prep time: 4 to 5 minutes

This delicious dressing makes any salad better, but it also works as a sauce over steamed vegetables or as a dip served with raw vegetables or gluten-free chips. I don't feel the least bit deprived eating food this good!

½ cup raw almonds
2 garlic cloves
3 tablespoons nutritional yeast
½ teaspoon ground cumin
½ teaspoon chili powder
¼ teaspoon ground coriander seed
¼ teaspoon paprika
½ teaspoon sea salt
¾ cup plus 2 tablespoons water
½ cup plus 2 tablespoons avocado oil
¼ cup plus 2 tablespoons freshly squeezed lemon juice
2 teaspoons Bragg Liquid Aminos or wheat-free tamari

In a high-powered blender, slowly blend all the ingredients for 1 minute. Turn the speed up to high and continue blending for 1 to 2 additional minutes or until the mixture is smooth and creamy.

Store the dressing in the refrigerator. It may separate, but anytime you want to use it, stir it up and it's as good as new.

EXPERIENCE: Clean was the most powerful choice I ever made. I have lost forty pounds and have such a sense of mastery over food now.

APPLE ONION CHUTNEY

C Cleanse

V Vegan

Makes: about 1 cup

Prep time: 5 minutes

Cooking time: 45 minutes

Sweet and savory, this is the perfect topping for just about anything you can think of that needs an extra "something." Warm or chilled, fresh or stored in the fridge for a few days, it's versatile and delicious. This chutney would also make wonderful gifts in small glass jars!

2 firm, tart apples (such as Granny Smith), peeled, cored, and diced into ¼- to ½-inch pieces
1 medium onion, diced into ¼- to ½-inch pieces
1 cup apple cider or water
¼ cup apple cider vinegar
¼ cup coconut palm sugar or honey
1 tablespoon minced fresh thyme
Sea salt and freshly ground black pepper to taste

In a medium saucepan, gently simmer the apples, onion, apple cider or water, vinegar, sugar or honey, and thyme over medium heat for 30 to 45 minutes, until all the liquid is absorbed. Once the mixture is a thick consistency, season it with a little salt and pepper.

Refrigerate the chutney in a container for up to one week.

Pairings: Serve the chutney with Crispy Roasted Chicken (page 169), Lemon Herb Chicken Burgers (page 156), or Savory Lentil Loaf (page 218).

SNAPPY CRACKERS

Ⓖ Gut

Vegetarian*

Makes: 2 to 3 dozen

Prep time: 20 to 30 minutes

Cooking time: 10 to 12 minutes

When we make healthy changes to our diets, it is often the potato chip / cracker / snack "crunch" that we miss. These crackers will quickly replace those salty, greasy options and become a healthy staple in your pantry.

3 cups almond meal/flour
1 cup ground raw sunflower seeds
2 tablespoons Italian seasoning
1 teaspoon sea salt
2 pasture-raised eggs, whisked
1 tablespoon extra-virgin olive oil

Preheat the oven to 350°F.

In a large mixing bowl, combine the almond meal/flour, sunflower seeds, Italian seasoning, and salt. Stir in the eggs and olive oil, and mix the dough until just combined. Then use your hands to form it into a ball.

Lay out a piece of parchment paper large enough to cover a baking sheet. Place the dough onto the parchment, then cover it with an additional piece of similar-size parchment. Use a rolling pin to roll out the dough between the parchment papers to about an ⅛-inch thickness. Peel off the top sheet of parchment. Use a dough cutter or knife to cut the dough into 1-inch-square crackers.

Place another sheet of parchment onto a baking sheet and move the cut crackers onto this parchment. Bake the crackers for 10 to 12 minutes, until crisp and golden brown.

Allow them to cool to room temperature before storing them in a container. They will keep one to two weeks.

*Contains eggs

ALMOND POPPY SEED CRACKERS

Ⓒ Cleanse

Ⓥ Vegan

Makes: about 2 dozen

Prep time: 20 to 30 minutes

Cooking time: 10 to 12 minutes

These will satisfy your crunchy cracker cravings. Packed with protein, rather than gluten and carbs, these are delicious alone, in soup, or with a dip or spread.

1 cup almond meal/flour
½ cup buckwheat flour
½ cup brown rice flour
¼ cup ground chia seeds
2 tablespoons poppy seeds
2 teaspoons sea salt
2 tablespoons extra-virgin olive oil
½ cup water

Preheat the oven to 350°F.

In a large mixing bowl, combine the almond meal/flour, buckwheat flour, brown rice flour, chia seeds, poppy seeds, and salt. In a small bowl, whisk together the olive oil and water, then stir them into the dry ingredients. Mix the dough until it is just combined, then use your hands to form it into a ball.

Lay out a piece of parchment paper large enough to cover a baking sheet. Place the dough onto the parchment, then cover it with an additional piece of similar-size parchment. Use a rolling pin to roll out the dough between the parchment papers to about an ⅛-inch thickness. Peel off the top sheet of parchment. Use a dough cutter or knife to cut the dough into 1-inch-square crackers, or leave it in one solid piece.

Place another sheet of parchment onto the baking sheet and move the cut crackers onto this parchment. Bake the crackers for about 10 to 12 minutes, until crisp and golden brown.

Allow them to cool to room temperature before storing them in a container. They will keep one to two weeks.

ROSEMARY DROP BISCUITS

Ⓒ Cleanse

Ⓥ Vegan

Makes: about 1 dozen

Prep time: 20 minutes

Cooking time: 20 minutes

The perfect quick breakfast on the go, snack, or side to any meal, these are gluten-free family-friendly savory biscuits. Make them into a dessert by adding berries and coconut cream!

1 cup sorghum flour
1 cup brown rice flour, plus a bit extra for dusting
1 tablespoon baking powder
1 tablespoon chopped fresh rosemary
½ teaspoon freshly ground black pepper
2 teaspoons sea salt
⅓ cup coconut oil, melted
¾ to 1 cup hot water

Preheat the oven to 350°F.

In a mixing bowl, combine the sorghum flour, brown rice flour, baking powder, rosemary, pepper, and salt. Pour the melted oil and hot water into the dry ingredients and mix until the dough is fully combined and holds together. You want it a bit on the wet side, because if it's too dry the biscuits will fall apart while baking. If the dough is too dry, add more hot water until it's slightly sticky.

Line a baking sheet with parchment paper, then spoon the dough onto the parchment in 12 equal-size biscuits, so they will bake evenly.

Bake the biscuits on the center rack of your oven for 8 to 10 minutes, then turn the baking sheet around in the oven and continue baking until they are uniformly golden and crisp, for another 6 to 8 minutes. Remove them from the oven and let them cool for a few minutes before serving them warm.

You can also let the biscuits cool completely and store them in the fridge in a container for up to two weeks.

CASHEW ALMOND NUT BUTTER

Alison Burger, health and fitness instructor

C Cleanse

G Gut

V Vegan*

I like to eat my cashew almond butter as a snack with something fresh and crunchy like apple slices or celery. It is also great mixed into dairy-free yogurt, cereal, or granola bowls (think acai bowl: berries, nuts, coconut flakes). It can be used in gluten-free baking too.

2 cups raw almonds
2 cups raw cashews
½ cup raw pecans
¼ teaspoon vanilla bean powder or ½ raw vanilla bean
1 tablespoon ground cinnamon, or to taste
½ teaspoon ground nutmeg
½ teaspoon sea salt, or to taste
1 tablespoon bee pollen (optional)
3 to 4 tablespoons coconut oil
3 droppers SweetLeaf hazelnut liquid stevia

In a food processor, combine the almonds, cashews, pecans, vanilla bean powder or vanilla bean, cinnamon, nutmeg, salt, and optional bee pollen. Process the mixture on high until everything is evenly combined. It will look like a powder within the first minute, but continue to blend it until it starts to look sticky, about 4 minutes. It may then need to be mixed or pressed down with a spatula, so stop the processor every few minutes to do so to keep the blending consistent. Continue processing the butter on high until it is fairly smooth and looks even.

Next, add the coconut oil and stevia. If your butter is already fairly smooth, you will not need to add as much coconut oil; if it is a little dry, add more coconut oil. It is important to note that using raw nuts will yield a drier butter and using soaked nuts will yield an oilier batch. Using toasted nuts will change the flavor of the butter and will yield a much oilier butter (plus, it will reduce the nutritional benefit of the butter).

Continue processing the butter until you have reached the desired consistency, then use the spatula to scrape the butter into a glass storage jar and refrigerate for three to four days.

*Omit bee pollen

SEEREAL BARS

Farshid Sam Rahbar, M.D., and Annie McRae, N.C.

Vegetarian*

Makes: approximately 24 bars

Prep time: 10 minutes

Cooking time: 15 minutes

The name "SeeReal" originates from the ingredients being a combination of seeds and cereal. Once you have made these bars, doing so will become a weekly habit! This recipe is easy and quick to make. They are especially good when you need a pre-workout power-packed snack to give you stamina and energy. They are also excellent for a post-workout "refill" of satisfying nutrition to give you continued energy without upsetting your blood sugar levels.

⅓ cup coconut butter
1 tablespoon honey
3 pasture-raised eggs
½ cup quinoa flakes
½ cup cooked brown rice
¼ cup raw sunflower seeds
¼ cup cracked or ground flaxseeds
¼ cup raw sesame seeds
¼ cup shaved unsweetened coconut
1 tablespoon ground cinnamon (optional)
¼ to ⅓ cup dried fruit, such as raisins, sultanas, cranberries, cherries, apricots, and/or dates, or ½ cup peeled and finely chopped apple

Preheat the oven to 300°F.

In a saucepan, gently melt the coconut butter over low heat. Remove the pan from heat, then stir in the honey. Then stir in the eggs one at a time. Set the mixture aside.

In a large bowl, mix together the quinoa flakes, rice, sunflower seeds, flaxseeds, sesame seeds, coconut, cinnamon, and dried fruit or chopped apple until everything is well combined. Pour in the egg mixture and blend thoroughly.

In either a nonstick or a parchment-lined 7 × 12-inch baking pan, spread the dough evenly and press it down. Bake it for about 15 minutes.

Let it cool, then cut it into 1½ × 2-inch bars. Store the bars in a container in the fridge. They travel well. Take them with you to work or when you are in the car and need a snack.

Variations:

Increase the quinoa flakes to 1 cup if you do not have the cooked rice.

For a real treat, replace the dried fruit with dark chocolate chips and walnuts pieces or, my favorite version, cranberries and pecans.

*Contains eggs

CRUNCHY MAPLE MESQUITE WALNUTS

C Cleanse

V Vegan

Makes: 1 pound

Prep time: 10 minutes

Cooking time: 30 minutes

On family travels, hikes, or days when you're on the go, recipes like this always make for happy and satiated people, especially kids. This delicious snack is one of the best garnishes for any kind of salad or roasted vegetables.

1 pound raw walnuts
2 tablespoons mesquite meal
1 teaspoon vanilla bean powder or ½ teaspoon vanilla extract
1 teaspoon ground cinnamon
1 teaspoon ground allspice
½ teaspoon ground clove
½ teaspoon sea salt
½ cup coconut nectar

Preheat the oven to 350°F.

Place the walnuts into a large bowl then toss with the mesquite meal, vanilla bean powder or extract, cinnamon, allspice, clove, salt, and coconut nectar, until they are evenly coated.

Spread the nuts in a parchment-lined baking dish and slowly roast the walnuts for about 30 minutes. Keep checking on them every 10 minutes so they do not burn. The walnuts are ready when they are golden brown and crisp. Remove them from the oven and allow them to cool to room temperature.

Store them in an airtight container for up to one month.

Chef Frank on Making Extra Food

Having healthy snacks around is a great way to keep you from making less than excellent food choices. Double or triple some recipes so you can have extra portions around for a few weeks. With soups, you can freeze any unused amounts in quart containers for reheating when you are too busy to cook. Snacks like crackers or spiced nuts guarantee that you'll always have something on hand to fill you up instead of grabbing sugary packaged foods.

FISH

From salmon and halibut to sea bass and fish sticks, you'll find lots of clean fish options here. Fish are a lean protein source that taste great oven-baked or grilled, as an entrée or added to soups and salads. We recommend eating smaller, cold-water fish both for their high level of nutrients and lower level of contaminants. We encourage you to check out Food & Water Watch (Foodandwaterwatch.org) for updates on sustainable fish where you live and to substitute with whatever is wild-caught and "okayed" at the moment.

OVEN-BAKED FLOUNDER WITH GARLIC AND GREEN OLIVES

C Cleanse

G Gut

Serves: 2

Prep time: 15 minutes

Cooking time: 10 minutes

Garlic and olives give a slight kick to the mild flavor of the fish.

1 pound flounder or sole fillets, cut into 2 portions
2 tablespoons extra-virgin olive oil
1 large garlic clove, thinly sliced
1 teaspoon capers, roughly chopped
¼ cup pitted green olives, sliced
1 cup chicken stock, vegetable stock, or water
2 tablespoons roughly chopped fresh oregano
Sea salt and freshly ground black pepper to taste

Preheat the oven to 425°F.

Arrange the flounder fillets in an oiled baking dish and set them aside.

Heat the olive oil in a small saucepan set over medium-high heat. When the oil is warm, sauté the garlic until it's golden brown. Stir in the capers and olives until the mixture is combined. Pour in the stock or water, and allow it to reduce by half before adding the oregano, salt, and pepper.

Pour the sauce over the fish and transfer the fish to the oven. Bake the fillets for about 10 minutes, or until they flake easily with a fork or knife.

Pairings: Serve this dish alongside sautéed dark, leafy greens with balsamic vinegar, roasted vegetables, mashed potatoes, or yams.

CHARRED LEMON-BROILED SOLE

C Cleanse

G Gut

Serves: 2

Prep time: 5 minutes

Cooking time: 5 minutes

Lemon is commonly paired with fish, but the charring on this dish makes it slightly crispy and extra tasty.

1 pound fresh sole fillets
Extra-virgin olive oil
2 pinches sea salt
Freshly ground black pepper to taste
4 to 6 sprigs fresh thyme
1 lemon, very thinly sliced

Preheat the broiler in your oven.

Line with parchment paper a baking dish large enough to hold all the fish.

Drizzle each fillet with a bit of olive oil then lay them on the parchment paper. Try not to let them overlap. Season them with salt and pepper, then scatter the sprigs of thyme on top.

Arrange the lemon slices over the thyme and drizzle everything with olive oil.

Broil the fish for about 5 minutes. The broiler will give the lemons a nice char and allow them to release their juices over the fish. Serve warm.

Dr. Junger on Food & Water Watch

Fresh, wild-caught fish is a great source for essential omega-3 fatty acids, easily digestible protein, and fair amounts of vitamin D and selenium. However, there are many factors to consider when buying fish, from contamination to overfishing. Food & Water Watch has created an invaluable seafood guide that explains where a fish has been caught, how it's been farmed, and whether it's contaminated. Check out the guide at Foodandwaterwatch.org.

COCONUT POACHED SALMON

Gwyneth Paltrow, actor and founder of goop.com

C Cleanse

G Gut

Serves: 2

½ cup vegetable or chicken broth
2 stalks lemongrass (inner bulbs), finely chopped
1 cup coconut milk
1 lime, juiced
2 ¼-pound pieces of salmon, seasoned with salt and pepper
Dark, leafy winter greens, finely chopped
1 to 2 anchovy fillets
Salt and pepper to taste

Add the broth to a large, deep pan over medium-high heat. Cook for a few minutes until it begins to boil and add the lemongrass, cooking it for a minute until fragrant. Reduce heat to medium, add the coconut milk and most of the lime juice, and place the salmon fillets into the liquid skin side down. Cover and poach for about 10 minutes until cooked through. Transfer fillets to a serving platter over dark, leafy winter greens.

Continue to cook the liquid for another minute or so until thick, adding in the anchovies and mashing them into the sauce with the back of a wooden spoon. Season the sauce with salt and pepper to taste and spoon over salmon and greens. Squeeze remaining lime over the salmon and serve.

Note: This recipe originally appeared on Goop.com.

PAN-ROASTED HALIBUT WITH ARTICHOKE AND CELERY SALAD AND LAVENDER VINAIGRETTE

C Cleanse

G Gut

Serves: 2

Prep time: 10 minutes

Cooking time: 15 minutes

This is an amazing flavor and texture combination. Halibut is one of the most delectable and crowd-pleasing fish, so this is an extra special way to impress dinner guests and show them how flavorful and gorgeous clean cooking is.

2 6- to 8-ounce halibut fillets
Pinch of sea salt
¼ teaspoon freshly ground black pepper
2 tablespoons avocado oil
A few edible flowers for garnish

For the Artichoke and Celery Salad
1 14-ounce can artichoke hearts, rinsed and drained
Inner core of 1 head of celery (with yellowish leaves intact), thinly sliced diagonally
¼ cup chopped fresh parsley or ⅛ cup dried parsley

For the Lavender Vinaigrette
⅓ cup extra-virgin olive oil
2½ tablespoons lemon juice
2 teaspoons lavender buds, ground in a mortar and pestle
Sea salt to taste

Preheat the oven to 350°F.

Season the fillets with salt and pepper.

Heat an ovenproof skillet over medium-high heat, and add the avocado oil. When the oil is hot (you should see some smoke), add the fillets, flesh side down. Sear the fish for 2 to 3 minutes, until golden brown, then flip them and transfer the pan to the preheated oven. Depending on the thickness of the fillets, roasting should take only 5 to 8 minutes.

Meanwhile, in a large bowl combine all the ingredients for the salad. In a small bowl, whisk together the olive oil, lemon juice, and crushed lavender buds, then pour about three-quarters of the mixture over the salad. Gently toss everything to combine, then season the salad with a little sea salt.

Remove the halibut from the oven and divide the fillets between two serving plates. Add half of the salad to each plate, then drizzle the remaining quarter of the vinaigrette over the fish and around the plate. Garnish each serving with the edible flowers.

LEMON AND THYME BAKED SEA BASS WITH BRUSSELS SPROUT HASH

C Cleanse

G Gut

Serves: 4

Prep time: 15 minutes

Cooking time: 30 to 45 minutes

With its use of a gorgeous method of cooking freshly caught fish, seen in France as well as over campfires, this dish is at home anywhere. It's wonderful served in the middle of the table, letting each person use a fork to peel away the skin then scoop out the flesh. We find that communal eating brings people closer together and results in the best conversations. Just be mindful of the bones, as they aren't fun to swallow.

1 whole sea bass (roughly 6 pounds), cleaned and scaled
¼ cup plus 1 tablespoon extra-virgin olive oil
1 cup fresh parsley leaves (about 1 bunch)
1 heaping tablespoon freshly chopped thyme
2 scallions
3 garlic cloves
1 lemon, sliced into thin rounds
1 cup organic dry white wine

For the Hash
2 tablespoons avocado oil
1 large onion, diced
8 ounces white mushrooms, roughly chopped
1 pound Brussels sprouts, grated
2 teaspoons sea salt

Preheat the oven to 400°F.

Rinse and dry the fish. Then, using a sharp knife, make three diagonal ½-inch-deep slices along both sides of the fish.

Use a food processor to grind the parsley, thyme, scallions, and garlic, or mince them together with a knife. Combine the minced herbs with enough olive oil to make a paste, then spread the herb-garlic paste all over the outside of the fish, pushing some down into each of the six diagonal cuts.

Transfer the fish to a lightly oiled baking dish and top it with the lemon slices, then pour the white wine over it. Bake the bass for 25 to 30 minutes, checking after 20 minutes to be sure it's not overcooking. It's ready when you can pull the flesh away from the bones.

While the fish cooks, make the hash. Heat the avocado oil in a large skillet set over medium-high heat. When the oil is hot, sauté the onion for 2 to 3 minutes, stirring occasionally until it's translucent. Lower the heat to medium, then add the mushrooms and Brussels sprouts, and continue sautéing and stirring for 10 to 12 minutes. (If the pan starts to dry up, add a few additional tablespoons of oil.) When all the vegetables are tender and the hash is a dark golden brown, remove it from the heat and season it with the salt, but keep it warm until the fish is ready to serve.

When the fish is cooked through, transfer it to a large serving platter and pour the liquid from the bottom of the pan over the fish. Serve it warm with the hash.

DILLY SALMON SALAD

C Cleanse   **Serves:** 2
G Gut   **Prep time:** 10 minutes

This summery salad is perfect for using up leftover salmon and can be served in a variety of ways. Enjoy over mixed greens, as a filling for deviled eggs, on top of cucumber slices, or in a panini or wrap.

1 12-ounce can wild-caught salmon
¼ cup minced red onion
2 celery stalks, thinly sliced
¼ cup chopped fresh dill
2 tablespoons lemon juice
Sea salt to taste

For the Mayonnaise
½ cup raw cashews
½ cup raw pine nuts
½ cup unsweetened coconut milk
1 teaspoon sea salt

Drain the salmon of any water and place it in a large bowl. Use a fork to mash it up, then stir in the onion, celery, and dill.

In a blender, purée all the mayonnaise ingredients until the mixture is light and airy. Add as much of the mayonnaise as needed to coat the salmon salad, then season further with a few splashes of lemon juice and salt to taste. Great to eat by itself or over leafy greens.

COD WITH ROASTED CHILI PEPPERS AND CAYENNE

Mark Hyman, M.D., chairman of the Institute for Functional Medicine and founder and medical director of the Ultra Wellness Center

Ⓖ Gut

Prep time: 20 minutes

Cooking time: 25 minutes

The peppers adorning this fish add a beautiful earthy color and a kick of fire. Choosing cod protects you from mercury and other toxins usually found in larger predatory fish, such as swordfish or tilefish.

4 teaspoons extra-virgin olive oil
1 medium poblano pepper
½ jalapeño pepper
1 garlic clove
½ shallot, chopped
¼ teaspoon cayenne
½ teaspoon sea salt
4 6-ounce skinless cod fillets

Preheat the oven to 350°F.

Grease a baking sheet with 1 teaspoon of the olive oil and set it aside.

Rub the poblano and jalapeño peppers with ½ teaspoon of the oil and roast them over an open flame, on a grill, or in a broiler until the skin is completely charred. Place the peppers in a bowl and cover the bowl tightly with plastic wrap. Let the peppers sit for 5 minutes, then uncover the bowl and peel away all the blackened skins and remove the seeds and stems.

In a food processor, combine the roasted peppers with the remaining 2½ teaspoons of olive oil, garlic, shallot, cayenne, and salt, and purée the mixture until it is completely smooth.

Place the cod on the prepared baking sheet and evenly spread each fillet with the roasted pepper mixture. Bake the fish until they flake easily when tested with a fork, 20 to 25 minutes. Transfer the fillets to a platter and serve.

Any leftover fish can be refrigerated overnight, but it's best when served the same day.

Dr. Junger on the Perfect Meal

Mark Hyman's cod is the perfect balance between culinary elegance and every-day simplicity. I love the flavorful punch the pepper purée provides with the meaty, flaky, and juicy cod. And it doesn't hurt that you get blood-sugar-stabilizing protein, heart-healthy fat, and metabolism-boosting phytonutri-ents all in one easy meal. When you want something that is quick and tasty yet offers loads of nutrition, make this dish.

FISH STICKS WITH TARTAR SAUCE

G Gut

Serves: 2

Prep time: 10 minutes

Cooking time: 15 to 20 minutes

Here's a classic New England meal with a healthy twist. Gluten-free breading and healthy coconut oil make this yummy and super kid-friendly.

½ cup or more almond flour
2 large pasture-raised eggs, whisked
½ cup or more coconut flour
2 tablespoons lemon pepper seasoning
1 pound flounder fillets, sliced into ¾-inch-wide strips
¾ cup coconut oil, divided
Sea salt and freshly ground black pepper to taste
1 lemon, cut into wedges

For the Tartar Sauce
1 batch Sour Cream (page 98) or Mayonnaise (page 91)
2 tablespoons minced shallot
1 dill pickle, minced

First, make the tartar sauce. In a medium bowl, fold into your choice of either Sour Cream or Mayonnaise the minced shallot and pickle. Set the sauce aside.

To bread the fish, place the almond flour, whisked eggs, and coconut flour into three separate bowls. Add the lemon pepper to the coconut flour, stirring to combine. Coat a fish fillet completely in the almond flour, then shake off the excess. Next, dip the fillet into the eggs, followed by the coconut flour mixture. Lightly pat the coconut flour into the fillet and set it aside (on a baking sheet is great and an easy cleanup). Repeat this with all the fillets.

Heat roughly half the coconut oil in a large skillet. When the oil is hot, add the fish (but don't overcrowd the pan). Fry the fillets until they are golden brown, flipping after 3 minutes so they cook about 3 minutes per side.

Transfer the cooked fish to a paper towel to drain any excess oil. Add more oil to the pan as needed to cook all the fish. Season the fillets well with salt and pepper, and serve warm with lemon wedges and tartar sauce.

COCONUT FISH SOUP

C Cleanse*

G Gut

Serves: 2

Prep time: 10 minutes

Cooking time: 15 minutes

We love a great fish stew—easy to make and so comforting and delicious to enjoy. This can be varied with different fish, depending on what you have at your local market (you can even try it with chicken!). The Red Boat fish sauce is delicious and the only clean version we've found, so it's a great staple to keep on hand.

2 tablespoons coconut oil
1 small onion, diced
1 medium carrot, roughly chopped (about 1 cup)
1 tablespoon freshly grated ginger
2 garlic cloves
2 Thai red chili peppers (optional)
1 tablespoon Red Boat fish sauce
1 13.5-ounce can unsweetened coconut milk
1 cup water or vegetable stock
1½ pounds wild-caught salmon or other wild-caught fish variety, skin removed, pin bones removed
1 lime, cut into wedges
Cilantro leaves for garnish

Heat the coconut oil in a large pot set over medium-high heat. When the oil is hot, add the onions and sauté them, stirring occasionally, until they are translucent, about 2 to 3 minutes. Add the carrot, ginger, and garlic, sautéing for a few extra minutes before adding the optional red chilies, fish sauce, coconut milk, and water or stock. Bring the mixture to a boil, then lower the heat to medium and add the fish. Continue cooking for 10 to 12 minutes.

Serve the soup steaming hot with a few lime wedges and garnished with cilantro leaves.

*Omit red chili peppers

ZUCCHINI-WRAPPED WHITEFISH WITH CHIVE OIL

C Cleanse
G Gut

Serves: 2

Prep time: 30 minutes

Cooking time: 10 minutes

This is a wonderful meal as is, or it can be sectioned into smaller, bite-size pieces and served as you would bacon-wrapped scallops, making it a lighter-flavored version of a classic wrapped seafood appetizer.

1 large zucchini
2 tablespoons extra-virgin olive oil
Zest of 1 lemon
2 teaspoons chopped fresh oregano
2 pinches freshly ground black pepper
1 teaspoon sea salt
2 6- to 8-ounce firm (fresh is better than frozen) whitefish fillets, such as striped bass, halibut, or cod

For the Chive Oil
1 bunch (about ½ cup chopped) fresh chives
½ cup extra-virgin olive oil
¼ teaspoon sea salt

First, make the chive oil. In a blender or food processor, purée all the chive oil ingredients until the mixture is smooth. Pour it through a fine-mesh strainer, and store it in an airtight container in the fridge until you're ready to use it.

Cut the ends from the zucchini, then slice it as thinly as possible lengthwise, about ⅛-inch thick. Place the slices in a glass bowl or dish and coat them with a few tablespoons of olive oil. Toss in the lemon zest, oregano, pepper, and salt. Mix well, then let the zucchini marinate for 10 to 15 minutes.

Preheat the oven to 350°F.

Lay about three to four zucchini slices horizontally on a work surface, each overlapping slightly along the lengthwise edges. Place a fish fillet at one end of the zucchini, then roll it until the fillet is completely wrapped in the zucchini. Repeat the steps for the second fillet.

Place the wrapped fish in an oiled baking dish or cast-iron pan with the ends of the zucchini tucked underneath so they don't curl up while the fish is roasting. Roast for 8 to 10 minutes, then serve them warm, each fillet drizzled with a few tablespoons of the chive oil.

Chef Frank on Flavored Oils and Vinegars

Flavored oils and vinegars can add a lot to a dish. They also look beautiful in the pantry and make wonderful homemade gifts, along with being a great way to use up extra herbs from the summer's harvest. By blending or infusing herbs and spices into oils, you not only add a beautiful color but also give it a deeply intense flavor. I often infuse fresh red chili peppers or cloves of garlic in apple cider vinegar for months at a time. You can use an infusion in a vinaigrette or simply as a garnish.

POACHED COD WITH SOBA NOODLES AND PONZU SAUCE

C Cleanse

Serves: 2

Prep time: 20 minutes

Cooking time: 5 to 6 minutes

This is a delicious, "clean" take on a traditional Asian dish. The sauce is amazing, and you'll probably want it on everything. It can be used to dress salads or noodles as well, so make more than you need for just this dish. Trust us, you'll want more.

2 6- to 8-ounce portions cod (striped bass, halibut, or hake will work as well)

For the Soba Noodle Salad
1 8.8-ounce package King Soba soba noodles
3 red radishes, thinly sliced
¼ cup julienned daikon radish
1 small carrot, julienned
Leaves from 4 to 5 cilantro sprigs, roughly chopped
1 tablespoon raw black sesame seeds
2 tablespoons toasted sesame oil

For the Poaching Liquid
4 cups water
2 tablespoons freshly sliced ginger
2 garlic cloves, minced
2 bay leaves
1 strip kelp
Juice of 1 lemon
2 tablespoons rice wine vinegar

For the Ponzu Sauce
½ cup wheat-free tamari
2 tablespoons rice wine vinegar
¼ cup water
1½ tablespoons lime juice
1 heaping tablespoon freshly grated ginger
1 scallion, thinly sliced

First, make the salad. Cook the soba noodles according to directions on the package, then rinse them under cold water to stop the cooking process. Toss the noodles in a large bowl with the radish, daikon radish, carrot, cilantro, sesame seeds, and sesame oil. Set the salad aside.

In a pot, combine all the poaching liquid ingredients and bring them to a gentle simmer. Slowly ease the fish into the liquid and poach it for about 5 to 6 minutes. Keep watch on it, as cooking fish too long can make it flake apart.

While the fish cooks, in a small bowl whisk together all the ingredients for the ponzu sauce.

To serve, divide the noodles between two large, wide bowls. Place the fish on top of each portion of noodles, then drizzle the ponzu sauce over everything.

FISH TACOS

Ⓒ Cleanse*

Serves: 4

Prep time: 20 minutes plus 20 to 30 minutes for marinating

Cooking time: 15 minutes

You can't beat fish tacos. The soft corn tortillas wrapped around perfectly seasoned and cooked whitefish; a bit of spice and lime with or without the mango salsa. These are a definite winner any time of year, but are especially great for summertime dinners.

¼ cup extra-virgin olive oil
Juice of 1 lime
1 tablespoon chipotle chili powder
¼ cup chopped fresh cilantro leaves
1 pound sea bass or whatever sustainable wild-caught fish is available
8 soft sprouted brown rice tortillas, warmed

For the Mango Sauce
1 ripe mango, peeled, pitted, and diced into ½-inch cubes
⅛ cup chopped fresh cilantro leaves
2 teaspoons freshly grated ginger
Juice and zest of 1 lime
1 tablespoon fish sauce (Red Boat is a Clean-approved brand)
3 tablespoons extra-virgin olive oil

For the Garnish
2 to 3 cups finely shredded purple cabbage
Cilantro leaves
Sliced red chili peppers (optional)

To prepare the fish, in a bowl whisk together the olive oil, lime, chipotle chili powder, and cilantro. Place the fish in a glass baking dish and pour the marinade over it. Let it marinate for 20 to 30 minutes in the refrigerator.

While the fish marinates, in a blender purée all the mango sauce ingredients until the mixture is smooth. Place the sauce in a bowl or a squeeze bottle and set it aside.

Preheat the oven to 375°F.

When the fish is ready, grill or bake it for 8 to 10 minutes, until it is firm to the touch. Remove it from the oven, lowering the temperature of the oven to 200°F. Wrap the corn tortillas in foil and warm them in the oven while you use a fork to flake the fish into smaller pieces.

To serve, place two warmed tortillas on each plate. Divide the fish between the eight tortillas, top with the shredded cabbage, cilantro leaves, and optional red chilies, then drizzle everything with the mango sauce.

*Omit red chili peppers

SPICED SALMON WITH BLUEBERRY VINAIGRETTE

C Cleanse

G Gut*

Serves: 2

Prep time: 10 minutes

Cooking time: 6 to 8 minutes

This is a very Northern dish that uses blueberries and salmon together. The colors are vibrant and the flavor melts in your mouth in sweet and slightly sour perfection. Northeast or Northwest dwellers will love this meal, which uses local and wild ingredients—the best way to eat, in our opinion.

2 6- to 8-ounce portions fresh, wild-caught salmon
2 tablespoons coconut oil

Spice Rub
2 teaspoons fennel seeds
6 cardamom pods
1 tablespoon coriander seeds
½ teaspoon ground ginger
½ teaspoon sea salt
Pinch of freshly ground black pepper

Blueberry Vinaigrette
1 cup fresh or frozen wild blueberries
2 tablespoons extra-virgin olive oil
Juice of ½ lime (about 1½ tablespoons)
1 tablespoon coconut nectar
3 tablespoons water
Pinch of sea salt

Preheat the oven to 350°F.

First, make the vinaigrette. In a blender, purée all the vinaigrette ingredients until the mixture is smooth. If it's too thick, add a bit of water to thin it out. Pour the vinaigrette into a jar and set it aside.

In a small bowl, combine all the spice rub ingredients, then spread the mixture generously over the top of each salmon fillet. Shake off any excess.

Heat the coconut oil in a large ovenproof skillet set over medium-high heat. When the oil is hot, add the salmon, spice side down. Cook for 2 to 3 minutes, until the undersides are golden brown. Flip the fillets and transfer the skillet to the oven for another 4 to 5 minutes. For the best flavor and texture, cook the fish to a medium-rare consistency, or to your preference.

Serve the salmon drizzled with the vinaigrette.

*Omit coconut nectar

SALMON STIR-FRY

C Cleanse

G Gut*

Serves: 2

Prep time: 20 to 25 minutes

Cooking time: 10 minutes

This dish is really fast to pull together once all your ingredients are prepped. Add it to cooked soba noodles or serve it over quinoa and mixed greens.

12 ounces fresh wild-caught salmon, cut into 1- to 1½-inch chunks
2 tablespoons sesame oil
1 large shiitake mushroom, stalk removed, diced
½ cup sliced daikon radish, cut into thin half-moons
6 cups chopped bok choy
2 tablespoons chopped scallions
1 teaspoon sesame seeds

For the Marinade
1 tablespoon freshly grated ginger
1 large garlic clove, minced
¼ cup toasted sesame oil
2 tablespoons rice wine vinegar
1 tablespoon whole-grain mustard
¼ cup wheat-free tamari
1 tablespoon coconut nectar (optional)

In a bowl, whisk together all the marinade ingredients. Set half of the marinade aside in another bowl and add the salmon to that portion to marinate for 15 to 20 minutes.

After the salmon has marinated, heat the sesame oil in a large wok or sauté pan until it is just smoking, then add the mushrooms. Use a wooden spoon to continuously stir the mushrooms to prevent burning. Cook for about 3 to 4 minutes before adding the salmon and stir to combine it with the mushrooms, then add the radish and bok choy. Continue to sauté and stir for 1 to 2 minutes. Add the remaining half of the marinade along with the scallions and sesame seeds. Allow the liquid to reduce and thicken, then serve.

*Omit coconut nectar

HARISSA-COATED HADDOCK

C Cleanse*

G Gut

Serves: 2

Prep time: 30 minutes

Cooking time: 10 to 12 minutes

Harissa is a spicy African chili paste that works well with a number of various ingredients. Paired with a mild whitefish, this dish is extra tasty alongside the Quinoa with Celery and Apples (see page 195). With harissa, a little bit goes a long way, so taste while preparing and save the extra paste for later use.

1 pound haddock fillet

For the Harissa

½ ounce dried New Mexico, ancho, or chipotle chili peppers (or dried red chilies)

1½ cups chopped carrots

4 garlic cloves, chopped

¼ cup fresh parsley leaves

¼ cup fresh mint leaves

2 to 3 tablespoons extra-virgin olive oil

1 tablespoon lemon juice

2 teaspoons sea salt

Preheat the oven to 350°F.

First, make the harissa. Place the dried chilies in a jar, then pour hot water over them and let them sit for 20 to 30 minutes. Strain them and set aside the soaking liquid.

In a blender or food processor, purée the chilies with the carrots, garlic, parsley, mint, olive oil, lemon juice, and salt until a thick paste is formed. Use the reserved chili soaking liquid, as needed, to thin out the paste slightly.

Smear a thin layer of the harissa over the top side of the haddock, then transfer it to an oiled baking dish. Bake the fish for about 10 to 12 minutes, and serve warm.

Note: Extra harissa can be kept in a container for up to one month. Store it in a jar topped with a layer of olive oil to preserve its freshness.

*Omit fresh chili peppers; dried seasoning is fine

OVEN-ROASTED COD

C Cleanse

G Gut

Serves: 4

Prep time: 10 minutes

Cooking time: 12 to 15 minutes

The buttery taste and delicate texture of cod perfectly pairs with the herbs and lemon in this dish. For long and busy days, this dish can be prepped ahead of time, kept in the fridge, then tossed in the oven after work or school and be on the table within 15 minutes.

About ½ cup fresh parsley
½ cup roughly chopped raw almonds
Zest of 1 lemon
1 large garlic clove
Sea salt
Freshly ground black pepper
1 medium red onion, sliced into ¼-inch-thick rounds
2 to 3 tablespoons extra-virgin olive oil
4 6- to 8-ounce cod fillets

Preheat the oven to 400°F.

Place the parsley, almonds, lemon zest, and garlic together on a cutting board. Using a sharp knife, chop the ingredients until they are well combined, though some chunky texture is okay. Stir in a pinch each of salt and pepper.

In a small baking dish, arrange the onion slices. Drizzle them with olive oil and sprinkle with sea salt.

Drizzle a touch of oil over each fish fillet, then coat each with the herb and almond mixture. Place the fillets onto the layer of red onions, herb side up. Bake the cod for 12 to 15 minutes, until it is firm.

Serve each fillet with a portion of the red onions, and drizzle any oil and juices from the pan over the fish.

TUNA NOODLE CASSEROLE

C Cleanse

Serves: 4 to 6

Prep time: 10 minutes

Cooking time: 30 minutes

Comfort food! This cooks in under 30 minutes, so it's the perfect meal to feed a hungry crowd, especially when you're short on time.

2 tablespoons coconut oil
½ cup sliced onions
2 cups chopped mushrooms (any variety)
3 cups unsweetened almond milk
1 cup broccoli florets
1 cup frozen peas
1 pound rice pasta
2 6- to 8-ounce cans wild-caught albacore tuna or wild-caught salmon
2 tablespoons kudzu root powder, dissolved in ¼ cup water
2 tablespoons nutritional yeast
2 heaping tablespoons dark miso (preferably soy free)

Preheat the oven to 350°F.

Melt the coconut oil in a large pot set over medium-high heat. Sauté the onions and mushrooms, stirring occasionally, for 3 to 4 minutes. Add the almond milk and bring the mixture up in temperature until it starts to simmer. Stir in the broccoli and peas, and continue to simmer for 5 minutes.

While the sauce cooks, bring 8 cups of salted water to a boil. Pour in the rice pasta and cook the noodles until they are tender, then strain them.

When the broccoli is also tender, add the tuna or salmon and the prepared kudzu root to the mixture. Continue stirring often as the sauce thickens. Add the nutritional yeast and miso, then remove the pot from the heat.

Gently incorporate the cooked pasta into the tuna-vegetable mixture to coat the noodles. Pour the mixture into a baking dish and bake for 20 minutes, using the last few minutes to stick it under the broiler to brown the top.

POULTRY

The key to creating great poultry dishes is selecting good-quality meat. We first start with hormone- and antibiotic-free varieties and then if we can find it, we use organic or pastured. Then we add lots of veggies to balance out the meal. In this section, you'll find quick 15-minute recipes for more festive dishes like Chicken Osso Bucco to impress your friends. The wide range of dishes will give you lots of clean options and make it easier to eat clean long term.

LEMON HERB CHICKEN BURGERS WITH THOUSAND ISLAND DRESSING

Ⓒ Cleanse*

Ⓖ Gut

Serves: 4

Prep time: 20 minutes

Cooking time: 15 minutes

There's really no other word for these burgers except: YUM. The flavoring and the satisfaction of a meal you can wrap your hands around is unmatched.

1 pound pasture-raised, skinless, boneless chicken breast, cut into large chunks (or you can use ground pasture-raised chicken or turkey)
1 medium onion, diced
1 garlic clove, minced
¼ cup chopped fresh parsley
2 teaspoons chopped fresh thyme
Zest and juice of 1 lemon
Sea salt to taste
2 tablespoons coconut oil
4 Sami's Bakery buns or other gluten-free option
1 handful mâche lettuce, baby spinach, or arugula

For the Thousand Island Dressing
1½ cups (about 4) quartered plum tomatoes
½ cup raw macadamia nuts or cashews
2 garlic cloves
⅛ cup lemon juice
⅛ cup extra-virgin olive oil
1 teaspoon sea salt
2 dill pickles, minced

For the Garnish
2 tablespoons coconut oil
1 large red onion, sliced into thin rounds

First, make the dressing. In a blender, purée the tomatoes, nuts, garlic, lemon juice, olive oil, and salt for 45 seconds, until the mixture is thick and creamy. Transfer the contents to a small bowl and stir in the minced pickles. Set it aside. (Any extra dressing can be stored in the fridge for up to three days.)

To prepare to garnish, heat the coconut oil in a skillet set over medium-high heat. Sauté the onions until they are slightly caramelized, then set them aside.

*Omit tomatoes

For the burgers, in a food processor purée the chicken, onion, and garlic until everything is well combined. Transfer it to a large bowl and add the parsley, thyme, lemon zest, lemon juice, and salt. Blend the mixture well with your hands, then form it into four equal-size burgers.

In a large skillet set over medium-high heat, melt the coconut oil, then add the burgers. Allow them to brown on one side for several minutes before flipping them and browning the other side. If you are not serving these right away, you can transfer them to a heated oven at this point to keep them warm.

When the burgers are ready, serve them on buns topped with the fresh greens and sautéed red onion, and with a side of Thousand Island Dressing.

CHICKEN AND BROCCOLI PAD THAI

Serves: 2

Prep time: 10 to 15 minutes

Cooking time: 10 minutes

This quick dish is the clean version of a traditional pad Thai. Have all your ingredients prepped and ready to go before you begin cooking, as this doesn't take long to cook.

4 to 6 ounces pasture-raised boneless, skinless chicken breast, cut into thin strips ¼ inch thick
1 package (8 ounces) King Soba rice noodles
Avocado or olive oil

For the Marinade
2 tablespoons fish sauce (Red Boat is a Clean-approved brand)
1 tablespoon coconut sugar
1 red chili pepper
1 tablespoon rice wine vinegar

For the Pad Thai
2 tablespoons coconut oil
2 garlic cloves, thinly sliced
1 head (about 2 cups) broccoli, cut into small florets
1 pasture-raised egg, whisked

For the Garnish
2 scallions, chopped
2 tablespoons roasted cashews, roughly chopped
1 lime, cut into wedges

Set the chicken breast strips into a glass bowl or small baking dish. Whisk together all the marinade ingredients in another bowl and pour the mixture over the chicken. Cover the dish and allow it to sit for 15 to 20 minutes so the flavors can mingle.

Prepare the rice noodles according to directions on the package. Once the noodles are cooked through, drain and rinse them under cold water. Drizzle them with a touch of avocado or olive oil and set them aside.

Heat a wok or large skillet and add the coconut oil for the pad Thai. When the oil is hot, sauté the garlic until it is fragrant. Strain the marinated chicken, then toss it into the skillet along with the broccoli florets. Stir-fry the mixture rapidly while shaking the pan, and continue until the chicken is completely cooked. Pour in the whisked egg and use a wooden spoon to slowly mix the egg with the other ingredients. As soon as the egg bits are set and cooked through, remove the pan from the heat.

On two serving plates, arrange a portion of rice noodles topped with the chicken and broccoli mixture and garnished with scallions, roasted cashews, and a few lime wedges.

MUSTARD-BAKED CHICKEN

C Cleanse

G Gut

Serves: 2

Prep time: 5 minutes

Cooking time: 20 to 30 minutes

A spicy kick to a delicious and easy baked chicken recipe. Any mustard works, but we love one available at health food stores that has apple cider vinegar in it.

2 whole pasture-raised chicken legs, thighs, and drumsticks separated
¼ cup extra-virgin olive oil
2 tablespoons whole-grain mustard
4 garlic cloves
1 teaspoon fennel seeds
1 teaspoon apple cider vinegar
2 teaspoons sea salt

Preheat the oven to 400°F.

In a large bowl, toss all the ingredients together and allow the chicken to marinate for 15 minutes in the refrigerator. Transfer the chicken to a baking dish and spoon any excess marinade over it. Bake for 20 to 30 minutes, or until a nice brown crust forms on top of the meat. Serve warm.

COCONUT CURRY

Amy Myers, M.D., founder and medical director of Austin UltraHealth

C Cleanse*

V Vegan†

Serves: 4

This is one of my all-time favorite go-to recipes. This dish reminds me of the time I spent in India, the flavors are so rich, inviting, and soul warming. Coconut curry is wonderful to share with family or serve at a dinner party, and my favorite part about making this dish is the leftovers for lunch the next day.

1 tablespoon extra-virgin olive oil
2 garlic cloves, chopped
1 medium onion, diced
½ tablespoon ground turmeric
½ tablespoon ground cumin
1 tablespoon ground coriander
½ teaspoon onion powder
1 sweet potato, peeled and chopped into ½-inch cubes
2 celery stalks, chopped
½ cup chopped scallions
1 cup water
1 teaspoon sea salt
1 pasture-raised chicken breast, cooked and cut into bite-size pieces
1 13.5-ounce can full-fat unsweetened coconut milk
Cooked brown rice
Flesh of 1 ripe avocado, sliced

Heat a large skillet over medium heat. Coat the pan with olive oil, and when the oil is hot, sauté the garlic until it's slightly browned. Add the onion, and add more oil if needed. Cover and cook the onions until they are translucent. Add the turmeric, cumin, coriander, and onion powder, and mix to coat the onions and garlic. Then add the sweet potatoes, celery, scallions, water, and salt. Let everything simmer until the sweet potatoes are soft. Stir in the cooked chicken and coconut milk, and continue simmering to mix the flavors.

Serve over cooked brown rice and top with the sliced avocado.

Variations: To make it grain-free, serve it without rice.

*Omit sweet potatoes
†Omit chicken

SLOW-COOKED CHICKEN WITH FENNEL AND WILD MUSHROOMS

Ⓒ Cleanse*

Ⓖ Gut

Serves: 4

Prep time: 15 minutes

Cooking time: 30 minutes

This dish is super easy to pull together and perfection every time it's made. The ingredients can be varied, but this version is definitely a favorite and a must-try. It has a perfect flavor combination, and the chicken is the most tender and juicy when cooked this way.

1 whole pasture-raised chicken, all parts separated
Sea salt and freshly ground black pepper to taste
2 tablespoons avocado oil
1 medium onion, cut into large chunks
4 ounces fresh wild mushrooms, thickly sliced
1 fennel bulb, tops and tough base removed, cut into large chunks
3 garlic cloves, minced
8 ounces organic dry white wine
1 quart chicken stock or water
1 bay leaf
2 medium red bell peppers, seeded and cut into large chunks
2 tablespoons chopped fresh thyme
2 tablespoons kudzu root powder
½ lemon

Cut the chicken breasts into large chunks and separate the thighs from the drumsticks. Season all the meat liberally with salt and pepper.

Heat a large Dutch oven over medium-high heat. Add the avocado oil, and when it's hot, add the chicken. Sear all the sides of the chicken until they are golden brown, then remove the chicken from the pan and set it aside.

If the pan seems dry, add a bit more oil, then add the onion, mushrooms, and fennel. Sauté the mixture, stirring occasionally, for 2 to 3 minutes before adding the garlic. When every-thing is fragrant, add the chicken again to the pot and pour in the wine. Allow the wine to reduce by half before adding 4 cups of chicken stock or water and the bay leaf. Bring the liquid to a boil, then cover the Dutch oven, reduce the heat to medium, and slowly simmer. After 10 minutes add the bell peppers and continue simmering for an additional 15 to 20 minutes. Add a touch more liquid if it seems to be evaporating too quickly.

To finish, stir in the thyme, kudzu root powder, a squeeze of lemon, and a few additional pinches of salt. Serve it over quinoa, millet, or brown rice.

Note: If you purchase a whole chicken, you can make a stock the day before you wish to pre-pare this dish and use the stock as your cooking liquid.

*Replace bell peppers with summer squash or zucchini

GARLIC-CRUSTED CHICKEN

G Gut

Serves: 2

Prep time: 10 minutes

Cooking time: 8 to 10 minutes

We made a version of this on the Clean blog and it was an instant hit. Kids go crazy for this meal, and we'd be surprised if there are leftovers, but if so, use them on a salad the next day.

1 pasture-raised egg
2 tablespoons unsweetened coconut or almond milk
1 cup almond meal
1 teaspoon garlic powder
1 teaspoon paprika or chili powder
1 teaspoon sea salt
1 large or 2 small pasture-raised boneless, skinless chicken breasts
¼ cup plus 3 tablespoons extra-virgin olive oil
1 tablespoon apple cider vinegar
5 garlic cloves, minced
1 tablespoon freshly ground black pepper
Fresh parsley leaves for garnish (optional)

Preheat the oven to 425°F.

Line a baking sheet with parchment paper (or be prepared to really scrub the baking sheet afterward).

In a small bowl, whisk together the egg and coconut or almond milk.

In a large plastic bag, combine the almond meal, garlic powder, paprika or chili powder, and sea salt. One by one, dip each chicken piece in the egg and milk mixture, then put it inside the plastic bag and shake each piece until it is well coated. Place the pieces on the baking sheet. When you have coated all the chicken, drizzle the pieces with ¼ cup of the olive oil and bake them for 8 to 10 minutes.

Meanwhile, in a small bowl mix the 3 tablespoons of olive oil with the vinegar, garlic, and pepper. Set it aside to let the flavors combine. This is the sauce you'll serve with the chicken.

When the chicken is ready, remove it from the oven, and arrange it in a deep serving dish. Drizzle the garlic-pepper sauce over the pieces, tossing them to coat, and sprinkle them with parsley if you wish.

Don't be surprised when there aren't any leftovers, but if by some chance there are, the chicken and the sauce are equally delicious cold, in wraps, or on salads.

THE MOST PERFECT CHICKEN BREAST

C Cleanse

G Gut

Serves: 2

Prep time: 5 minutes

Cooking time: 15 to 20 minutes

This chicken is so simple and perfect, and is a staple of many clean recipes. Just remember, the overall taste and health benefits of any piece of meat or animal product depend on how it was raised and what it ate. Choose pasture-raised chickens. And don't forget to offer up your gratitude for any animal that gives its life for our bodies' nourishment.

2 6- to 8-ounce pasture-raised chicken breasts (skin on)
1 teaspoon sea salt
¼ teaspoon freshly ground black pepper
2 tablespoons avocado oil

Preheat the oven to 350°F.

Season each chicken breast liberally on both sides with salt and pepper.

Heat the avocado oil in a large ovenproof skillet set over medium-high heat. When the oil is hot, add the chicken breasts skin side down. Allow the skin to render its fat and brown nicely, lowering the heat to medium if it begins to smoke too much. Cook the chicken on the stovetop for about 8 to 10 minutes, until you notice the breasts look about halfway cooked through, then flip each breast and transfer the skillet to the oven for an additional 4 to 6 minutes.

Remove the skillet from the oven and let the chicken cool on a cutting board for 2 minutes. Use a sharp knife to make thin slices against the grain. Serve!

THAI MARINATED TURKEY BREAST

C Cleanse

Serves: 4

Prep time: 30 minutes minimum to overnight (for the marinade)

Cooking time: 30 minutes

Thai spice makes things so delicious. Turkey with Thai seasoning isn't a common combination but it's fantastic.

1½- to 2-pound pasture-raised turkey breast, sliced into ½- to ¾-inch-thick slices against the grain
½ batch Thai Dipping Sauce (page 88)
Juice of 1 lime
¼ cup chopped cilantro
2 to 3 tablespoons avocado oil, for cooking
1 bunch scallions

Arrange the turkey slices in a baking dish and pour the Thai Dipping Sauce over the top. Use your hands or a pair of tongs to mix the turkey and the marinade. Let it stand for a minimum of 30 minutes or in the fridge for up to 8 hours (overnight).

When the turkey is ready, prepare a grill or heat a heavy-bottom skillet. Brush the grill with oil or add a few tablespoons of oil to the skillet. Cook the turkey for 3 to 4 minutes on one side before flipping and continuing to cook until each piece is firm to the touch, approximately 30 minutes. Use a brush or a turkey baster to frequently cover the meat with more of the marinade.

As the turkey cooks, grill or sauté the scallions until they are lightly charred (if you're using a grill) and soft. Set them aside.

When the turkey is cooked through, allow the meat to rest for a few minutes before slicing it. Top with chopped cilantro and lime juice. Serve the slices over greens or with your favorite vegetables.

DUCK BREAST WITH CRANBERRY PEAR CHUTNEY

Ⓒ Cleanse

Serves: 2

Prep time: 10 minutes

Cooking time: 30 minutes

This is a wonderful holiday meal, gorgeous in the middle of the table and mouthwateringly tasty. The slightly sweet sauces pair perfectly with duck. You could also use chicken or turkey, if you can't find duck locally.

2 4- to 6-ounce pasture-raised boneless duck breasts (skin on)
Pinch of sea salt
¼ teaspoon freshly ground black pepper

For the Chutney
4 cups fresh cranberries
1 pound ripe pears, any variety, peeled, cored, and roughly chopped
½ teaspoon chopped fresh rosemary
1 cinnamon stick
½ teaspoon vanilla extract
1 cup water
¼ cup or more coconut nectar or raw honey (when not on cleanse)

Preheat the oven to 350°F.

First, make the chutney. In a heavy-bottom saucepan, heat the cranberries, pears, rosemary, cinnamon stick, vanilla, and water over medium heat until the water begins to simmer and the cranberries begin to break down. Continue to simmer for about 15 to 20 minutes, stirring the mixture often. If the chutney gets too thick, add a touch more water ¼ cup at a time.

Once the cranberries and pears are well cooked and the flavors have developed, stir in the coconut nectar or honey to taste. Cook for just a few more minutes, then transfer the chutney to a serving bowl and set it aside.

While the chutney is cooking, use a sharp knife to score the duck breasts. Make four or five ¼-inch-deep slices across each breast.

Set a large, ovenproof skillet over medium-high heat and, when it's hot, add the breasts, fat side down. Allow the fat to render and become crisp, about 5 minutes. Carefully flip each breast and cook them for an additional 1 to 2 minutes before transferring the skillet to the oven. Cook for 3 to 4 minutes, then remove the pan from the oven and let the duck rest on a cutting board for a minute before thinly slicing it on a 45 degree angle.

To serve, fan out the slices of duck divided between two serving plates and top each arrangement with a portion of the chutney. Season the duck with a pinch of salt and fresh ground pepper.

Pairings: Serve alongside Root Vegetable Hash (page 60).

CHICKEN OSSO BUCCO

Ⓖ Gut

Serves: 2

Prep time: 20 minutes

Cooking time: 1 hour

A perfect osso bucco should fall off the bone without a knife. It's a simple way to impress your guests, as they won't know that it wasn't an entirely complicated and difficult process. Your secret about how easy it really was is safe with us.

4 to 6 pasture-raised chicken thighs (either bone-in or boneless)
Sea salt and freshly ground black pepper to taste
2 tablespoons avocado oil
1 large onion, diced
1 carrot, diced
2 celery stalks, diced
4 garlic cloves, minced
1 tablespoon tomato paste
½ cup flat-leaf parsley leaves
4 sprigs fresh thyme
1 bay leaf
8 ounces dry white wine
1 cup water

Preheat the oven to 325°F.

Season the chicken thighs with salt and pepper.

Heat a large 6-quart Dutch oven set over medium-high heat. Add the avocado oil and, when it's hot, brown the thighs for 4 minutes on each side. When all the thighs are browned, remove them from the pan and set them aside.

Stir the onion, carrot, and celery together in the same pan, scraping up any bits on the bottom of the pan left over from the chicken, until the vegetables are soft, about 10 minutes. Stir in the garlic, cook for another minute, then add the tomato paste and cook an additional 2 to 3 minutes.

Tie the parsley and thyme together with kitchen twine into a bouquet garni, and add it to the pan along with the browned chicken thighs, bay leaf, white wine, and water. Bring the mixture to a simmer, cover the pan, and place it in the oven. Cook the mixture for another 45 minutes.

Serve the chicken over brown rice and sautéed greens with spoonfuls of the cooking liquid.

CURRIED COCONUT CHICKEN WITH CUCUMBER MANGO SALAD

Ⓒ Cleanse*

Serves: 2

Prep time: 10 minutes

Cooking time: 15 minutes

The spice is cut with cold sweetness in this salsa-type salad, for a winning combination no matter what the season or occasion.

½ cup shredded unsweetened coconut
2 tablespoons curry powder
2 teaspoons sea salt
¼ cup unsweetened coconut milk
2 4- to 6-ounce pasture-raised chicken breasts
2 tablespoons coconut oil
1 lime, cut into wedges

For the Salad
1 ripe mango, peeled, pitted, and cut into large chunks
1 medium cucumber, peeled, sliced ⅛-inch thick
¼ red onion, thinly sliced
1 red chili pepper, minced
2 tablespoons roughly chopped fresh mint
Sprinkle of sea salt
Juice of 1 lime

Preheat the oven to 350°F.

Combine the coconut, curry powder, and salt in a small bowl. Set the mixture aside. Pour the coconut milk in a separate small bowl. One by one, dip each chicken breast into the coconut milk, coating it evenly and shaking off any excess. Then dip it into the coconut-curry mixture, pressing the coating onto the chicken evenly.

Heat a large ovenproof skillet over medium-high heat. Add the coconut oil, and when the oil is hot, carefully place the chicken into the pan. Cook the breasts for about 2 to 3 minutes, until they are lightly browned on one side, then flip them and transfer the skillet to the oven for another 5 minutes.

While the chicken cooks in the oven, in a medium bowl toss together all the ingredients for the mango salad until everything is well combined. Set the bowl aside.

Remove the chicken from the oven and squeeze some lime juice over the top. Allow the breasts to rest for a few minutes before slicing and serving them with a good-size portion of the mango salad.

*Omit red chili pepper

SHREDDED CHICKEN

C Cleanse*
G Gut

Serves: 2 to 4

Prep time: 5 minutes

Cooking time: 25 minutes

Use this recipe as a base for chicken salad, "pulled pork"–type sandwiches and wraps, chicken soup, and tacos.

4 cups water
2 4- to 6-ounce pasture-raised boneless, skinless chicken breasts
1 tablespoon onion powder
2 garlic cloves
½ cup tomato purée (fresh or canned)
1 bay leaf
1 teaspoon dried thyme
1 tablespoon sea salt

Place all the ingredients in a medium pot set over medium-high heat and cover it with a lid. Bring the mixture to a boil, then lower the heat to medium and simmer it for 20 minutes. Remove the lid and allow the chicken to cool, then shred it using your fingers.

*Replace tomato with ¼ cup apple cider vinegar

Chef Frank on Using Spices

I love using spices! They add deep flavor, are medicinal, and help to bring ingredients together. When spices are ground, they begin to oxidize and lose their flavor. With a few exceptions, I like to buy my spices whole and grind them fresh as needed. Doing so will yield a much more complex flavor and add so much more to your meals. You can use a mortar and pestle or a coffee grinder to grind small batches. For maximum flavor, toast the spices in a dry pan before grinding to release their essential oils.

CRISPY ROASTED CHICKEN

C Cleanse

G Gut

Serves: 4 to 6

Prep time: 5 minutes

Cooking time: 1 hour and 10 minutes

This is such a wonderfully comforting and sensual meal. Food is best when it's a blend of taste and texture. This chicken is a classic that satisfies cravings and provides immune-boosting properties. Meat is more easily digested when it's cooked in a whole and saturated fat, so don't worry. Our bodies need some cholesterol and healthy fats to be properly fueled and to promote optimal brain function.

1 whole pasture-raised chicken
1 tablespoon sea salt
½ teaspoon freshly ground black pepper
2 to 3 tablespoons coconut oil (or another saturated fat, such as lard or duck fat)
Zest of 1 lemon
2 tablespoons chopped fresh thyme

One hour before cooking, remove the chicken from the fridge. It cooks more evenly if it's closer to room temperature.

Preheat the oven to 425°F.

In a small bowl, combine the salt, pepper, coconut oil, lemon zest, and thyme. Use a brush or your hands to spread the mixture all over the skin of the chicken, getting it into all the nooks and crannies.

Place the seasoned chicken in a cast-iron pan or baking dish and roast it for 20 minutes, then lower the oven temperature to 325°F and continue cooking for about another 45 minutes.

There are two ways to tell if your chicken is done. You can make a piercing in the lower thigh with a sharp knife. If the liquid runs clear and not pink, it's done. Or you can twist the drumstick. If it pulls away from the rest of the chicken, it's done. Remove the chicken from the oven and let rest for 5 minutes before slicing it. Don't forget to save the bones for making Chicken Stock (page 224).

CHICKEN WITH KALE AND OLIVES

C Cleanse

G Gut

Serves: 1

Prep time: 10 minutes

Cooking time: 20 minutes

Easy and quick, this is a definite weeknight winner when you're crunched for time, and the leftovers taste great over mixed greens the next day. It's also a wonderful weekend or dinner party meal.

1 pasture-raised boneless, skinless chicken breast (4 to 6 ounces), cut into thin strips
½ to 1 teaspoon sea salt
1 tablespoon coconut oil
2 garlic cloves, minced
1 large shallot, sliced into thin circles
2 teaspoons capers
1 bunch kale, stemmed and roughly chopped
½ lemon (for the juice)
¼ cup roughly chopped and pitted olives
Extra-virgin olive oil

Lightly season the chicken breast strips with salt and set them aside.

Melt the coconut oil in a sauté pan set over medium-high heat. (Having your pan nice and hot will help prevent the chicken from sticking.) Add the chicken breast pieces and cook them for 1 minute, then flip them over. Add the garlic, shallots, and capers, and toss everything together gently. Cook the mixture for an additional 1 to 2 minutes, then add the kale and squeeze a bit of lemon over everything. Give the pan a quick stir and cover. Steam the mixture until the kale is wilted, another 2 to 3 minutes. Toss in the olives, drizzle in a bit of olive oil, and add an additional pinch of salt. Serve warm.

CHICKEN WITH PRESERVED LEMONS AND FRAGRANT SPICES

C Cleanse

G Gut

Serves: 4

Prep time: 15 minutes

Cooking time: 1 hour

This has a beautifully elegant presentation and the smells are out of this world. It's a great way to treat yourself to something special and make your entire house smell insanely good.

¼ cup coconut oil
4 whole pasture-raised chicken legs
2 teaspoons sea salt
Freshly ground black pepper
2 large yellow onions, sliced
1½ tablespoons ground coriander
2 teaspoons ground ginger
1 teaspoon ground turmeric
6 to 8 saffron threads
1 cup chicken stock
2 tablespoons coconut butter
2 teaspoons minced fresh cilantro
1 whole preserved lemon, cut into thin strips (available at specialty stores or at Whole Foods Market)

Preheat the oven to 350°F.

Heat the coconut oil in a 7- to 8-quart Dutch oven set over medium-high heat. Season the chicken legs with salt and pepper, then cook them in the pan, turning them until all their sides are browned, about 10 to 12 minutes. Transfer the chicken to a plate.

Sauté the onions in the pan with the leftover chicken juices for 5 to 6 minutes, stirring occasionally, until they are golden brown. Add the coriander, ginger, turmeric, and saffron, further sautéing until it's fragrant.

Return the chicken legs to the pan and add the stock. Bring the mixture to a boil, then transfer the pan to the oven. Bake the chicken covered until it's tender, 30 to 40 minutes. Stir in the coconut butter, cilantro, and lemon strips, and bake again covered for 5 additional minutes. Serve the chicken over steamed brown rice, millet, or quinoa.

ROASTED CAULIFLOWER AND CHICKEN SAUSAGE CASSEROLE

Janet Goldman Weinberg, Clean community member

Ⓖ Gut   **Serves:** 4, as a main course

Cauliflower, the star of the show in this dish, makes a perfect companion for your clean lifestyle. It's easy to digest, low in sugar, and provides a powerhouse of nutrition, along with healthy doses of vitamins C, K, and B. In addition, it's loaded with antioxidants, which support the body's natural detox system. Serve this as an entrée and get plenty of vegetables, protein, and healthy fat.

1 medium head cauliflower (roughly 2 pounds)
4 garlic cloves, minced
2 tablespoons extra-virgin olive oil, plus extra for the baking dish
½ pound raw organic Italian chicken sausage, nitrate- and sugar-free, removed from casings
1 medium onion, diced
Leaves of 2 sprigs fresh thyme
1 28-ounce can whole organic peeled tomatoes, drained and the liquid reserved (the reserved liquid can be omitted to achieve less tomato flavor)
Sea salt and freshly ground black pepper to taste
⅔ cup almond meal
¼ cup nutritional yeast or Cashew Cheese (page 97); you can use Parmesan cheese if you're not on a Clean program

Preheat the oven to 350°F.

Lightly coat a 9 × 13-inch baking dish with olive oil.

Cut the cauliflower head into quarters. Slice away the leaves and stem and, with an angled cut, remove the core from each quarter. Chop the quarters into roughly bite-size florets, each about 1 inch across, then chop the florets in half or quarters to achieve flat surfaces that encourage browning in the oven.

In a large bowl, toss the cauliflower pieces with half of the minced garlic and 1 tablespoon of the olive oil. Spread the seasoned cauliflower on a baking sheet and roast the pieces in the oven, turning them frequently, for about 15 minutes or until they are evenly browned. Remove the pan from the oven and set it aside.

Heat the remaining tablespoon of olive oil in a 10-inch sauté pan set over medium-high heat. When the pan is quite hot, add the sausage. Use a spoon to break up the meat, and cook it for 8 to 12 minutes, or until the sausage is cooked through and beginning to get crispy. Since the sausage will stick, as you sauté use your spoon to scrape bits from the bottom of the pan. This will add wonderful flavor to the dish.

Lower the heat to medium-low and add the onion, the remaining half of the garlic, and the thyme. Sauté the mixture for about 5 minutes, stirring frequently and continuing to scrape up any bits that stick to the pan.

Crush the tomatoes and add them to the pan. Stir thoroughly, then add the reserved tomato sauce, if desired, and sauté for about 5 more minutes. Turn off the heat and taste the sauce. Add salt and pepper to taste, and stir in the roasted cauliflower.

In the prepared baking dish, distribute the cauliflower and sausage mixture evenly. In a small bowl, combine the almond meal and nutritional yeast (or cashew or Parmesan cheese), and sprinkle this over the cauliflower and sausage.

Place the baking dish in the middle of the oven and bake the casserole for 25 minutes, or until the topping has browned and the sauce is bubbling. Remove it from the oven and let it stand for 5 minutes before serving.

SLOW-COOKED CHICKEN

C Cleanse

G Gut

Serves: 2

Prep time: 10 minutes

Cooking time: 3 to 4 hours

This is another low-maintenance dish with extra protein and incredible flavor. Put it in the slow cooker, go do something fun, and come back to a wonderful-smelling hot meal.

2 carrots, roughly chopped
3 celery stalks, roughly chopped
1 large onion, roughly chopped
1 whole pasture-raised chicken
3 tablespoons extra-virgin olive oil
1 lemon, zested and cut in half
2 tablespoons lemon pepper seasoning
1 tablespoon sea salt
1 garlic bulb, peeled and all the cloves crushed
3 sprigs fresh thyme

Turn the slow cooker on high, then add the carrots, celery, and onion.

Coat the chicken skin with the olive oil, then rub it with the lemon zest, lemon pepper, and salt. Stuff the chicken cavity with the lemon halves, crushed garlic, and thyme.

Cook the chicken in the slow cooker for 3 to 4 hours. Use a fork to flake apart the meat when it's ready.

MEAT

These meat dishes were created to be clean, hardy, and nutrient-dense. While meat isn't the primary food category of a clean diet, it also isn't something to fear. In general, we recommend reducing your overall intake of meat and adding more fruits and vegetables. When you do make these delicious dishes, look to use hormone- and antibiotic-free, organic, grass-fed, or pastured animal products.

LAMB AND WILD MUSHROOM STUFFED EGGPLANT

G Gut

Serves: 4 to 6

Prep time: 30 minutes

Cooking time: 20 minutes

This dish is richly seasoned and universally appealing. Even for those of you who aren't crazy about mushrooms or eggplant, you may want to give this recipe a try.

2 equal-size eggplants, up to a pound each
Extra-virgin olive oil
1 tablespoon sea salt, plus a few pinches for the filling
Freshly ground black pepper to taste
2 or more tablespoons avocado oil
3 cups roughly chopped mushrooms
½ pound ground pasture-raised lamb
1 cup diced onion
2 garlic cloves
2 tablespoons chopped fresh oregano
2 tablespoons chopped fresh mint
1 teaspoon ground coriander
½ teaspoon ground cumin
2 teaspoons paprika
½ teaspoon ground cinnamon
¼ teaspoon ground allspice
1 cup chicken stock or water
1 tablespoon kudzu root, dissolved into 2 tablespoons of water
Splash of lemon juice

Preheat the oven to 400°F.

Cut the eggplants in half lengthwise. Using a spoon, scoop out the flesh, leaving about a quarter to half of the flesh so the eggplants will hold their structure when baked. Reserve the scooped-out flesh.

Place the hollowed-out eggplants in an oiled baking dish. Drizzle them with olive oil, and sprinkle them with salt and pepper. Bake them for 15 minutes, just enough to soften up the remaining flesh. Remove the dish from the oven and set it aside.

Reduce the oven temperature to 350°F.

Heat a large sauté pan set over medium-high heat. Add the avocado oil, and when the oil is hot, sauté the mushrooms for 3 to 4 minutes. Scoop the mushrooms into a bowl and set the bowl aside for the moment.

Roughly chop 1 cup of the reserved eggplant flesh and sauté it in the same pan until it is lightly browned. (You will need to add a bit more avocado oil to the pan.) Then add the eggplant flesh to the reserved cooked mushrooms.

Again add a few more tablespoons of oil to the pan and brown the lamb with the onion, garlic, oregano, mint, coriander, cumin, paprika, cinnamon, and allspice. Stir the mixture often to prevent the spices from burning. When the lamb is halfway cooked through, return the reserved mushrooms and eggplant flesh to the pan. Pour in the chicken stock or water and bring the mixture to a simmer. Allow the filling to continue to cook for a few minutes, then add the dissolved kudzu root. Add a few pinches of salt and a splash of lemon juice. By this point the liquid should have cooked down and thickened up a bit. Remove the pan from the heat.

Spoon the filling into the hollowed-out eggplant halves, then bake them for 20 minutes. Serve them with your favorite chutney.

MOROCCAN LAMB KEBABS

C Cleanse

G Gut*

Makes: about 12 kebabs

Prep time: 20 minutes plus 30 minutes for marinating

Cooking time: 15 minutes

There are lots of ingredients but they come together very easily. This is a must-try for a spiced dinner paired with sides dishes, or served as an appetizer at a dinner party. Look for local meat that's been pastured and not grain-fed. Where your food comes from is of the utmost importance, and how the animals we consume were treated is something we all should consider with each meal.

You will need 10 to 15 wooden skewers for this recipe, soaked in water for 30 minutes or longer.

2 pounds pasture-raised boneless leg of lamb, cut into 1-inch pieces
Sea salt to taste
3 to 4 tablespoons extra-virgin olive oil
1 large red onion, halved, then cut into wedges (cut so that some of the root is part of each wedge)
2 Granny Smith apples, cut into large chunks

For the Spice Rub
2 teaspoons paprika
½ teaspoon ground cumin
2 teaspoons ground coriander
1 teaspoon ground cardamom
2 teaspoons ground cinnamon
½ teaspoon freshly ground nutmeg

For the Tzatziki Sauce
1 cup raw sunflower seeds, soaked for 2 hours in 4 cups of water, strained, and rinsed
2 tablespoons extra-virgin olive oil
3 tablespoons lemon juice
2 to 3 teaspoons sea salt
¼ cup roughly chopped fresh parsley
¼ cup roughly chopped fresh cilantro
1 cup minced cucumber

In a small bowl, combine all the ingredients for the spice rub. Place the lamb chunks in a separate bowl and pour in enough of the spice mixture to fully coat all the pieces. Sprinkle with salt to taste, and drizzle with the olive oil. Cover the lamb and allow it to marinate for 30 minutes or longer.

*Substitute peppers or other veggies for apples

Skewer 3 or 4 chunks of the lamb along with the red onion wedges and apple chunks. Prepare as many skewers as will use all the lamb, onion, and apple pieces, which should be about 12.

Prepare a grill or cast-iron grill pan and cook the skewers for 3 to 4 minutes on one side, then flip them and cook for a few additional minutes.

While the lamb cooks, prepare the tzatziki sauce. In a blender, purée the sunflower seeds, olive oil, lemon juice, and salt until the mixture is creamy, about 30 seconds. Use some water if you need to thin out the sauce, although it should be nice and thick. Transfer the sunflower seed purée to a bowl and fold in the parsley, cilantro, and cucumber.

When all the lamb is cooked, place the skewers on a serving platter with a bowl of the tzatziki sauce in the middle.

BRAISED LAMB SHANKS

C Cleanse*
G Gut

Serves: 2

Prep time: 25 minutes

Cooking time: 3 to 4 hours

As always, choose your meat wisely. Eating pasture-raised meat from local farms, raised on grass and in the fresh air, not only ensures that we respect the circle of life and take a great deal of responsibility for our place in the food chain but also that the meat will be healthier for you, with more usable protein and the best possible fat content.

2 pasture-raised lamb shanks
2 teaspoons fennel seeds, ground
Sea salt to taste
¼ to ½ teaspoon freshly ground black pepper
2 to 4 tablespoons coconut oil
2 carrots, diced
3 celery sticks, diced
1 large onion, diced
4 garlic cloves, minced
2 tablespoons tomato paste
8 ounces organic red wine
1 bay leaf
1 tablespoon chopped fresh rosemary
1 2-inch cinnamon stick
1 quart chicken stock or water

Preheat the oven to 325°F.

Season the lamb shanks with the freshly ground fennel seeds and a generous amount of salt and pepper.

Heat a 6-quart Dutch oven (or any deep ovenproof pot) over high heat. Add the coconut oil, and when the oil is hot, add the lamb shanks. Brown them well on all sides, then remove them from the pot and set them aside.

Add a few more tablespoons of oil to the same pot, then sauté the carrots, celery, onion, and garlic for 8 to 10 minutes, stirring occasionally to prevent burning. Stir in the tomato paste and cook for a few more minutes. Pour in the wine, scrape the bottom of the pan, and allow the mixture to reduce by half.

Return the shanks to the pot and add the bay leaf, rosemary, cinnamon stick, and chicken stock or water. Salt and pepper to taste. Allow the liquid to come to a boil, then turn off the heat, cover the pot, and place it in the oven.

Cook covered for 3 to 4 hours. At this point, the shanks should be fall-off-the-bone tender and ready to eat.

To create a sauce, strain the leftover liquid into a separate pot and bring it to a boil. Allow the flavorful stock to reduce until it's thick enough to coat the back of a spoon.

*Omit tomato paste

CAMBRIDGE FRIED RICE

Paul Jaminet, Ph.D., and Shou-Ching Jaminet, Ph.D., authors of Perfect Health Diet

Serves: 6 to 8

Prep time: 15 minutes to gather and chop ingredients, if leftovers are used

Cooking time: 15 minutes

Fried rice is a classic dish of China and the primary way Chinese eat leftovers. There are many fried rice recipes in China; the most famous and popular, Yangzhou fried rice, features barbecued pork, shrimp, and scrambled egg. When we adjusted this recipe to use ingredients endorsed by our *Perfect Health Diet* (Scribner, 2012), we renamed it for our hometown, Cambridge, Massachusetts.

Fried rice is best made with leftover white rice, so that it has had a day (or three) since cooking to dry out. Include any leftover meats or vegetables in your refrigerator; this is how the Chinese make it. Be creative about flavors. Fried rice can be made with a different set of ingredients every time!

2 tablespoons extra-virgin olive oil
1 cup diced scallions
1 cup diced shiitake mushrooms
1 cup grated carrot
1 cup fresh snow peas
1 cup diced cooked shrimp
6 tablespoons coconut oil
6 pasture-raised eggs
4 cups previously cooked long-grain white rice
½ cup leftover diced or ground beef or lamb (if you are using uncooked beef or lamb, brown the meat in the wok first)
Sea salt, freshly ground black pepper, and ground turmeric to taste

The key to a good fried rice is to "fry" (really, warm and coat in oil) the ingredients separately, to get a good diffusion of oil throughout the rice and food.

You'll need a large wok for the frying, and plates or bowls to hold the ingredients as they are cooked. All the cooking can be done at medium heat.

Heat the olive oil in the wok, then stir-fry the scallions and set them aside. Then stir-fry the shiitake mushrooms, then the carrots and peas. Stir-fry the shrimp last.

Add 2 tablespoons of the coconut oil to a heated small sauté pan and scramble the eggs. Add the scallions as the eggs are cooking. When the eggs are firm but not dry, set them aside too.

Add the remaining 4 tablespoons of coconut oil and the white rice to the wok. Stir the rice until it is uniformly coated and has absorbed the oil. Now add all the previously cooked ingredients—the vegetables, shrimp, eggs, and meat—and stir to combine everything well. Add salt, pepper, and turmeric to taste. That's all there is to it!

Transfer the mixture to a large serving plate, and enjoy it while it's still warm.

POMEGRANATE-GLAZED LAMB CHOPS

Serves: 2

Prep time: 5 minutes

Cooking time: 10 minutes

A secret ingredient in one of the most delicious sweet yet tart sauces, pomegranate molasses is amazing and one of those condiments that you'll pull out over and over, especially to delight and impress.

6 pasture-raised lamb chops
1 to 2 tablespoons extra-virgin olive oil
1 tablespoon ground coriander seeds
2 teaspoons sea salt
¼ teaspoon freshly ground black pepper
¼ cup pomegranate molasses
2 tablespoons julienned fresh mint leaves

Place the lamb chops in a shallow dish. Coat them with olive oil and generously season them with the coriander seeds, salt, and pepper.

Heat a grill pan over high heat. When it is very hot, sear the lamb chops on one side for 2 to 3 minutes before flipping them and cooking the other side for an additional 2 to 3 minutes. As soon as you remove the chops from the pan, brush or drizzle them with the pomegranate molasses and sprinkle them with the fresh mint.

Pairings: Serve these with Sweet and Spicy Squash and Apple Purée (page 116).

ROASTED LAMB LOIN WITH MINT PESTO

C Cleanse

G Gut

Serves: 2

Prep time: 15 minutes

Cooking time: 10 minutes

Mint is a classic and wonderful pairing with lamb. Definitely use fresh mint if you can. You'll want to use this pesto over and over, so you may want to make a large batch!

1 pound pasture-raised lamb loin chops
2 tablespoons extra-virgin olive oil
1 tablespoon sea salt
2 tablespoons chopped fresh oregano

For the Mint Pesto
2 garlic cloves
¼ cup raw pistachios
2 cups fresh mint
½ cup fresh flat-leaf parsley
¼ cup extra-virgin olive oil
1 teaspoon sea salt
½ teaspoon freshly ground black pepper

Place the chops in a baking dish. Drizzle them with olive oil and season them with salt and oregano. Use your hands to thoroughly combine the ingredients. Let the chops marinate at room temperature for 10 minutes.

While the lamb is marinating, prepare the pesto. In a food processor, pulse the garlic and pistachios until they are roughly chopped. Add the mint and parsley, and process them until they too are roughly chopped, then leave the machine running while slowly adding the oil in a steady stream. Keep processing until it reaches a desired thickness, then season the pesto with salt and pepper and set it aside.

Grill or pan-sear the marinated lamb chops on high for 2 to 3 minutes on each side. This will achieve a medium-rare temperature internally, but cook them longer if you desire.

Serve each lamp chop with a scoop of the pesto.

Pairings: Enjoy this dish with Roasted Pears and Parsnips (page 117).

COCONUT ZUCCHINI NOODLES AND SPICED MEATBALLS

C Cleanse*

G Gut

Serves: 2 to 3

Prep time: 15 minutes

Cooking time: 30 minutes

This meatball and noodle dish is amazingly flavored and is a family-friendly dish to make. Kids will love helping you shape the meatballs and create the veggie noodles.

2 to 3 tablespoons coconut oil
½ cup sliced onions
2 garlic cloves
2 tablespoons minced lemongrass
1 red chili pepper, minced (optional)
1 13.5-ounce can unsweetened coconut milk
¼ cup water
1 broccoli crown, cut into small florets (about 2 cups)
¾ to 1 pound zucchini, ends removed and sliced lengthwise with a peeler or mandoline into long pappardelle-like "noodles"
Sea salt to taste
½ cup roughly chopped fresh cilantro
1 lime, cut into wedges

For the Spiced Meatballs
1 pound ground pasture-raised lamb
1 tablespoon freshly grated ginger
2 scallions, sliced paper-thin
1 teaspoon ground turmeric
1 tablespoon wheat-free tamari
1 tablespoon fish sauce (Red Boat is a Clean-approved brand)
1 tablespoon lime juice

First, prepare the meatballs. In a large bowl, combine all the ingredients for the meatballs and mix them thoroughly with your hands or a wooden spoon. Wet your hands, then form even-size balls. I usually go for about the size of a golf ball.

Heat a 4-quart Dutch oven over medium-high heat. Melt the coconut oil, and once it's nice and hot, add the meatballs. Cook them for 30 to 45 seconds on each side, until they are all nicely browned. When they are about halfway done browning, make some space in the center of the pan and add the onions, garlic, lemongrass, and optional red chili. Continue to cook the mixture for 1 to 2 minutes, then move the meatballs back into the center of the pan and add the coconut milk and water. Cover the pan and simmer for about 5 more minutes before adding the broccoli. Within a few minutes the broccoli should be tender and the

*Omit red chili pepper

coconut milk reduced and starting to thicken. Carefully fold in the zucchini noodles and allow them to cook in the liquid. Cook them just until the zucchini is tender. Salt to taste.

Serve with a garnish of cilantro and a squeeze of lime.

GINGERED BEEF RAMEN

Serves: 4

Prep time: 15 minutes

Cooking time: 15 minutes

Quick and easy, this is a hearty and healthy variation on the traditional packaged ramen. It has a gingery kick and helps digestion and circulation. Watch everyone wolf this down and ask for seconds.

2 to 3 tablespoons avocado oil
2 to 3 tablespoons toasted sesame oil
12 ounces top round pasture-raised beef, thinly sliced (about ¼-inch thick) against the grain
2 tablespoons freshly grated ginger
2 garlic cloves, minced
1 quart vegetable or beef stock
2 tablespoons rice wine vinegar
1 package (8 ounces) King Soba ramen noodles
1 cup daikon radish, thinly sliced
1 bunch scallions, both greens and whites thinly sliced
1 to 2 teaspoons red pepper flakes (optional)

Heat a large wok or skillet over high heat. Add 1 tablespoon each of the avocado and sesame oils. Working in three small batches (don't overcrowd the pan), quickly cook the beef with a third of the ginger and a third of the garlic for 2 to 3 minutes. Set the mixture aside and continue, adding another tablespoon of each of the oils and another third of the ginger and garlic, until all the beef is cooked.

While you cook the beef, heat the vegetable or beef stock with the vinegar in a pot set over medium heat. Add the ramen noodles to the hot stock and cook them just until they are tender.

Divide the cooked noodles between four serving bowls and stir in the beef mixture. Garnish each bowl with radish slices, scallions, and optional red pepper flakes.

SPAGHETTI AND MEATBALLS WITH THIRTY-MINUTE MARINARA

Serves: 4

Prep time: 15 minutes

Cooking time: 45 minutes

Just because you don't eat gluten, it doesn't mean you can't have a classic spaghetti-and-meatball dish. Satisfy your pasta cravings with this. Trust us, you'll be glad you did.

1 pound gluten-free spaghetti

For the Marinara
2 tablespoons avocado oil, plus another few tablespoons for cooking the meatballs
1 small onion, roughly chopped
2 garlic cloves, minced
2 teaspoons Italian seasoning
1 cup red wine
1 28-ounce can whole peeled tomatoes, blended into a purée
1¾ cups water

For the Meatballs
1 pound grass-fed ground beef
¼ cup minced onion
1 pasture-raised egg
1 tablespoon ground chia seeds
2 tablespoons almond flour
¼ cup chopped fresh parsley
2 teaspoons sea salt
¼ teaspoon freshly ground black pepper

Preheat the oven to 350°F.

First, make the marinara. Heat a Dutch oven over medium-high heat. Add 2 tablespoons of the avocado oil, and when it's warm, sauté the onion until it's translucent, about 3 to 4 minutes. Add the garlic, stir to combine, and sauté the mixture until it is fragrant. Add the Italian seasoning followed by the wine, and reduce the mixture by half. Pour in the tomato purée and the water, then lower the heat and simmer the sauce for 20 minutes, stirring occasionally and allowing it to condense and thicken.

While the sauce thickens, in a large bowl stir together all the ingredients for the meatballs until they are well combined. Using your hands, form even-size balls, about the size of golf balls, and set them aside. Heat another few tablespoons of avocado oil in an ovenproof sauté pan. When the oil is hot, add the meatballs and brown them about 2 minutes on each side before transferring the pan to the oven. Cook them for about 10 more minutes.

Bring 3 quarts salted water to a boil. Cook the spaghetti until it's tender, then drain the noodles and toss them with the meatballs and the sauce. Serve immediately.

HERBED BUFFALO BURGERS

Ⓒ Cleanse*
Ⓖ Gut

Serves: 4

Prep time: 5 minutes

Cooking time: 10 minutes

If you can't find buffalo, or any other wild game, try grass-fed beef for an equally tasty burger. This herb mix isn't a traditional burger flavoring, but it's absolutely incredible.

1 pound ground buffalo
½ cup mixed fresh herbs, such as parsley, sage, thyme, and/or rosemary, roughly chopped
1 tablespoon sea salt
1 pasture-raised egg

In a large bowl, mix all the ingredients thoroughly until they are well combined. Portion the mixture into 4 evenly shaped patties. Grill, bake, or pan-sear them on the stovetop to however you like your burgers.

*Omit egg

Chef Frank on Using Herbs

Herbs play an important role in my cuisine. Freshly picked and chopped, they add pop to any dish. When cutting back on salt intake, the best way to increase flavor is to use herbs. As a general rule of thumb, I use dried herbs for long cooking procedures like soups, stews, or anything in a slow cooker. Fresh herbs are best when added at the last moment before serving so you get all the flavors and aromas in the dish. If a recipe calls for fresh herbs and you only have dried, halve the amount called for. When blending fresh herbs into a dressing or soup, try not to overprocess, as it can make your dish too bitter.

I like to change the herbs I use with the seasons. In the summer, I use lots of basil, cilantro, parsley, and mint. Once the weather gets colder, I switch to more sage, rosemary, and thyme. Have fun growing your own in containers inside, a wonderful way to bring medicinal and culinary foods right into your home.

SHEPHERD'S PIE

C Cleanse

Serves: 4

Prep time: 15 minutes

Cooking time: 1 hour (including roasting time)

There's nothing quite like digging into warm comfort food when it's cold outside. This meal is the perfect warming winter lunch when you're on a cleanse, but it's a great dinner anytime of the year. We've given you this classically delicious recipe, but feel free to try any other variations you come up with. Venison or grass-fed beef are incredible in this too, or add more vegetables and make it entirely vegetarian if you wish. The pomegranate seeds on top add a super antioxidant punch, perfect for cold and flu season. They can also help ease muscle pain, so this would be a great meal after being outside all day, working or playing, or after a long cold-weather run.

For the Mashed Root Vegetables
2 medium parsnips, peeled and cut into large chunks
1 large celery root, peeled and cut into large chunks
2 tablespoons coconut oil
½ cup unsweetened almond milk
Sea salt to taste
¼ teaspoon ground white pepper

For the Filling
2 tablespoons coconut oil
1 pound ground pasture-raised lamb
1 large carrot, chopped into small pieces
1 large onion, chopped into medium pieces
2 celery stalks, chopped into medium pieces
1 tablespoon Mediterranean seasoning; or 2 teaspoons dried oregano, 2 teaspoons onion
    powder, and 1 teaspoon dried thyme
3 tablespoons millet or brown rice flour
2 cups chicken or vegetable stock
Sea salt to taste

Preheat the oven to 375°F.

To make the mashed root vegetables, place the parsnips and celery root into a medium-size pot. Add an inch of water, cover the pot, and cook the vegetables over high heat until they are tender when pierced with a fork. Strain them thoroughly.

Put the strained root vegetables back into the same pot. Drizzle them with the coconut oil and, using a hand masher, mash them until the mixture is smooth. Add the almond milk, and season with salt and white pepper. Cover the pot and set it aside.

Next, prepare the filling. Heat a large sauté pan with the coconut oil. When the oil is hot, sear the lamb until it is fully browned, stirring frequently, then add the carrot, onion, and celery, stirring to combine. Cook the mixture until everything's soft. Sprinkle in the Mediterranean seasoning and flour, and continue to stir to prevent any burning. After a few minutes, add the stock. Slowly simmer the mixture until it gradually thickens, then season it with salt and remove the pan from the heat.

Pour the lamb and vegetable filling into a large baking or pie dish (any shape works—round, oval, square, rectangle), spreading it evenly. Using a spatula, layer the root vegetable mash over the entire surface of the filling. Bake the pie for 20 minutes, until warmed through and lightly browned on top. Serve warm.

VEGETABLES

The quality of our health has a lot to do with the amount of plant food in our diet. A common trait of the world's longest-lived peoples is a slant toward eating more plants. The rich diversity of vegetables in their diet provides the phytonutrients and antioxidants needed to help reduce inflammation, oxidative stress, and free radical damage. That's why we have placed a lot of attention on creating vegetable-based meals chock-full of nutrients that taste great.

SPINACH PATTIES

Peggy and Megan Curry, founding partners of Curry Girls Kitchen

C Cleanse*

G Gut†

Spinach patties are great as a hearty meal or as a grab-and-go snack. Our favorite way to eat them is on a bed of spicy mixed greens and roasted vegetables. Top each patty with a dollop of red pepper hummus and avocado slices. They are also terrific served on a bun or crumbled inside a wrap.

4 teaspoons extra-virgin olive oil
½ to 1 cup finely chopped shiitake mushrooms
1 onion, diced, or 1 leek, green part only finely chopped
2 to 3 garlic cloves, minced
1 bunch fresh or frozen spinach
2 scallions, finely chopped
1 egg or 3 tablespoons chia seeds, ground and soaked in ¼ cup water for 15 minutes
½ to 1 cup cooked quinoa or brown rice
¼ cup raw sunflower seeds, toasted and ground
¼ cup grated Pecorino or Romano cheese (optional)
¼ cup crumbled sheep or goat feta (optional)
1 teaspoon Italian seasoning
Sea salt and freshly ground black pepper to taste
2 to 3 tablespoons coconut oil

In a medium skillet, heat 2 teaspoons of the olive oil, then sauté the mushrooms, onion or leek, and garlic. Transfer the mixture to a medium bowl and set it aside.

In the same pan, heat the remaining 2 teaspoons of olive oil and add the spinach. Cover and steam the spinach for 1 to 2 minutes, until the leaves are wilted, then drain it, pressing it against the edge of a strainer to remove any excess liquid. Chop the cooked spinach, and add it to the mushroom, onion, and garlic mixture. Add the scallions, egg or soaked chia seeds, quinoa or rice, ground sunflower seeds, optional cheeses, Italian seasoning, salt, and pepper, and combine everything thoroughly. The mixture should hold together when formed into a patty.

Again in the same pan, heat the coconut oil over medium heat until it's hot. Form the spinach mixture into patties and sauté each patty until it's browned on both sides, about 5 minutes per side.

Serve the patties warm as a meal or at room temperature on top of a salad.

Note: The patty mixture can be made a day ahead and refrigerated. Also, the patties can be baked for 30 minutes instead of pan-frying, if you prefer. If you wish to store the cooked patties, wrap each one in parchment paper and store them in a freezer bag in your freezer.

*Without egg or dairy
†Without brown rice

SESAME NOODLES

C Cleanse

V Vegan

Serves: 2

Prep time: 20 minutes

Cooking time: 15 minutes

This warm and slightly nutty noodle dish combines the snappy flavor of ginger with the earthiness of toasted sesame oil. Enjoy these on their own or paired with lamb, fish, or chicken.

1 package King Soba black rice noodles
1 medium carrot, grated
½ cup finely shredded purple cabbage
½ cup roughly chopped fresh cilantro
2 tablespoons raw sesame seeds

For the Vinaigrette
¼ cup toasted sesame oil
1 tablespoon rice vinegar
2 tablespoons wheat-free tamari
1 red chili pepper (optional)
2 garlic cloves
1-inch chunk ginger, grated

Have all the vegetables prepared and the dressing blended before cooking the rice noodles, so the noodles will still be warm when you combine everything.

In a blender or small bowl, purée or whisk together all the ingredients for the dressing. Set it aside.

Cook the rice noodles according to the directions on the package, then drain them well and transfer them to a large bowl. Toss the warm noodles with the carrot, cabbage, cilantro, and sesame seeds, and dress the salad with enough vinaigrette to coat everything thoroughly. Serve immediately.

LENTILS SEASONED IN DOMINICAN SOFRITO

Zoe Saldana, actress

Sofrito is usually the first thing to go into the pot when we make soups, stews, beans, and rice dishes. You can use it right away or store it in the refrigerator for later use.

For the Sofrito
2 red onions, peeled and diced
2 large green bell pepper, seeds removed, and diced
1 head of garlic, cloves peeled and minced
1 jar (4 ounces) diced pimentos, drained
1 can (8 ounces) tomato sauce
½ teaspoon dried oregano
½ teaspoon dried thyme
1 tablespoon apple cider vinegar
1 tablespoon ground annatto (aka achiote)

For the Lentils
½ cup olive oil
1 garlic clove
2 tablespoons lemon juice
1 tablespoon of sofrito. Or more if you want it savory!
1 small red bell pepper, seeded and chopped
1 small green pepper, seeded and chopped
1 small white onion, chopped
1 tablespoon apple cider vinegar
1 16-ounce package dried brown lentils, rinsed and drained

First, make the sofrito. Chop and blend all the ingredients in a food processor or blender. Place the mixture in a glass jar with a tight lid. Refrigerate up to two weeks.

Place lentils in a large pot with enough water to cover by a few inches. Bring to a boil, and cook until lentils are tender, about 15 minutes. Drain and rinse with cold water in a colander to cool. Let stand for a few minutes to drain well.

In a large pan, sauté olive oil and garlic. Wait for the garlic to turn brown but don't burn it! Add lemon juice and sofrito, and sauté for a minute. Add the red pepper, green pepper, and onion and sauté until it is cooked to your liking. Add the vinegar and the lentils, and stir everything for 2 to 4 minutes. Voila!

You can eat this dish hot or cold, anytime of the day or night. These lentils taste better the longer they sit. I always pour a little bit of olive oil over the dish every time I serve myself a bowl. I sometimes even add some cayenne pepper to spice it up.

You can substitute the olive oil for coconut oil or almond oil. And substitute the peppers as well for any vegetable to your liking. My mom sometimes adds chayotes because they are my favorite vegetable. Bon appetit!

QUINOA WITH CELERY AND APPLES

C Cleanse

V Vegan

Serves: 2

Prep time: 20 minutes

Cooking time: 15 minutes

This is a delicious side dish and a great meal to bring to a gathering, as it travels and keeps well without needing to be warmed up. It's also an excellent salad topper throughout the week—a wonderful recipe to make ahead of time and use for several days.

1½ cups quinoa
3 cups water
4 celery stalks, thinly sliced
2 medium crisp apples, diced
¼ cup extra-virgin olive oil
2 to 3 tablespoons apple cider vinegar
3 scallions, thinly sliced
Sea salt and freshly ground black pepper to taste

Heat the quinoa and water in a small covered pot. Simmer the quinoa for 15 minutes, then remove the pot from heat and let it stand for 5 minutes. Uncover the pot and allow the quinoa to cool to room temperature. Or to speed up the process, spread the quinoa in a baking dish and set it in the fridge for 20 minutes.

When the quinoa has cooled, transfer it to a large bowl and stir in the celery, apples, olive oil, vinegar, and scallions. Season the mixture generously with salt and pepper, and serve.

SAVORY STUFFED VEGETABLES

Ⓖ Gut

Makes: 3 to 4 cups of stuffing

Prep time: overnight plus 30 minutes

A lovely addition to any meal, these vegetables look pretty on the table, and they can be easily adjusted to each family member's preference. It's fun to let kids fill their own.

Vegetables to Stuff
Red bell peppers, stems and seeds removed, then cut in half
Cucumber, cut lengthwise, seeds removed
Roma tomatoes, cut in half, seeds and pulp removed
Romaine or Bibb lettuce leaves

For the Stuffing
1 cup raw almonds, soaked for 6 to 8 hours, strained and rinsed well
1 cup raw sunflower seeds, soaked for 2 hours, strained and rinsed well
2 shallots, roughly chopped
2 garlic cloves, minced
½ cup sun-dried tomatoes, soaked until soft (about 20 minutes)
1 large red bell pepper, finely diced
2 celery stalks, finely diced
¼ cup extra-virgin olive oil
Juice of 1 lemon
½ cup chopped fresh parsley
1 tablespoon chopped fresh thyme
½ teaspoon chipotle chili powder
Sea salt to taste

In a food processor, grind the almonds into a coarse meal, then put them into a large bowl. Process the sunflower seeds, shallots, and garlic together just until they are broken up, then add them to the almonds. Process the sun-dried tomatoes until they are well blended, and add them to the almond mixture too.

Stir into the bowl the bell peppers, celery, olive oil, and lemon juice, then fold in the parsley, thyme, and chipotle. Season the stuffing to taste with the salt. It should be crumbly yet moist.

Stuff your preferred selection of uncooked vegetables and serve.

ZUCCHINI MANICOTTI

G Gut

V Vegan

Serves: 2

Prep time: overnight plus 1 hour

This is a clean version of an Italian favorite. You'll be surprised it's cashew cheese and not ricotta! The dish is perfect for feeding a large group and a great summertime meal since it involves minimal cooking.

3 large zucchini (about 2 pounds)
2 to 3 tablespoons extra-virgin olive oil
Sea salt and freshly ground black pepper to taste
1 batch Cashew Cheese (page 97)
½ cup chopped fresh herbs, such as basil, thyme, parsley, and/or rosemary

For the Tomato Sauce
1 red bell pepper, seeded and quartered
4 Roma tomatoes, quartered
½ cup sun-dried tomatoes, soaked in 2 cups warm water for 30 minutes, then strained with
    the soaking liquid reserved
½ cup raw cashews
¼ cup raw hemp seeds
¼ cup extra-virgin olive oil
2 garlic cloves
1 tablespoon Italian seasoning
½ teaspoon sea salt

If you would like your manicotti warm, preheat the oven to 250°F.

First, prepare the tomato sauce. In a blender, purée all the sauce ingredients until the mixture is thick and creamy. Use some of the reserved sun-dried tomato soaking liquid to help achieve a sauce-like consistency. The sauce is best made the day you wish to make this dish, but it can be made 1 day in advance and stored in the fridge for up to four days.

Use a mandoline or a long, sharp knife to slice the zucchini lengthwise into ¼-inch-thick strips. Gently toss the strips in a large bowl with 2 tablespoons of the olive oil and a sprinkle of salt and pepper. Let them marinate for 5 minutes.

In a separate bowl, fold the fresh herbs into the prepared Cashew Cheese, then set the bowl aside.

To prepare the manicotti, lay 2 to 3 marinated zucchini strips on a work surface, slightly overlapping them lengthwise. Spread a generous amount of the cheese mixture along one end. Similar to sushi, roll the zucchini strips up until you form a "manicotti" roll. Continue until all the zucchini and cheese are used up.

Either divide the manicotti between two serving plates or, if you would like to bake them, set them in a baking dish. Top them with the tomato sauce and either serve them as is or bake them in the oven for 15 to 20 minutes before serving.

CLEAN SUSHI

Ⓒ Cleanse

Ⓥ Vegan*

Serves: 4

Prep time: 45 minutes

Cooking time: 30 minutes

Instead of plain white rice, this sushi is made with brown rice and other protein-packed grains. If you want to add sushi-grade fish (sashimi) or cooked salmon, feel free. The possibilities here are endless, limited only by your imagination. We've given you the basics so you can make it your own.

Note: You will need a bamboo mat to roll these sushi. Although bamboo mats aren't essential, they are traditional and really do help make your rolls even and symmetrical.

4 to 6 asparagus spears
1 broccoli crown, cut into small florets
1 large carrot, sliced into thin strips
Flesh of 2 ripe avocados, sliced
10 nori sheets
Prepared wasabi
Wheat-free tamari for dipping

For the Sushi Rice
¼ cup quinoa
¼ cup millet
¼ cup amaranth
¼ cup short-grain brown rice

For the Dressing
⅛ cup ume plum vinegar
2 teaspoons coconut nectar or raw honey (when not on cleanse)
Sea salt to taste

First, prepare the sushi rice. Combine the quinoa, millet, amaranth, and brown rice in a pot with 2 cups of water. Bring the pot to a boil, cover it, and lower the heat to simmer them for about 20 minutes. Check the liquid, as you may need to add approximately ¼ cup more water. Once the grains are cooked and most of the water is absorbed, set the pot aside and let it rest for 5 minutes.

While the grains cook, in a small bowl whisk together all the ingredients for the dressing. When the grains have cooled a bit, gently stir in the dressing and combine the mixture well. Transfer the dressed rice to a parchment-lined baking sheet and place it in the fridge for 15 minutes.

---

*Without any added fish; if using coconut nectar

In a pot of simmering, salted water, quickly blanch both the asparagus and the broccoli florets until they are just tender, 1 to 3 minutes, then submerge them in cold water to immediately stop the cooking. Set the vegetables aside.

To make the sushi rolls, lay a sheet of nori on a bamboo mat. Make sure the creases in the nori sheets are lined up in the same direction as the strips of bamboo in your mat—both running horizontally. With moistened hands to prevent any sticking, lightly spread ½ cup of the cooled rice-and-grain mixture over the bottom half of the nori sheet. The key is not to press the mixture very hard onto the nori sheet but to lay it lightly on top. Portion some asparagus, broccoli, carrot, and avocado in an even row across the middle of the layer of grains.

Starting from the bottom, roll the nori away from you into a roll, as tightly formed as possible. When you near the end, with your finger moisten the full length of the edge of the nori sheet with water, then complete the roll, sealing the nori to itself.

Once all the rolls are complete, cut each roll into 6 pieces and serve them with wasabi, tamari, and any other condiments you like.

MEDITERRANEAN RICE NOODLES

C Cleanse*

V Vegan

Serves: 2

Prep time: 20 minutes

Cooking time: 15 minutes

We love King Soba noodles on the Clean team and could easily find hundreds of uses for them. This is a delicious Mediterranean-flavored version of a noodle bowl, quick and easy, and perfect for those meals you need to have on the table as fast as possible.

1 package King Soba rice noodles
2 to 3 tablespoons extra-virgin olive oil
½ pound fresh green beans, ends snipped off
About 10 cherry tomatoes, halved
¼ cup pitted olives
8 to 10 fresh basil leaves, torn
Zest and juice of 1 lemon
1 to 2 teaspoons sea salt
Freshly ground black pepper

Cook the rice noodles according to the directions on the package, then run them under cold water, and drain them well. In a medium bowl, toss the noodles with the olive oil.

While the noodles are cooking, bring 4 cups of salted water to a boil. Have a bowl of ice water ready nearby. Blanch the green beans in the boiling water until they are tender and bright green, about 2 minutes, then remove them from the hot water and immediately submerge them in the ice water to stop the cooking. Drain them, and cut each bean into thirds.

Stir the beans, tomatoes, olives, basil, lemon zest, lemon juice, salt, and pepper into the bowl of noodles. Adjust the seasonings to taste, and serve.

*Replace tomatoes with other vegetables, like thinly sliced fennel bulb or sautéed summer squash

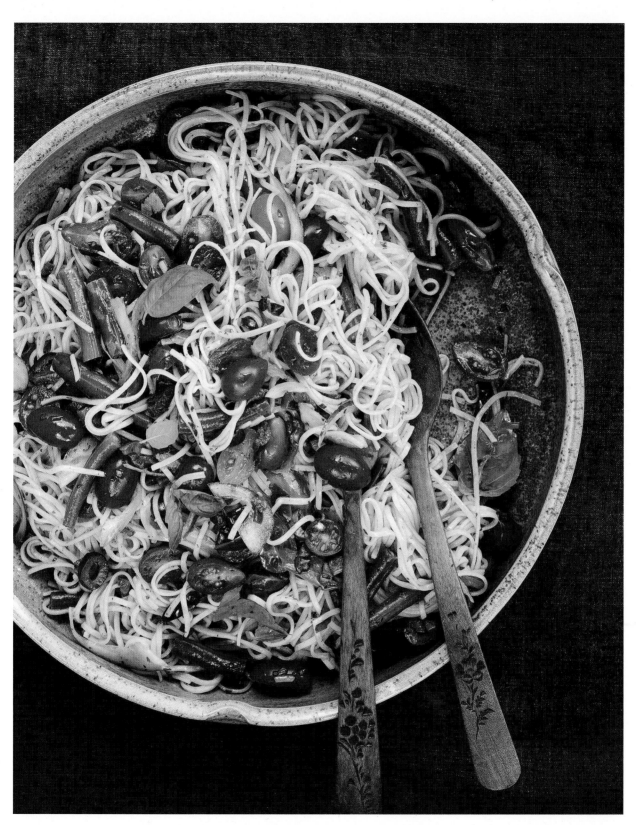

Mediterranean Rice Noodles, page 200

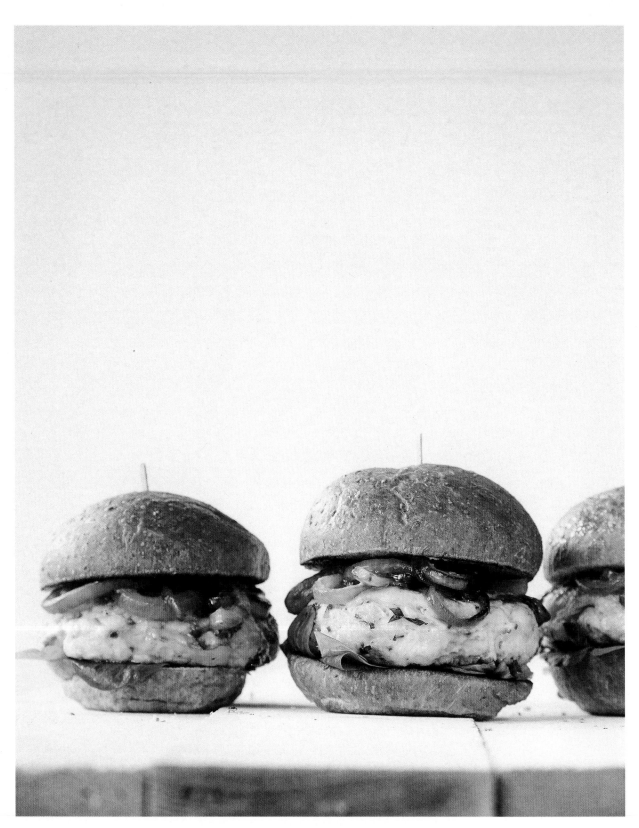

Lemon Herb Chicken Burgers with Thousand Island Dressing, page 156

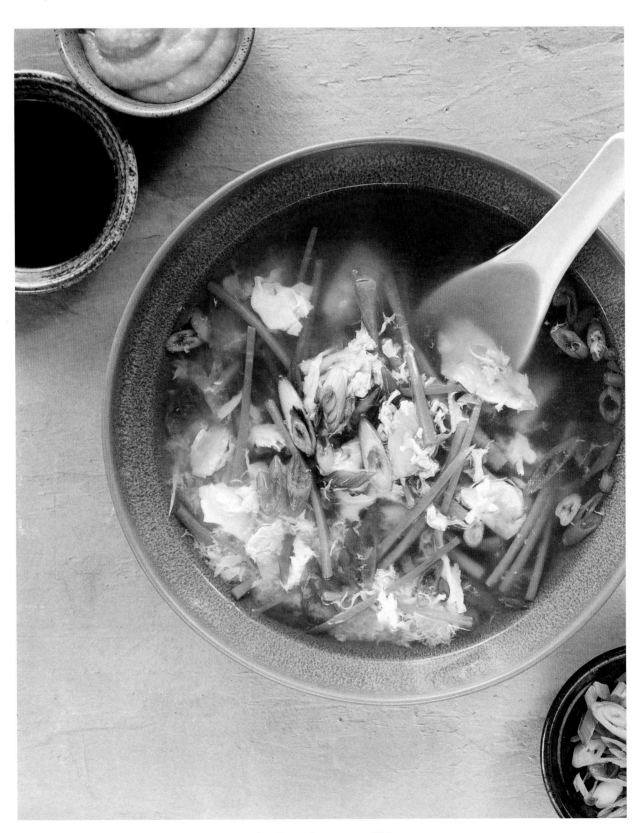

Egg Drop Soup, page 236

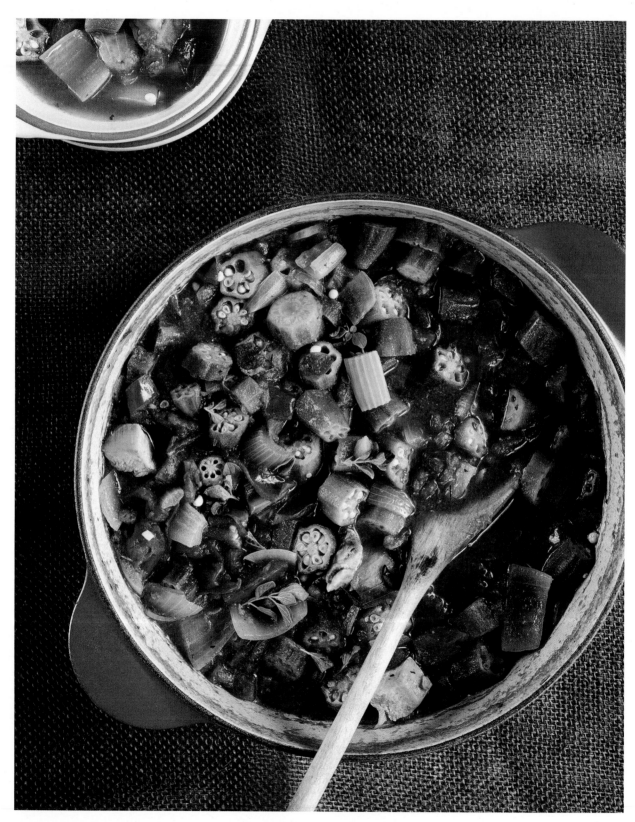

Maw Maw's Gumbo, page 238

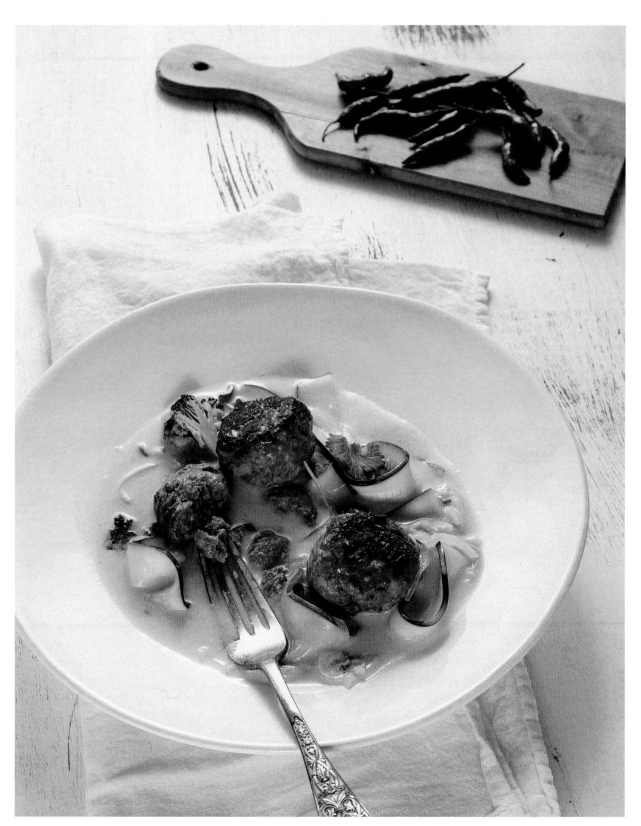

Coconut Zucchini Noodles and Spiced Meatballs, page 184

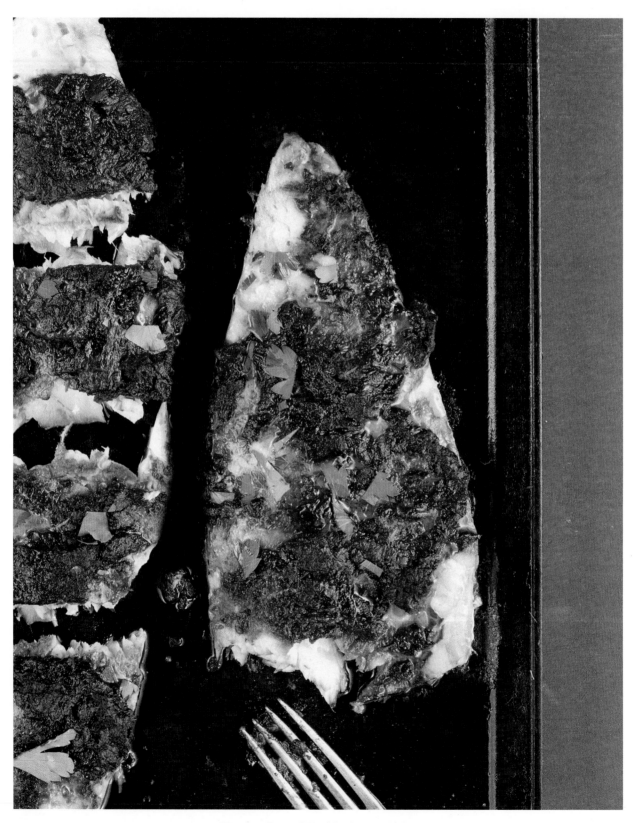

Harissa-Coated Haddock, page 151

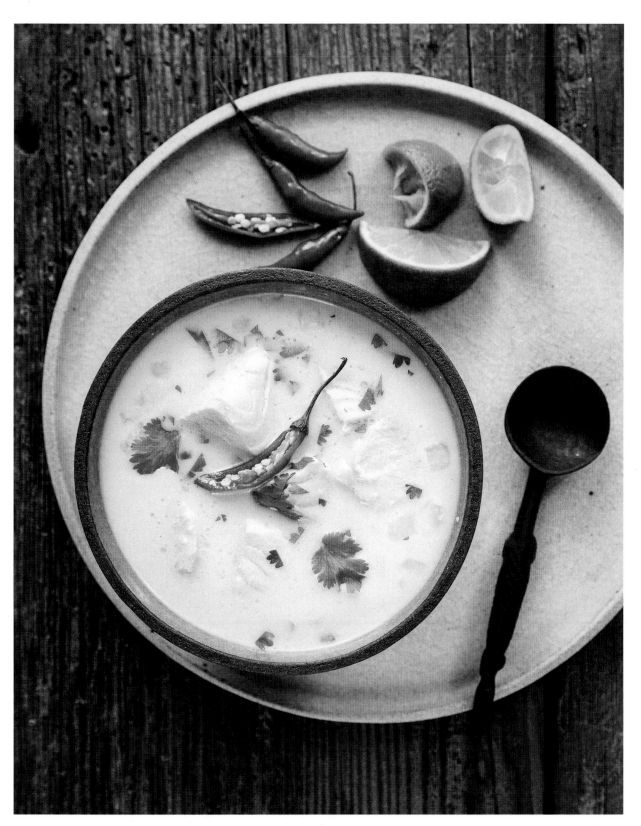

Coconut Fish Soup, page 143

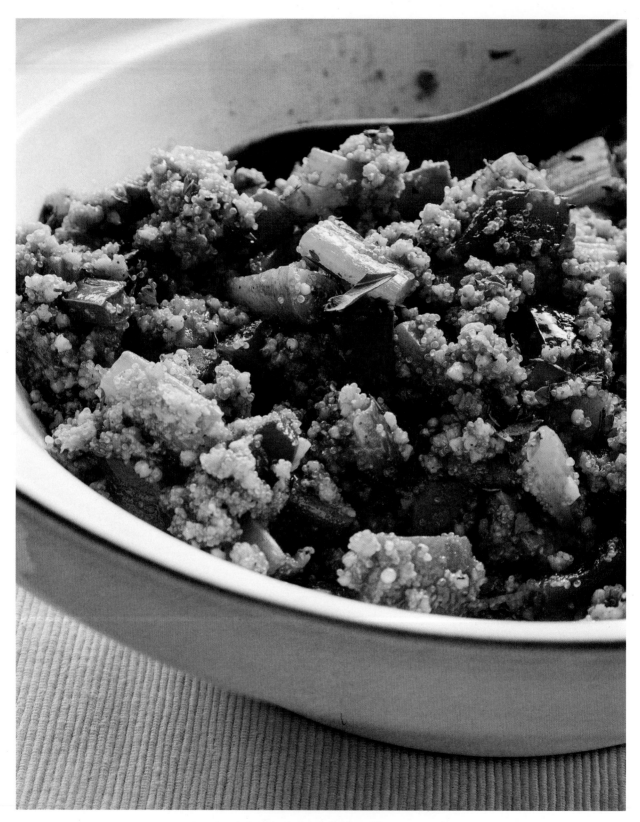

South-of-the-Border Vegetable Millet, page 201

SOUTH-OF-THE-BORDER VEGETABLE MILLET

C Cleanse*
V Vegan

Serves: 2
Prep time: 10 minutes
Cooking time: 30 minutes

Spicy and protein-packed, this is great on its own, but feel free to add chicken, serve it over dark, leafy greens, or put it in a wrap.

2 tablespoons coconut oil
1 medium onion, diced
½ cup small-diced carrot
1 celery stalk, diced small
1 cup cauliflower florets
½ cup chopped red or yellow bell pepper
1 garlic clove, minced
½ cup millet
½ cup amaranth
2 cups vegetable stock or water
1½ tablespoons Mexican seasoning
2 teaspoons sea salt
¼ cup roughly chopped fresh cilantro
Flesh of 1 ripe avocado, cut into chunks
1 red chili pepper, minced (optional)

Heat a medium-large Dutch oven (one that holds at least 8 cups) over medium-high heat. Add the coconut oil, then sauté the onion for 2 to 3 minutes, stirring occasionally. Once the onion is translucent, add the carrot, celery, cauliflower, bell pepper, and garlic. Continue to sauté for a few more minutes before adding the millet and amaranth. Stir the grains, allowing them to slightly toast in the pan. After 2 to 3 minutes, stir in the stock or water and the Mexican seasoning. Cover the pot, lower the heat to medium, and allow the mixture to cook on the stovetop for 12 to 15 minutes. Almost all the liquid should be absorbed, but if not, let it cook a few more minutes. When it's ready, turn off the heat and it let stand, covered, for 5 minutes.

Stir in the salt and divide the mixture between two serving bowls. Garnish each bowl with the cilantro leaves, avocado, and optional red chili.

Variations: For a cleanse-friendly version, omit the red chili pepper and replace the bell peppers with summer squash or zucchini.

*With the variation

GREEK QUINOA WITH HEARTS OF PALM

C Cleanse*
G Gut
V Vegan

Serves: 2
Prep time: 15 minutes
Cooking time: 20 minutes

We love our quinoa dishes since they are a great way to get quick and meatless protein. Hearts of palm and Kalamata olives give this a wonderful texture, and the whole thing has an incredible flavor. Plus, it fills you up without weighing you down.

1 cup quinoa
2 cups water
1 can (14 ounces) hearts of palm, drained, rinsed, and cut into ¼-inch-thick slices
½ cup diced red onion
1 large, ripe tomato, roughly chopped
½ cup chopped Kalamata olives
1 garlic clove, minced
2 tablespoons chopped fresh oregano
¼ cup extra-virgin olive oil
2 tablespoons red wine vinegar
2 to 3 teaspoons sea salt

In a medium pot, combine the quinoa and water. Cover and bring it to a boil, then lower the heat and simmer the quinoa for 15 minutes. Remove the pot from the heat and let it stand, covered, for an additional 5 minutes. Remove the lid and let the quinoa cool to room temperature.

In a large bowl, combine the hearts of palm, onion, tomato, olives, garlic, oregano, olive oil, vinegar, and salt. When the quinoa has cooled sufficiently, stir it into the vegetable mix and serve.

*Omit tomato

ROASTED CAULIFLOWER WITH PISTACHIO DRESSING

C Cleanse

G Gut

V Vegan

Serves: 2

Prep time: 10 minutes

Cooking time: 20 minutes

Roasted cauliflower is one dish that not everyone has tried, but once they do they'll be hooked for life. This dressing is also something you're going to want to make and have on hand all the time. It's likely to become one of your favorite salad dressings by far.

1 head cauliflower, cut into small florets (about 4 cups)
1 small red onion, sliced into ¼-inch-thick rounds
¼ cup extra-virgin olive oil
Pinch of sea salt
2 teaspoons curry powder

For the Dressing
½ cup raw pistachios
1½ tablespoons sherry vinegar
¼ cup loosely packed fresh cilantro leaves, plus additional for garnish
¼ cup extra-virgin olive oil
¼ cup water
Sea salt to taste

Preheat the oven to 375°F.

In a large bowl, toss the cauliflower and red onion with the olive oil, salt, and curry powder. Spread the mixture into a baking dish, and roast the vegetables for 15 to 20 minutes, or until the cauliflower is fork-tender and slightly browned.

While the cauliflower is cooking, heat a heavy-bottom skillet over medium-high heat. Add the pistachios and toast them in the dry pan, shaking the pan often, until the pistachios turn golden brown. Transfer the pistachios to a blender or a food processor, and add the vinegar, cilantro, olive oil, water, and salt. Pulse the mixture, leaving it still chunky, then pour it into a small serving bowl.

When the cauliflower is ready, remove it from the oven and transfer it to a serving dish. Garnish with cilantro. Personally, I like to dip the cauliflower into the sauce, but you can drizzle the sauce over it too, or toss everything together in a large bowl before serving.

CHILE RELLENOS STUFFED WITH MUSHROOMS, SWEET POTATOES, AND CHIPOTLE CASHEW CREMA

Mary Karlin, Clean community member

 Vegan   **Serves:** 4 to 8, depending on the size of the peppers

Clean and complementary flavors that shine are what I consider when creating ingredient components of a recipe. Seasonal and organic ingredients (whenever possible) provide the optimum nutrition and flavor. This is the basic criteria for my daily menus and for those I teach to others in my books and cooking classes.

Rather than fried, these are wonderful grilled for a smoky flavor. If you don't have a grill, bake them in an oven at 375°F for 30 minutes. You can substitute cooked red or tricolor quinoa for half or all of the potato if you prefer.

8 large poblano peppers
½ teaspoon sea salt, plus more for the sweet potatoes or yams
2 large sweet potatoes or yams, peeled, cooked, and mashed
1½ teaspoons achiote paste (or some kind of curry or chili paste, if you can't find achiote), crumbled
Zest of 1 lime
3 tablespoons extra-virgin olive oil, plus extra for brushing
1 small white onion, diced
4 garlic cloves, minced
½ pound shiitake mushrooms, stems removed, coarsely chopped
¼ cup mirin or dry white wine
¼ cup coarsely chopped fresh cilantro

For the Chipotle Cashew Crema
1 cup raw cashews or other nuts, soaked and drained
1 teaspoon nutritional yeast flakes
½ teaspoon chipotle chili powder (optional)
½ teaspoon sea salt
¼ cup water
¼ cup coconut or other nut milk

First, make the crema. In a blender, purée all the crema ingredients until smooth. Add up to ¼ cup more water, if you prefer a thinner consistency. The crema can be stored in the fridge up to one week.

To prep the peppers, cut a 3-inch-long slit down one side of each poblano to allow for stuffing. Remove the white part and most of the seeds, and lightly salt the inside. Repeat with all the peppers, and set them aside on a baking sheet.

In a large bowl, combine the mashed sweet potato, achiote paste, and lime zest. Season to taste with salt and set aside.

Heat 3 tablespoons of the olive oil in a large skillet set over medium heat. Sauté the onions until they are translucent, then add the garlic and mushrooms, and continue sautéing for 5 more minutes. Add the mirin or white wine, and continue to cook the mixture until the mushrooms are soft and the liquid has been absorbed. Remove the pan from the heat and stir in the cilantro.

Preheat the oven to 450°F. Alternately, preheat a stovetop cast-iron griddle pan, rib side up, or use an outdoor grill according to the manufacturer's instructions.

Using a spoon, fill each poblano pepper halfway (roughly ¼ cup or more for each pepper) with the sweet potato mixture. Follow this with a generous spoonful of the mushroom mixture, and push it down to pack the pepper well.

Return the stuffed peppers to the baking sheet and lightly brush each with olive oil for cooking in the oven, or place the peppers over direct heat on the prepared grill. Turn the peppers occasionally while cooking until the skins are blistered and slightly charred. If you're grilling them, move them to indirect heat to finish. Cook the peppers until they are soft, about 10 more minutes.

Transfer them to a platter to serve them while they are still hot. Serve 1 chile relleno per person, drizzled with the crema.

VINCENT ARPINO'S CLEAN BROOKLYN SICILIAN PIZZA PIE

Howie Greene, Clean community member

G Gut

Serves: approximately 2

Prep time: 15 minutes

Cooking time: 25 to 30 minutes

1½ cups almond flour
½ cup coconut flour
1 teaspoon baking soda
½ teaspoon sea salt
2 pasture-raised eggs
2 tablespoons extra-virgin olive oil, plus more for forming the crust
1 cup organic tomato purée or tomato sauce (I use Sclafani brand, but any brand with clean ingredients works, or make your own)
Fresh or dried basil and oregano leaves to taste
Daiya mozzarella vegan cheese, raw cheese (if not cleansing), or a homemade nut cheese
Optional additions: spinach, mushrooms, olives, onions, tomatoes, chicken sausage, anchovies, etc.

Preheat the oven to 425°F.

In a large bowl, combine the almond flour, coconut flour, baking soda, and salt. In a small bowl, beat the eggs, then fold them into the dry ingredients. Slowly add the olive oil and water. Knead the mixture with your hands, forming it into a big ball. Let it sit for 10 minutes.

Line a baking sheet with parchment paper and coat the paper lightly with either olive oil or coconut oil spray. Coat your hands with a little olive oil too. Using your hands, spread the dough on the parchment to form a rectangle about ¼-inch thick (don't use a rolling pin!). Bake it in the oven for 9 minutes.

Remove the pan from the oven and let it cool for 5 minutes. Then, holding the parchment paper with both hands, carefully slide it off the baking sheet. Line the baking sheet with an additional piece of parchment paper and, again carefully, flip the crust over onto the fresh sheet of parchment paper.

Using a soup ladle, spread the tomato sauce over the crust. Sprinkle the pizza with basil and oregano and dot it with your preference of cheese. Bake it for 3 minutes. Turn the pan around 180 degrees in the oven, to cook the crust evenly, and bake it for another 3 minutes.

Remove the pan from the oven and, if desired, add any additional ingredients. Drizzle the pizza with olive oil and return it to the oven for another 12 minutes.

Remove it from the oven, let it cool for 3 minutes, then slice it with a pizza cutter. Enjoy!

EXPERIENCE: The Clean program and Clean Gut diet have changed my life and the lives of so many others in my world. They have taught me how to improve my health and well-being, and given back to me years of lost energy and productivity. I look and feel years younger, and because of Clean, I've been able to pass on so many great ideas, lessons, and recipes to those around me. Thank you, Dr. Junger and the Clean team!

SUMMER SQUASH PUTTANESCA

Ⓖ Gut

Makes: 1 quart

Prep time: 10 minutes

Cooking time: 45 minutes

Puttanesca is traditionally a tangy and salty dish from Italy with a storied past and multiple theories about its name. We've cleaned up this dish a bit by avoiding any additional salt, relying on the already brined anchovies, capers, and Kalamata olives. It's still a very easy meal, especially if you have premade sauce. Make the sauce ahead of time and freeze it for this meal, or if you're using a high-quality premade sauce, simply warm it up and skip right to making the squash noodles.

2 large summer squash or zucchini (about 2 pounds total)
¼ cup extra-virgin olive oil
1 cup finely chopped onion
6 garlic cloves, minced
2 tablespoons tomato paste
48 ounces canned whole peeled tomatoes, broken up in your hands, juice reserved
1 cup tightly packed, pitted, and halved Kalamata olives
2 tablespoons capers
½ teaspoon dried basil
½ teaspoon red pepper flakes
2 tablespoons minced anchovy fillets (about 8 fillets)

Use a spiralizer or a peeler to slice the summer squash or zucchini into ¼-inch-thick "noodles." Set them aside.

Heat the olive oil in a large skillet set over medium-high heat. When the oil is hot, sauté the onions for 2 to 3 minutes, stirring occasionally until they become translucent. Add the garlic and cook, stirring frequently, until the mixture is fragrant. Stir in the tomato paste and continue to cook, stirring constantly, for another 2 minutes. Add the tomatoes with their juice, plus the olives, capers, basil, red pepper flakes, and optional anchovy fillets. Lower the heat to medium and simmer the sauce for 30 to 40 minutes, allowing it to reduce and thicken.

When the sauce is the consistency you want it, fold in the squash noodles and cook them until they are just warmed through. Serve immediately.

CONFETTI VEGETABLES WITH SPICY SAUCE

Ⓒ Cleanse

Ⓖ Gut

Ⓥ Vegan

Serves: 2

Prep time: 20 minutes

Cooking time: 10 to 15 minutes

This confetti is quick, fun, and tasty. Kids will love helping with this brightly colored meal and the pseudo-Thai peanut sauce.

1 tablespoon coconut oil
1 broccoli crown, cut into florets
2 teaspoons freshly grated ginger
3 cloves garlic, peeled and minced
3 medium carrots, peeled and julienned
2 summer squash, peeled and julienned
About 1 cup (¼ pound) snap peas, cut at an angle into thin strips
2 scallions, thinly sliced, for garnish
Fresh cilantro leaves for garnish

For the Sauce
½ cup unsalted almond butter
1 tablespoon freshly minced ginger
1 tablespoon miso (we generally use South River chickpea, but any brand is fine)
2 garlic cloves, minced
1 teaspoon chili powder, or to taste
2 teaspoons ground coriander
1¼ cups unsweetened coconut milk

First, make the sauce. In a blender, blend all the sauce ingredients until the mixture is smooth and creamy. Taste it and adjust the seasonings as desired. Set the sauce aside.

Heat a large wok or sauté pan over medium-high heat. Melt the coconut oil, then stir in the broccoli florets. Sauté them for a few minutes, then stir in the ginger and garlic. Cook the mixture until it's fragrant, then add the carrots, summer squash, and snap peas, continuing to cook until everything is warmed through.

Pour into the pan roughly half the sauce, gently tossing the mixture with a pair of tongs or two serving spoons. When the mixture is well coated, remove it from the heat and divide it between two serving plates. Garnish each plate with the scallions and cilantro leaves. Any excess sauce can be stored in the fridge for up to a week.

WILD RICE WITH MIDDLE EASTERN FLAVORS

Ⓒ Cleanse*

Ⓥ Vegan

Serves: 2

Prep time: 24 hours for soaking plus 10 minutes

Cooking time: 20 minutes

With crazy-delicious flavors and extra calcium in the sesame seeds, this is another protein-packed meal to fuel you up, while remaining light and versatile. Wild rice is easy to digest, as it's not technically a grain but a sea grass.

1 cup wild rice, soaked in 3 cups water for 24 hours, strained, and rinsed well
1 bunch flat-leaf parsley, roughly chopped, about ½ cup
2 shallots, sliced into thin rounds
1 teaspoon ground cumin
3 tablespoons raw sesame seeds
10 to 12 cherry tomatoes, halved
2 tablespoons lemon juice
¼ cup extra-virgin olive oil
Sea salt to taste

Place the freshly rinsed wild rice into a small pot, cover the rice with water (2 parts water to 1 part rice), and cook the rice until it is soft and fluffy. Remove the lid and allow the rice to cool to room temperature.

When the rice has cooled, combine it in a large bowl with the parsley, shallots, cumin, sesame seeds, tomatoes, lemon juice, and olive oil until everything is well coated. Season the dish with salt to taste, and serve it at room temperature.

*Omit tomatoes

CLEAN KITCHARI

C Cleanse

V Vegan

Serves: 4

Prep time: 15 minutes

Cooking time: 45 minutes

A traditional healing and cleansing dish in the ayurvedic tradition, this is wonderfully spiced and anti-inflammatory, and it boosts circulation. Feel free to use ghee (clarified butter) in place of, or along with, the coconut oil for a more traditional version.

3 tablespoons coconut oil
2 teaspoons yellow mustard seeds
2 teaspoons cumin seeds
2 teaspoons fennel seeds
1½ cups chana dahl beans (found in most ethnic sections of supermarkets)
6 or more cups water
1 large yellow onion, diced small
1 cup chopped carrots
1 cup brown basmati rice
1 teaspoon ground turmeric
2 teaspoons sea salt, or to taste
¼ cup chopped fresh cilantro

Heat 2 tablespoons of the coconut oil in a large pot set over medium-high heat. Add the mustard seeds, cumin seeds, and fennel seeds, and stir them continuously until they turn light brown and begin to pop. Add the chana dahl along with the water and bring the pot to a boil. Reduce the heat to medium, cover the pot, and simmer the mixture until the water is about halfway gone, about 15 minutes.

While the dahl cooks, in a separate pan heat the remaining 1 tablespoon of coconut oil and sauté the onion and carrots until they are tender, then add them to the pot of chana dahl along with the rice and turmeric. Stir to combine everything and continue to simmer the mixture until both the rice and dahl are tender, adding more water as needed. Keep simmering until all the water is absorbed and everything is cooked through. Add salt to taste, and sprinkle with chopped cilantro before serving.

VEGETABLE NAPOLEON

G Gut

V Vegan

Serves: 2

Prep time: 20 minutes

Cooking time: 30 minutes

This results in a lovely stack of vegetables. The dish is completely worth the effort it takes to prep, but turn it into a fun family event with kids who are old enough to wield a knife. The effort will become as beautiful as the finished stacks.

1 fennel bulb
1 medium onion
2 portobello mushrooms
1 large zucchini
1 medium eggplant (about 8 to 10 ounces)
1 large summer squash (up to 1 pound)
Extra-virgin olive oil, sea salt, and freshly ground black pepper to taste

For the Tomato Basil Vinaigrette
1 large ripe tomato
2 garlic cloves, minced
2 tablespoons minced shallot
2 tablespoons red wine vinegar
¼ cup torn fresh basil leaves
1 teaspoon chopped fresh oregano leaves
¼ cup extra-virgin olive oil
Pinch of sea salt

First, prepare all the vegetables. Cut the fennel and onion in half, keeping their cores intact, then cut both halves into wedges, leaving a section of the core in each wedge so the pieces stay together. Remove the stems of the portobellos and use a spoon to scoop away the gills. Cut the zucchini in half lengthwise, then slice it into ¼-inch-thick half-rounds. Slice the eggplant and summer squash into ¼- to ½-inch rounds.

Combine the vegetables in a baking dish or spread them on a baking sheet. Drizzle olive oil over all the vegetables and sprinkle them with salt and pepper. Allow them to marinate for 10 minutes.

Either grill the vegetables, roast them in a 350°F oven, or sauté them in a heavy-bottom skillet with coconut oil until they are tender.

While the vegetables cook, make the vinaigrette. Cut the tomato in half, then run it over a box grater until only the skin remains. Discard the skin. In a small bowl, combine the tomato with the minced garlic, shallot, basil, and oregano. In another small bowl, whisk the oil, vinegar, and salt together, then combine with the tomato mixture. Set the vinaigrette aside.

Build a tower on each serving plate, stacking the vegetables on top of each other. It may take some time to find pieces that stack, but it's like putting together a puzzle! Drizzle the vinaigrette over each stack before serving.

ROASTED VEGETABLES WITH SILKY HUMMUS

C Cleanse

V Vegan

Serves: 4

Prep time: 15 minutes

Cooking time: 30 to 40 minutes

This is a comforting and super simple mix. Just chop the vegetables, quickly flavor, and put them in the oven. Blending the sauce is just as easy, and the finished meal is satisfying and pleasing to the whole family. Adjust with the vegetables you have on hand during each season.

3 pounds root vegetables, such as beets, carrots, parsnips, and/or rutabaga, cut into large, even-size chunks
4 teaspoons sea salt
½ cup extra-virgin olive oil, plus additional for coating the vegetables
3 cups cooked chickpeas (2 15-ounce cans)
2 teaspoons ground cumin
2 to 3 garlic cloves
¼ cup tahini
3 tablespoons lemon juice
2 teaspoons sea salt
½ to ¾ cup water
¼ cup chopped fresh parsley

Preheat the oven to 350°F.

In a large bowl, toss the chopped root vegetables with 2 teaspoons of the salt and enough olive oil to coat everything. Place the vegetables on a baking sheet and roast them until they are lightly browned and tender, about 30 to 40 minutes.

While the vegetables are roasting, make the hummus. In a food processor, blend the chickpeas, cumin, and garlic until the chickpeas stick to the edge of the container. Use a spatula to scrape the sides clean.

Add the tahini, lemon juice, salt, and the ½ cup olive oil, then process again while drizzling in the water to achieve a thick, smooth consistency.

Transfer the hummus to the center of a large serving plate. When the vegetables have finished roasting, position them around the hummus. Garnish with parsley and serve.

ROASTED CABBAGE WITH CHIPOTLE AND CARAWAY SOUR CREAM

C Cleanse   **Serves:** 2

G Gut   **Prep time:** 15 minutes

V Vegan   **Cooking time:** 25 minutes

Cooked cabbage is easily digested and has many health benefits. It's really tasty roasted with a slightly spicy kick and a creamy sauce.

1 green cabbage (2 pounds or less)
2 tablespoons extra-virgin olive oil
Sea salt
½ teaspoon chipotle chili powder (optional)
Sour Cream (page 98)
1 teaspoon freshly ground caraway seeds

Preheat the oven to 400°F.

Peel away the outer leaves of the cabbage, then cut the head into wedges, doing your best to include the core in each wedge. Arrange the cabbage wedges on a lightly oiled baking sheet. Sprinkle each wedge with salt and a touch of chipotle powder if desired. Place them in the oven and roast them until their edges get crisp. Depending on the size and thickness of the cabbage, this may take 15 to 25 minutes.

Meanwhile, prepare the Sour Cream recipe with the addition of the caraway seeds. Place the sour cream in a small serving bowl and set it aside.

Remove the cabbage from the oven and transfer it to a serving platter. Dollop some of the cream over the cabbage or dip the cabbage into the bowl of sour cream as you eat it.

Chef Frank on Root Vegetables

I'm a big fan of root vegetables, not only because of their great taste but also because they're so versatile. You can roast them, mash them, purée them, or add them to soups. Because some roots can be on the sweet side, they work well in both sweet and savory items.

MEXICAN TOSTADAS

C Cleanse*

V Vegan

Serves: 4

Prep time: overnight

Cooking time: 1 hour

Although this recipe is a bit involved, the end results are well worth the effort. The Tomato Salsa, Sour Cream, and pinto beans can all be done in advance.

1 cup dry or 1 can (15-ounce) pinto beans
1 tablespoon apple cider vinegar (optional)
½ batch Tomato Salsa (page 124)
1 batch Sour Cream (page 98)
Up to ½ cup avocado oil (coconut oil will also work)
1 cup minced onions
1 teaspoon garlic powder
2 teaspoons ground cumin
1 teaspoon paprika
¼ teaspoon ground cinnamon
2 teaspoons sea salt
2 zucchini or summer squash, cut into thin rounds (1½ to 2 pounds)
4 brown rice tortillas
2 hearts of romaine lettuce, shredded (about 4 cups shredded)
Flesh of 2 to 3 ripe avocados, sliced

If you are using dried pinto beans, prepare them first. Soak them in 4 cups of water with 1 tablespoon of apple cider vinegar overnight (8 to 12 hours). Drain them, rinse them well, then cook them in another 4 cups of water until they are very tender, about 20 minutes. Drain them and set them aside.

Prepare the Salsa and Sour Cream recipes beforehand or make them while the beans cook.

Heat 2 to 3 tablespoons of the avocado oil in a large skillet set over medium heat. Add the onions and sauté them until they are translucent, about 3 to 4 minutes. Stir in the cooked beans along with the garlic powder, cumin, paprika, cinnamon, and salt, plus ¼ cup water. Stir well to combine everything. Once the mixture is heated through, use a potato masher to mash up the beans. I like them to have a bit of texture, but make them as smooth as you wish. Continue stirring to keep them from burning, then set them aside and keep them warm, in the oven or on top of the stove.

In a medium skillet, sauté the zucchini or summer squash in the remaining 1 to 2 tablespoons of avocado oil until they are lightly browned and tender. Set them aside.

Crisp the corn tortillas in either a preheated 400°F oven or in a skillet with a little coconut oil.

Place a crisp tortilla on each serving plate, then spread it with a quarter or so of the refried beans. Top it with some of the shredded romaine, a few slices of avocado, some sautéed zucchini or summer squash, and a few dollops of the salsa. Drizzle each tostada with the sour cream and serve.

*Omit salsa

BAKED SPAGHETTI SQUASH WITH AUTUMN PESTO

C Cleanse

G Gut

V Vegan

Serves: 2

Prep time: 15 minutes

Cooking time: 45 minutes to 1 hour

This is a quintessential autumn dish. As the weather gets colder, the squash get sweeter and we look for ways to use the last of the dark, leafy-green harvest. This yummy meal combines the two perfectly.

1 spaghetti squash
1 cup raw pumpkin seeds
2 to 3 cups fresh spinach (1 large handful)
3 garlic cloves
½ teaspoon sea salt
¼ cup pumpkin seed oil or extra-virgin olive oil

Preheat the oven to 350°F.

Place the spaghetti squash in a baking dish and cook it in the oven until it's tender, roughly 45 minutes to 1 hour.

While the squash cooks, dry-roast the pumpkin seeds (or you can use them raw, if you wish). Place the pumpkin seeds into a dry, heavy-bottom sauté pan set over medium-high heat. Allow the seeds to warm and gently roast. Once you can smell pumpkin seeds in the air, lower the heat and gradually stir them to allow for even roasting. Some of the seeds will pop a bit like popcorn; that means you're close to done.

Continue until the seeds are golden brown, being careful not to burn them, then place them into a bowl and allow them to cool to room temperature.

Once the nuts have cooled, make the pesto. I make this in a mortar and pestle, but feel free to use a food processor or blender. Process the pumpkin seeds, spinach, garlic, and salt together until the mixture forms a chunky paste. Then drizzle in the pumpkin seed oil or olive oil until the mixture becomes spreadable. Set the pesto aside.

When the squash is tender, remove it from the oven and allow it to cool enough so you can handle it with your bare hands. Cut the squash in half and remove the seeds. Scoop out the noodle-like flesh and place it in a large bowl. Stir in some pesto, enough to coat all the squash evenly. Season it with more salt to taste, and serve.

BAKED TURNIP CASSEROLE WITH WALNUT SAGE CREAM

C Cleanse

G Gut

V Vegan

Serves: 4, as a side

Prep time: 15 minutes

Cooking time: 45 minutes to 1 1 hour

This dish is a delicious way to serve an often underused root vegetable. It's perfect for fall or winter with a side of roasted chicken, or on its own—a healthy comfort food.

1½ pounds turnips, peeled, ends removed
1 tablespoon coconut oil
1 medium onion, thinly sliced
2 tablespoons (3 to 4 cloves) minced garlic
1 bunch kale, stems removed, leaves roughly chopped

For the Walnut Sage Cream
2 cups walnuts, roasted
3 tablespoons apple cider vinegar
¼ cup extra-virgin olive oil
½ cup water
2 teaspoons sea salt
¼ teaspoon freshly ground black pepper
4 fresh sage leaves

Preheat the oven to 325°F.

Using a mandoline or a sharp knife, slice the turnips into thin rounds. If a turnip is large, cut each slice in half so all the slices are roughly the same size. Set them aside.

Heat the coconut oil in a sauté pan set over medium-high heat. Sauté the onion for 3 to 4 minutes, stirring occasionally, then add the garlic and continue sautéing until the mixture is fragrant. Add the kale, about 2 tablespoons of water, and a pinch of salt, stirring everything quickly until the kale is wilted. Set the vegetables aside.

To make the walnut sage cream, in a blender purée the walnuts, vinegar, olive oil, water, salt, and pepper until the mixture reaches a smooth and creamy consistency. Add the sage, blending it until it is just incorporated. Set the cream aside.

In either a 6 × 6-inch casserole pan or a 6-inch cast-iron pan, spread 2 tablespoons of the walnut sage cream over the bottom. Top the cream with a thin layer of turnips. Spread another layer of 2 to 3 tablespoons of cream. Top with a layer of about ¼ cup of the kale mixture. Repeat the alternating layers until you reach the top of the pan, or until you use up your ingredients, ending with a layer of the walnut sage cream.

Bake the casserole for 45 minutes to 1 hour, until the turnips easily slice with a knife. Serve immediately.

SAVORY LENTIL LOAF

Ⓒ Cleanse*
Ⓥ Vegan

Serves: 4
Prep time: 30 minutes
Cooking time: 1 hour

This hearty dish will satisfy all your friends and family who tend to want meat at every meal. You can plan ahead and prepare this the day before you want to serve it. You can place the mixture into a parchment-lined loaf pan and keep it in the fridge for up to two days until you're ready to bake it.

1 cup brown or wild rice
1 cup green lentils
Up to ¼ cup avocado oil
1 small onion, diced small
2 celery stalks, diced small
1 medium carrot, diced small
1 cup small-diced mushrooms
½ cup chopped fresh herbs, such as parsley, rosemary, chives, sage, and/or thyme
1 tablespoon sea salt, or to taste
Freshly ground black pepper to taste
¼ cup ground chia seeds
¼ cup nutritional yeast
Tomato or barbecue sauce of your choice

Place the rice in a small saucepan, and add 2 cups of water. Cover the pan, bring it to a boil, then lower the heat and simmer it for about 12 to 15 minutes, or until just about all the water has been absorbed. Remove it from heat and allow it to stand covered for an additional 10 minutes. Spread the rice into a baking dish to cool it.

Place the lentils in a small saucepan with 2½ cups of water. Cover the pan and bring the mixture to a boil, then lower the heat and simmer it until the lentils are tender, 15 to 20 minutes. Drain off any excess water, then allow the lentils to cool, uncovered, to room temperature.

While the lentils and rice are cooking, prepare your vegetables. Heat the oil in a large sauté pan set over medium-high heat. Sauté the onion, celery, carrot, and mushrooms until they are tender. If your pan is not large enough, you may need to do this in batches. When all the vegetables are cooked, allow them to cool to room temperature too.

Preheat the oven to 350°F.

In a food processor, place 1 heaping cup each of the cooked lentils, rice, and vegetables. Blend them until the mixture begins to form a ball and gets sticky. Use a rubber spatula to scrape down the sides while processing.

*Omit tomato or barbecue sauce

Place the processed mixture into a large bowl and add all the remaining cooked lentils, rice, and vegetables, plus stir in the fresh herbs, salt, pepper, chia seeds, and nutritional yeast. You may need to use your hands for this part. Once the mixture is evenly incorporated, taste and adjust the seasonings.

Scoop the mixture into a lightly oiled baking dish and use your hands to form it into a loaf about 2½ inches in height. Drizzle tomato or barbeque sauce over the top of the loaf, then bake it for 30 minutes. The outside should have a slight crunch to it.

Remove it from the oven and serve immediately.

MUSHROOM RISOTTO

Ⓒ Cleanse

Ⓥ Vegan*

Serves: 2

Prep time: 10 minutes

Cooking time: 30 to 45 minutes

Creamy and comforting, this classic buttery dish is well worth the time it takes to make. Standing over a warm pot stirring it frequently is incredibly meditative and a great chance to have a conversation with a loved one or catch up on an informative or soul-nurturing podcast.

2 tablespoons avocado oil, plus extra for the mushrooms
½ cup minced onion
2 garlic cloves
1 cup short-grain brown rice
4 ounces red wine
Up to 1 quart vegetable stock or water kept warm in a small pan on the stove
4 cups (about ½ pound) chopped fresh mushrooms (any variety you prefer), cut into
    bite-size pieces
1 to 2 tablespoons nutritional yeast
1 sprig fresh rosemary, finely chopped
Sea salt to taste
2 teaspoons olive oil or 1 teaspoon truffle oil (if you're not opposed to dairy, try butter from
    grass-fed cows, like a traditional risotto)

Melt 2 tablespoons of the avocado oil in a 2-quart saucepan set over medium-high heat. Sauté the onion and garlic until they are translucent, about 2 minutes, then reduce the heat to medium and stir in the rice. Sauté the mixture for an additional 2 minutes. This toasts the rice and gives it a wonderful nutty flavor.

Pour in the red wine and allow it to reduce by half before adding 1½ cups of the stock. Stir the mixture often and allow the rice to absorb most of the liquid before adding more. Continue cooking and stirring the rice, adding the liquid in ½-cup increments and remembering to stir often.

While the rice cooks, prepare the mushrooms. In a medium skillet set over medium-high heat, sauté the mushrooms in avocado oil until they are lightly browned. Set them aside.

When the rice feels just about fully cooked, at this point, the mixture should be thick and creamy. Stir in the sautéed mushrooms, nutritional yeast, rosemary, and salt. Finish with the olive or truffle oil, and serve immediately.

*Omit butter

PORTOBELLO STEAKS WITH MASHED CELERY ROOT

C Cleanse

G Gut

V Vegan

Serves: 2

Prep time: overnight plus 15 minutes on serving day

Cooking time: 1 hour

These are earthy, hearty, and an elegant medley of flavors that please not just vegetarians who want something more "meaty" for their meal, but meat-lovers as well. A definite crowd-pleaser.

½ batch Rosemary Mustard Marinade (page 94)
2 large portobello mushrooms

For the Mashed Celery Root
2 pounds celery root
2 tablespoons prepared horseradish
3 tablespoons coconut butter
2 teaspoons sea salt
¼ to ½ cup unsweetened almond milk
2 scallions, thinly sliced

Preheat the oven to 350°F.

Overnight, or several hours in advance, make the marinade and set it aside.

Remove the stems from the mushrooms, then use a fork to remove the gills. Do so by gently scraping in the direction of the gills about ⅛-inch deep. Set the mushrooms top side down in a baking dish and pour the marinade over them. Let them sit for at least 20 minutes or up to 8 hours.

While the mushrooms marinate, place the whole celery root into a glass baking dish with about ¼ inch of water in the bottom. Cover the dish with tinfoil and roast the root in the oven for 45 minutes to 1 hour. Remove the tinfoil and allow the root to cool until you can handle it with your hands.

Use a knife to peel away the celery root skin, then roughly chop the root and place the pieces into a food processor. Purée the root with the horseradish and coconut butter, and add enough almond milk for the mixture to reach a mashed potato–like texture and consistency. Season with sea salt then fold in the chopped scallions. Set aside and keep warm.

Place the mushrooms onto a baking dish and cook in the oven until tender, about 10 to 12 minutes.

Slice the mushrooms then set them on top of mounds of the celery root mash. Enjoy with garlicky greens or roasted asparagus.

MINTED PEA AND ASPARAGUS RISOTTO

Ⓒ Cleanse

Ⓥ Vegan*

Serves: 2

Prep time: 10 minutes

Cooking time: 30 minutes

This spring-themed dish works perfectly as an entrée or as a side dish. The trick with any risotto is to stir often to allow the rice to cream up once it's done cooking. This is certainly a dish that requires a lot of love and attention, but your efforts will be well-received.

1 tablespoon coconut oil
½ cup small diced onion
1 cup short grain brown rice
8 ounces organic Chardonnay
About 32 ounces chicken or vegetable stock
½ cup (about 4 to 5 stalks) asparagus, cut into ½ inch pieces
½ cup frozen (thawed) or fresh shucked peas
½ teaspoon smoked sea salt
2 teaspoons sea salt
½ teaspoon fresh black pepper
2 teaspoon fresh chopped mint
2 to 3 tablespoons coconut butter

Heat a 2-quart sauce pot over medium-high heat. Melt the coconut oil, then add the onion, cook until translucent, about 2 minutes. Reduce the heat to medium, stir in the rice and cook for an additional 2 minutes. This toasts the rice and gives it a wonderful nutty flavor. Pour in the white wine and allow it to reduce by half before adding 12 ounces of stock. Stir often and allow the rice to absorb most of the liquid before adding more. Continue cooking the rice, adding the liquid in 4-ounce increments and remembering to stir often.

When the rice feels just about fully cooked add the asparagus and continue to cook. At this point the rice should be thick and creamy. Add the peas, stir to combine, and heat through. Season with the salts, black pepper, and stir in the mint and coconut butter. Serve immediately.

*Use vegetable stock

SOUPS AND STEWS

We love soups and stews because they are warming and easily digestible. They are great meal options for all of our Clean programs and work well as an entrée, side, or quick snack. We've included stocks, gazpachos, gumbos, and more, all Clean-approved and waiting for your own personal touch. As Chef Franky says, "Don't be afraid to use what you have on hand and experiment with textures and spices." We give you permission to do the same. Have fun.

CHICKEN STOCK

C Cleanse

G Gut

Makes: 1 gallon

Prep time: 15 minutes

Cooking time: 3 to 4 hours

A wonderful healing base for a myriad of recipes, chicken stock is always good to have, fresh or frozen, on hand at all times.

1 whole pasture-raised chicken or chicken carcass
2 cups roughly chopped onions
1 cup chopped carrots
1 cup chopped celery
1 splash apple cider vinegar
2 bay leaves
1 tablespoon whole black peppercorns
2 garlic cloves, chopped
2 teaspoons dried thyme
Up to 4 cups vegetable scraps, such as leek tops, parsley stems, carrot ends, onion peels
Water, enough to cover everything

Place all the ingredients into a heavy-bottom stockpot. Include enough cold water to cover the contents of the pot by about 1 inch. Bring the mixture to just under a boil, then lower the heat and simmer it for 3 to 4 hours. While it's simmering, skim off any discolored foam that rises to the top.

If you are using a whole chicken, remove it from the pot after about 1 hour and pick all the meat off the bones. Set aside the meat for soups or other desired recipes.

When the stock is ready, carefully strain it through cheesecloth or a fine-mesh strainer. Cool it as quickly as possible, and store it in the fridge until needed. Any leftover stock can be frozen for future use, but it's best used within three months.

Dr. Junger on Healing Bone Broth

My team and I see many digestive disorders in a wide variety of people. Bone broths (made from marrow bones of pasture-raised animals and wild-caught fish) can be a wonderful digestive tonic. They help nourish and support the repair of the digestive tract. Plus, they contain glycine, an amino acid necessary for working with and balancing out methionine (an amino acid) found in muscle meat. Bone broths are also a great way to get your money's worth from your food purchases and stock your freezer with bases for soups all year long.

VEGETABLE STOCK

C Cleanse   **Makes:** 3 to 4 quarts

G Gut   **Prep time:** 10 minutes

V Vegan   **Cooking time:** 30 minutes to 1 hour

This stock is a versatile liquid that can be used in many recipes. An easy and sustainable method of making it is to save your vegetable scraps in the freezer until you have enough to make a pot of stock. But avoid using any brassicas, such as cabbage, turnips, Brussels sprouts, broccoli, and cauliflower, because they will turn the stock bitter.

2 tablespoons avocado oil
2 medium onions, roughly chopped (peels are fine, if organic)
2 large carrots, roughly chopped
6 celery stalks, roughly chopped
1 whole bulb garlic, roughly chopped (peels are fine to include, if organic)
2 bay leaves
1 strip kelp
10 whole black peppercorns
4 cups vegetable and herb scraps, such as parsley, thyme, and mushroom stems
1 gallon water

Heat the avocado oil in a large pot set over medium-high heat. Sauté the onions, carrots, and celery for about 3 to 4 minutes. Stir the vegetables occasionally and allow them to brown slightly. This will enhance the overall flavor of the stock. Add the garlic, and cook it until it's aromatic, then add the bay leaves, kelp, peppercorns, vegetable scraps, and water. Bring the mixture to a boil, then lower the heat and simmer it for 30 minutes to 1 hour. The longer it simmers, the more flavorful it will be.

Strain the stock through cheesecloth or a fine-mesh sieve, then store it in the fridge in air-tight containers for up to four days. Any leftover stock can be frozen for future use for up to three months.

MUSHROOM STOCK

Ⓒ Cleanse

Ⓖ Gut

Ⓥ Vegan

Makes: ½ gallon

Prep time: 15 minutes

Cooking time: 1 hour and 30 minutes

With a deep earthy taste, this recipe is a perfect base for savory soups and sauces. Choose wild mushrooms that have healing properties and immune-boosting benefits for a truly medicinal stock you can use all year long.

2 to 3 tablespoons avocado oil
1 pound mushrooms, such as portobello, shiitake, button, and/or crimini, thickly sliced
½ to 2 cups mushroom stems
½ ounce dried mushrooms
1 large leek, including green top, roughly chopped
4 garlic cloves, chopped
2 bay leaves
2 teaspoons dried thyme
1 tablespoon dried sage
1½ cups dry white wine
1 gallon water

Heat the avocado oil in a large pot set over medium-high heat. Sauté the mushrooms, mushroom stems, and dried mushrooms for about 4 minutes, stirring often, until they are lightly browned. Add the leek and garlic, and continue to sauté for 3 to 4 more minutes. Stir in the bay leaf, thyme, and sage, then deglaze the pan with the white wine. Simmer to reduce the liquid by half, then pour in the water. Bring the mixture to a boil, and reduce the heat to medium. Simmer the mixture for 1 hour and 30 minutes or until the liquid is again reduced by half. Strain the stock through cheesecloth or a fine-mesh strainer. Cool it, and use it within three days, or freeze any leftover stock for future use for up to three months.

MINESTRONE

V Vegan

Makes: about 1 gallon

Prep time: 15 minutes

Cooking time: 45 minutes

This is a classic and an easy way to pull together a meal when soup is wanted and vegetables abound.

2 tablespoons extra-virgin olive oil
1 medium red onion, chopped
2 medium carrots, peeled and diced
1 large celery stalk, diced
3 garlic cloves, minced
1 14.5-ounce can whole peeled tomatoes, crushed by hand or lightly chopped in a food processor
8 cups water
2 cups sliced green cabbage
1 15-ounce can cannellini beans, rinsed and drained
½ pound green beans, trimmed and cut into 1-inch pieces
¼ cup torn basil leaves
1 teaspoon chopped fresh rosemary
Sea salt and freshly ground black pepper to taste

Heat the olive oil in a large pot set over medium heat. Sauté the onion, carrots, and celery until they are tender, about 4 to 5 minutes. Add the garlic, stir to combine, and sauté for an additional 1 to 2 minutes. Pour in the tomatoes and bring the mixture to a boil, allowing the liquid to reduce slightly before adding the water and cabbage. Again bring the mixture to a boil, then lower the heat, and let it simmer for 20 minutes before adding the cannellini and green beans. Simmer for an additional 10 minutes, then fold in the fresh basil and rosemary and season the soup with salt and pepper.

ONION SOUP

C Cleanse

G Gut

V Vegan*

Serves: 4

Prep time: 10 minutes

Cooking time: 1 hour

Absolutely delicious, this is a slight twist on a traditional French soup, and we promise you won't even notice the missing hunk of bread or cheese.

2 tablespoons avocado oil

2 pounds yellow onions, thinly sliced

2 cups thinly sliced leeks

4 garlic cloves, sliced

8 ounces dry white wine

2 bay leaves

1 strip kelp

1 teaspoon wild mushroom powder or 1 ounce ground dried mushrooms

1 tablespoon dried thyme

8 cups water or chicken, beef, or vegetable stock

2 teaspoons sea salt, or chickpea miso to taste (South River brand is good)

Heat the avocado oil in a large pot set over medium-high heat. Sauté the onions, leeks, and garlic, stirring occasionally, until the onions are very soft and caramelized, about 20 minutes. Add the white wine, bay leaves, kelp, mushrooms, and dried thyme, and simmer to reduce the liquid by half. Pour in the water or stock of choice, partially cover the pot, and bring the mixture to a simmer. Cook for about 30 more minutes. Taste the soup and season with the salt or miso before serving.

*Use water or vegetable stock

HEARTY WINTER SOUP

Susana Belen, founder, We Care Spa

C Cleanse

G Gut*

V Vegan

This warming soup contains loads of vegetable protein and fiber. The carbohydrates included here are slowly released into the blood, making you feel full. The nut butter adds omega-3 fats and a great taste. I've included lots of different veggies and spices, so play around with the ones you prefer. I like to make large amounts and store it in the refrigerator or freezer.

1 cup lentils, split peas, or chickpeas
Chopped or shredded veggies: onions, garlic, celery, zucchini, squash, radishes, beets, carrots
Basil, oregano, ginger
Finely chopped leafy greens: choose from Swiss chard, collard greens, kale, bok choy, and
    spinach
Herbs and spices to flavor: cumin, rosemary, saffron, coriander, turmeric, sea salt or
    Himalayan salt
Organic raw tahini or nut butter

Soak 1 cup of lentils, split peas, or chickpeas for a couple of hours. If you use beans (black, pinto, black-eyed peas, etc.), soak them overnight. Rinse and cook in fresh water until well done.

In a separate pot with 2 cups of water, add chopped or shredded veggies and basil, oregano, and ginger to flavor. Cook and then blend veggie mixture in a Vitamix or blender. Add blended veggies to the bean soup. This makes soup for several meals. Divide into portion size and refrigerate or freeze.

At the time of serving, add finely chopped leafy greens to the cooked soup and cook for 3 to 4 minutes.

Then add healthy herbs and spices to flavor and 1 tablespoon of nut butter per cup to thicken.

*Omit beans; use lentils or split peas

MUSHROOM PARSNIP STEW

Ⓒ Cleanse

Ⓖ Gut

Ⓥ Vegan

Serves: 4 to 6

Prep time: 15 minutes

Cooking time: 1 hour

Earthy mushrooms and sweet parsnips pair so well in this lovely stew. It's easy to make year-round, especially fall through spring when parsnips are easily accessible to most people in their local markets.

2 to 3 tablespoons avocado oil
6 cups sliced fresh mushrooms (any variety you love)
2 cups chopped onion
1 cup chopped celery
2 large parsnips, cut into small chunks (about 4 cups)
3 garlic cloves
½ gallon Mushroom Stock (page 227)
1 bay leaf
1 strip dried kelp
3 tablespoons kudzu root powder
6 tablespoons water
¼ cup wheat-free tamari
1 to 2 teaspoons sea salt
1 tablespoon chopped fresh thyme
¼ cup chopped fresh parsley

Heat the avocado oil in a large pot set over medium-high heat. Sauté the mushrooms, stirring occasionally until they brown, about 4 to 5 minutes. Stir in the onion, celery, parsnips, and garlic, and sauté another 4 to 5 minutes. Pour in the mushroom stock and add the bay leaf and kelp. Bring the mixture to a boil, then lower the heat, partially cover the pot, and gently simmer for about 45 minutes.

Dilute the kudzu powder in the water, then stir it into the soup. Raise the heat a bit to bring the liquid to a boil. Once the soup begins to thicken, add the tamari and salt. Stir in fresh thyme and parsley before serving.

CARROT, CUMIN, AND CAULIFLOWER SOUP

C Cleanse

G Gut

V Vegan

Serves: 4

Prep time: 10 minutes

Cooking time: 20 minutes

Healthy for the skin, carrots blend perfectly with healthy-for-the-heart cauliflower. Cumin is a subtle spice with a lovely nutty flavor, and it has been shown to have health benefits of its own.

2 tablespoons coconut oil
1 medium red onion, chopped
2 garlic cloves, minced
2 teaspoons ground ginger
2 teaspoons freshly ground cumin seeds
1 teaspoon freshly ground coriander seeds
1 teaspoon freshly ground fennel seeds
1 pound carrots, chopped (about 4 cups)
2 cups chopped cauliflower
5 to 6 cups water
1 bay leaf
2 to 3 teaspoons sea salt
¼ cup coconut butter
¼ cup raw or roasted pumpkin seeds
2 to 3 tablespoons chopped fresh parsley

Melt the coconut oil in a large pot set over medium-high heat. Sauté the onion until it is translucent, about 3 to 4 minutes. Stir in the garlic and ginger followed by the cumin seeds, coriander seeds, and fennel seeds. Cook until the mixture is very fragrant, then add the carrots and cauliflower. Pour in the water and add the bay leaf. Partially cover the pot, bring the soup to a boil, then lower the heat to medium and let it simmer for 15 to 20 minutes before seasoning it with the salt.

Before serving, pour half the soup into a blender and purée it with the coconut butter until the mixture is creamy. Then stir it back into the pot.

Garnish each serving of soup with pumpkin seeds and fresh parsley.

Variations: For a heartier (and cleanse-friendly) version, add 1 cup cooked chickpeas in the last 10 minutes of simmering.

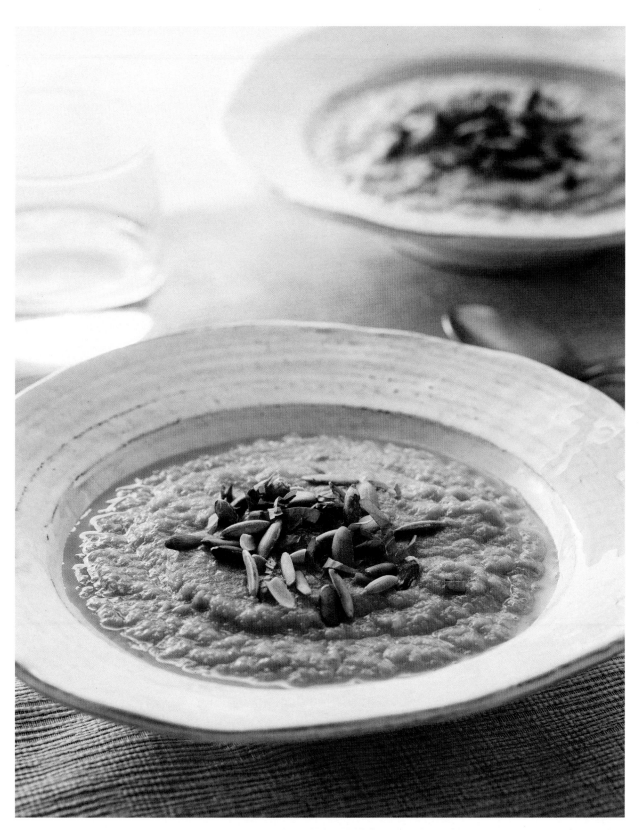

Carrot, Cumin, and Cauliflower Soup, page 232

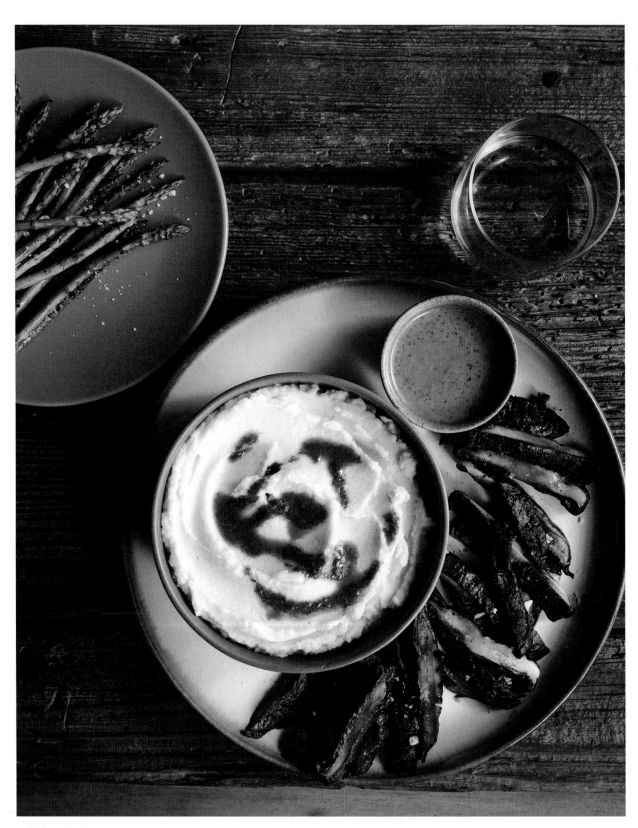

Portobello Steaks with Mashed Celery Root, page 221

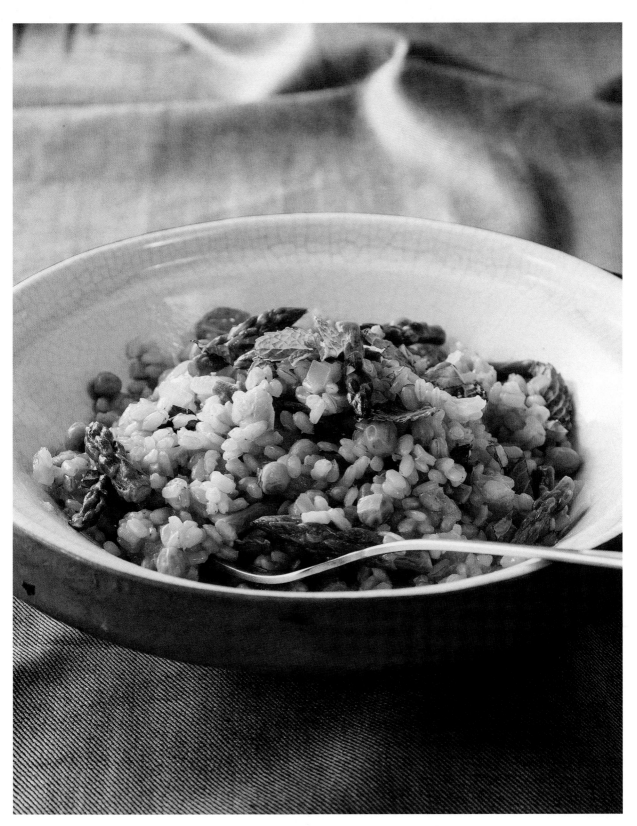

Minted Pea and Asparagus Risotto, page 222

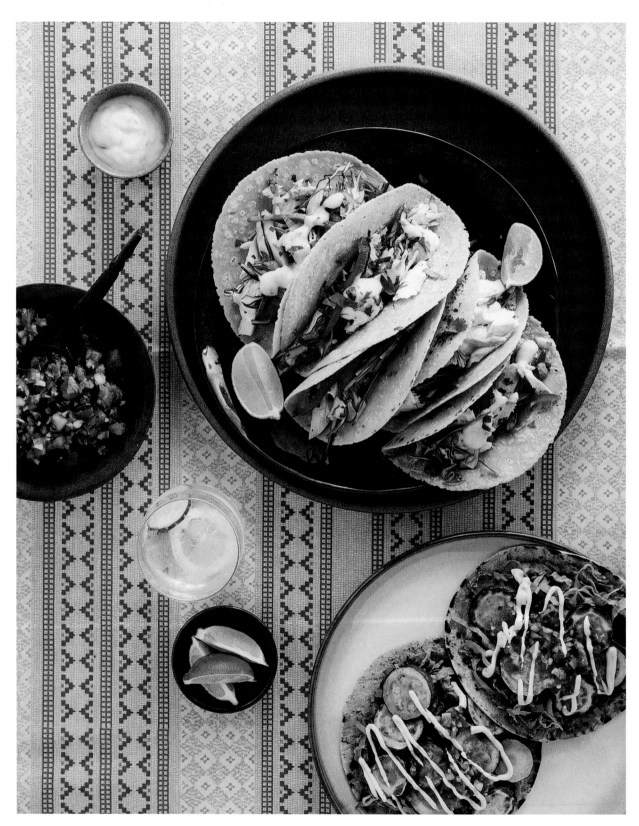

Fish Tacos and Mexican Tostadas, pages 148 and 215

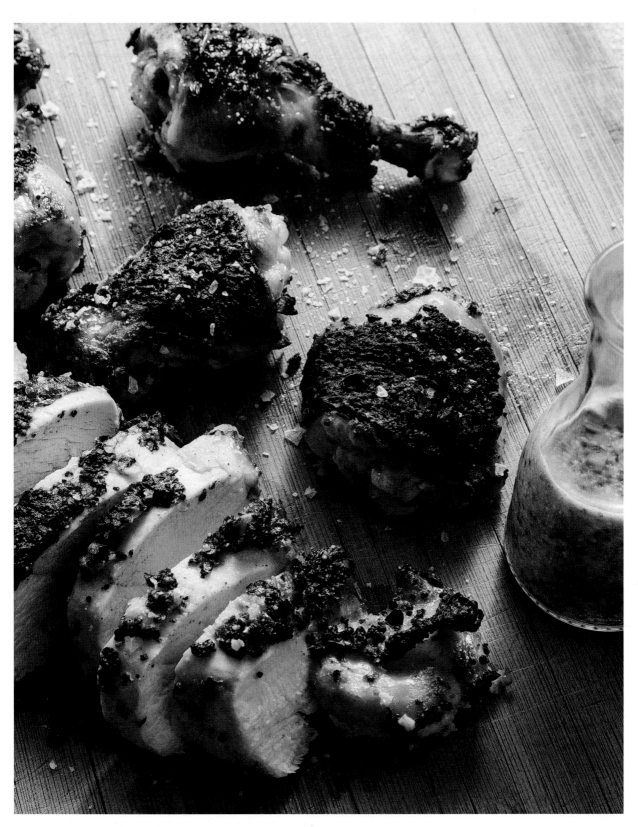

Mustard-Baked Chicken, page 159

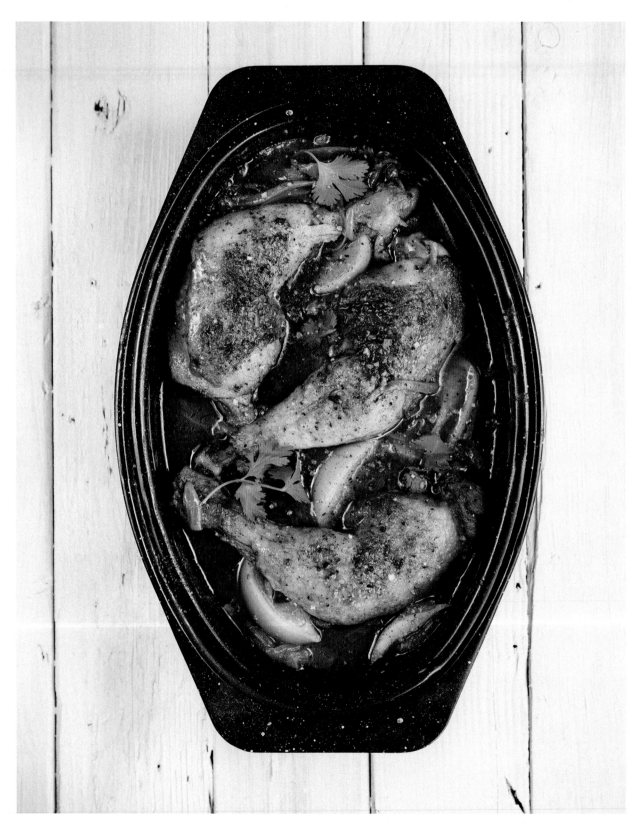

Chicken with Preserved Lemons and Fragrant Spices, page 171

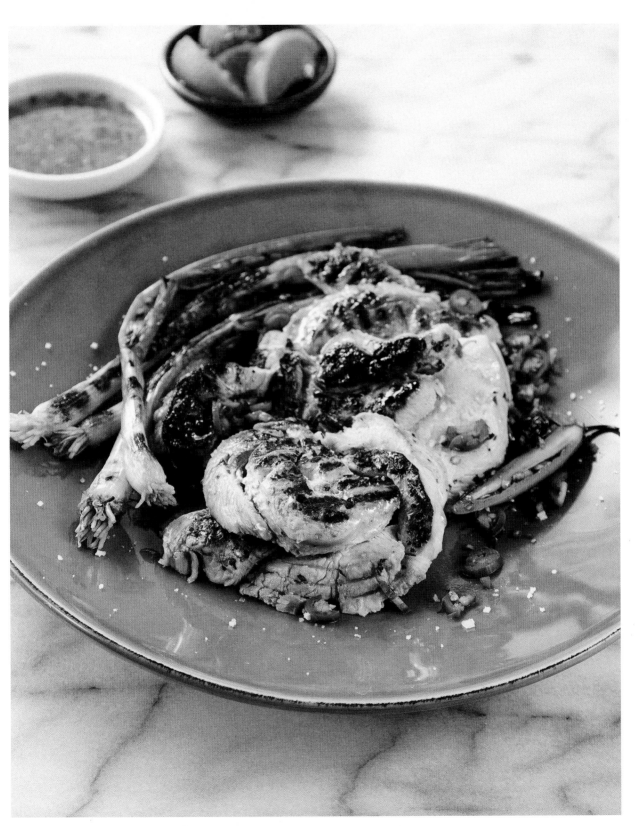

Thai Marinated Turkey Breast, page 164

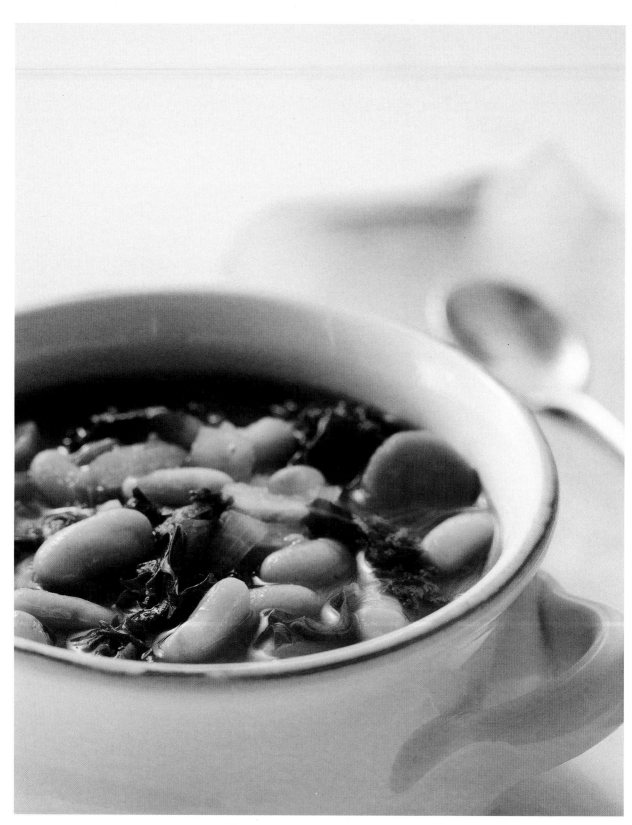

White Bean and Kale Soup, page 233

WHITE BEAN AND KALE SOUP

Ⓒ Cleanse

Ⓥ Vegan

Serves: 4

Prep time: overnight

Cooking time: 1 hour

Kale and white beans are a traditional pairing. If you want more protein or another take on this classic soup, feel free to add chicken or any sausage of your choice. Just remember, local and free-range/pastured is best.

2 tablespoons avocado oil
1 medium carrot, cut into large chunks
2 celery stalks, cut into large chunks
1 large onion, cut into large chunks
2 garlic cloves, minced
1½ cups dry cannellini (white) beans, soaked overnight (8 to 12 hours) in 4 cups water and
    1 teaspoon apple cider vinegar, then drained and rinsed well
6 or more cups chicken or vegetable stock
1 bay leaf
4 cups (about 1 bunch) roughly chopped kale
2 teaspoons sea salt, or to taste
2 teaspoons chopped fresh rosemary

Heat the avocado oil in a large pot set over medium-high heat. Sauté the carrots, celery, and onions, stirring occasionally, until the vegetables are slightly tender, about 4 to 5 minutes. Stir in the garlic and cook the mixture until it is fragrant. Add the cannellini beans, stock, and bay leaf, and bring the pot to a boil. Lower the heat, partially cover the pot, and gently simmer the soup about 20 minutes. Stir in the kale and continue to simmer another 10 minutes, until the beans are tender. If the soup begins to get quite thick, add more stock.

Before serving, season the soup with salt and stir in the fresh rosemary.

Variation: For a creamier version, purée a quarter to half of the soup in a blender until it's smooth, then stir it back into the pot.

MULLIGATAWNY SOUP

Wanda LeBlanc-Rushmer, Clean community member

Serves: approximately 6

This hearty Indian soup with curried chicken, apples, and brown rice is a great way to warm the belly when the leaves begin to fall. Definitely a favorite in our home!

1 tablespoon coconut oil
1 cup chopped celery stalks
1 cup chopped white or yellow onions
1 cup chopped carrots
1 garlic clove, minced
2 pasture-raised boneless, skinless chicken breasts, cut into 1-inch cubes
3 teaspoons curry powder
1 teaspoon chili powder
1 teaspoon ground cumin
2 whole cloves
6 cups chicken broth
1 19-ounce can diced tomatoes
½ cup uncooked brown basmati rice
1 teaspoon sea salt
½ teaspoon freshly ground black pepper
2 cups peeled, cored, and diced Granny Smith apples
¼ cup chopped fresh parsley
1 tablespoon lemon juice (optional)

Melt the coconut oil in a large soup pot set over medium heat. Sauté the celery, onions, carrots, and garlic, stirring occasionally, for 3 to 4 minutes, until the vegetables begin to soften. Add the chicken and cook it until it is no longer pink. Add the curry powder, chili powder, cumin, and cloves, and continue stirring for another 2 minutes before adding the chicken broth, tomatoes, rice, salt, and pepper. Bring the mixture to a boil, cover, then reduce the heat and simmer for 15 minutes. Stir in the apples and parsley, and simmer for an additional 10 minutes, then remove the pot from the heat and stir in the lemon juice if desired. Enjoy!

EXPERIENCE: I completed the Clean Cleanse several months ago and have continued to follow the program. I enjoy a healthy shake every morning, a full lunch, and a light dinner, along with snacks. I have lost some unwanted pounds, I feel more energetic, and my digestive system loves me for it! I highly recommend this program.

CHILLED CUCUMBER AVOCADO SOUP

C Cleanse

G Gut

V Vegan

Serves: 2

Prep time: 10 minutes

Chilling time: 30 minutes (optional)

Soups are one of the easiest and most soul-satisfying things to make and savor. But they don't have to be winter-only meals. Summer soups made from fresh ingredients, when a blender is the only tool you need, are wonderful when the weather is too hot to prepare large meals. Avocados make everything creamy and add essential saturated fat, which is anti-inflammatory and keeps your metabolism fired up.

2 large cucumbers, peeled, seeded, and roughly chopped (about 3 cups)
Flesh of 2 ripe avocados
1 cup raw cashews
Juice of 1 lemon
2 garlic cloves
2 teaspoons sea salt
1 cup water

For the Garnish
1 tablespoon chopped fresh mint, tarragon, or cilantro
Pinch of smoked sea salt or smoked paprika

In a blender, purée all the soup ingredients until the mixture is smooth and creamy. Serve it immediately, garnished with the fresh herbs and a pinch of the smoked salt or smoked paprika, or place the soup in an airtight container and chill it for 30 minutes before serving.

EGG DROP SOUP

Ⓖ Gut

Serves: 2 to 4

Prep time: 3 hours

Cooking time: 10 minutes

The Chinese translation for this is "egg flower soup." It's a beautiful and comforting bowl of egg wisps and immune-boosting chicken stock (preferably homemade).

2 tablespoons freshly sliced ginger
1 star anise
4 cups chicken stock (preferably homemade; page 224)
1 clove garlic, peeled and minced
2 pasture-raised eggs
2 scallions, thinly sliced
2 to 3 tablespoons chickpea miso or 2 to 3 tablespoons wheat-free tamari

Place the ginger, star anise, and garlic in a tea ball or sachet. Slowly bring the chicken stock to a simmer, with the herb ball or sachet. Let the herbs infuse for 3 hours then remove before whisking in the 2 eggs. Add chopped scallions, and serve the soup with the miso or tamari as a condiment.

LEMONY LENTIL SOUP

V Vegan

Serves: 4

Prep time: overnight plus 10 minutes

Cooking time: 3 to 4 hours

A citrus flavor brings a light loveliness to the earthy lentils. A bowl of this soup is protein-packed and wonderful anytime a hearty yet easily digestible meal is required.

1 cup green lentils
1 large leek, white section sliced into ¼-inch-thick rounds
1 medium onion, roughly chopped
1 medium carrot, chopped
1 celery stalk, chopped
½ cup roughly chopped fresh cilantro leaves
1 bay leaf
2 tablespoons cumin seeds, toasted and ground
Pinch of chipotle chili powder
2 tablespoons extra-virgin olive oil
4 to 6 cups vegetable stock or water
2 large sweet potatoes, peeled and cut into large chunks
1 bunch Swiss chard, stems removed, cut into bite-size pieces
Zest and juice of 1 lemon
Sea salt and freshly ground black pepper to taste

Soak the lentils overnight in 4 cups of water. Drain and rinse them, then add them to a slow cooker with the leek, onion, carrot, celery, cilantro, bay leaf, cumin seeds, chipotle powder, olive oil, and stock or water. Cook on high for 2 hours and 30 minutes before adding the sweet potatoes and chard. Cook 1 additional hour. Add the lemon zest and juice, and season with salt and pepper before serving.

MAW MAW'S GUMBO

Makes: ½ gallon

Prep time: 15 minutes

Cooking time: 1 hour

This traditional soup from New Orleans is perfect anytime of the year but best when fresh tomatoes are in season. Although our version ideally contains chicken, you can adjust the ingredients for any dietary need and make it vegetarian with chickpeas, sweet potatoes, or eggplant. Fish works just as well in this zesty soup: use whitefish or salmon.

2 tablespoons coconut oil
1 onion, diced
3 celery stalks, diced
4 garlic cloves, chopped
1½ pounds fresh okra, sliced
2 pounds fresh tomatoes (or 2 48-ounce cans), roughly chopped
2 tablespoons dried oregano
¼ teaspoon cayenne
1 tablespoon onion powder
1 tablespoon garlic powder
1½ tablespoons paprika
1½ tablespoons gumbo filé (easily found in spice aisles of any market)
4 cups water
1 pound pasture-raised chicken, sweet potatoes, or whitefish (your choice), cubed
4 cups cooked brown rice

Heat the coconut oil in a large Dutch oven set over medium-high heat. Sauté the onion, celery, and garlic for about 2 to 3 minutes. Stir in the okra followed by the tomatoes, oregano, cayenne, onion powder, garlic powder, paprika, and gumbo filé. Allow the liquid to start getting bubbly, then add the water. Once the soup comes to a boil, reduce the heat, and gently simmer it for 15 minutes, remembering to stir it occasionally. At this point add the chicken, sweet potatoes, or fish. Continue simmering for another 15 to 20 minutes before adjusting the seasoning.

Serve over steamed brown rice.

GAZPACHO

G Gut

V Vegan

Makes: about 1 quart, 2 servings

Prep time: 30 minutes

Cold soups are usually just the thing on a sweltering hot summer day. This soup is loaded with tomatoes, so it's the most delicious at the height of summer when tomatoes are literally falling off the vines.

2 cups roughly chopped tomatoes
¼ cup sun-dried tomatoes, soaked in 1 cup hot water for 20 minutes, then strained
1 garlic clove
¼ cup extra-virgin olive oil
8 cherry tomatoes, halved
¼ cup diced red onion
Flesh of 1 ripe avocado, cut into small pieces
1 medium cucumber, peeled, seeds removed, cut into small pieces
¼ cup roughly chopped fresh cilantro
2 tablespoons roughly chopped fresh mint
1 teaspoon ground cumin
1 teaspoon ground coriander
½ teaspoon chipotle chili powder
Juice of 1 lime
1 tablespoon sea salt

In a blender, purée the chopped tomato, sun-dried tomatoes, garlic, and olive oil until the mixture is smooth and creamy, then pour it into a large bowl. Add the cherry tomatoes, onion, avocado, cucumber, cilantro, mint, cumin, coriander, chipotle chili powder, lime juice, and salt. Stir well to combine everything. Taste and adjust the seasonings with extra salt, lime juice, or olive oil as needed. Allow the gazpacho to sit at room temperature for 15 to 20 minutes to develop its flavors before serving.

HARVEST SOUP WITH PUMPKIN MISO

C Cleanse

G Gut*

V Vegan

Serves: 6

Prep time: 15 minutes

Cooking time: 1 hour

Miso is packed with wonderful healing properties, enzymes, and such. It's good to get fermented foods into your diet, and this is a delicious way to do it. Remember not to boil the miso, as it destroys the live elements, which is why we add it at the end.

2 tablespoons avocado oil
2 medium leeks, sliced
2 cups chopped carrots
2 cups chopped beets
4 cups chopped cabbage
1 tablespoon Italian seasoning
1 bunch Swiss chard, stemmed and roughly chopped
Sea salt to taste

For the Pumpkin Miso
1 cup raw pumpkin seeds
5 tablespoons soy-free miso
1 tablespoon chopped fresh sage

Heat the avocado oil in a large pot set over medium-high heat. Sauté the leeks, stirring occasionally, for 2 to 3 minutes. Add the carrots, beets, and cabbage, stir to combine, and cook the vegetables for an additional 2 to 3 minutes. Stir in the Italian seasoning, then cover the mixture by 1 inch with water.

Bring the soup to a boil, then lower the heat, cover the pot, and simmer it for 30 minutes. Add the Swiss chard and continue to simmer for an additional 10 minutes. Season to taste with a few pinches of sea salt.

While the soup is cooking, toast the pumpkin seeds in a dry, heavy-bottom skillet set over medium-high heat. Shake the pan often to keep the seeds from burning. Once they are golden brown, transfer them to a food processor and grind them until they are crumbly. Add the miso and sage, and continue to process the mixture until it forms a ball.

To serve, ladle the soup into bowls and top each with a large dollop of the pumpkin miso.

*Omit beets

TURKEY CHILI

Makes: ½ gallon

Prep time: overnight, plus 10 minutes

Cooking time: 1 hour

Not a lot of foods say "comfort" and "warming" like chili. Here's a somewhat lighter and different version of a classic dinner, post-skiing or sledding meal, or sporting event dish.

2 tablespoons coconut oil
2 medium onions, diced
1½ teaspoons ground cumin
1½ teaspoons ground oregano
1½ pounds ground pasture-raised turkey
3 tablespoons chili powder
1 teaspoon ground cinnamon
1 tablespoon cacao powder
2 bay leaves
½ cup black beans, soaked overnight with a small strip of kelp, then strained and rinsed
1 28-ounce jar tomato purée (Bionaturae brand is preferred)
1 tablespoon tomato paste (Bionaturae brand is preferred)
3 to 4 cups chicken stock or water
2 celery stalks, diced
1 medium zucchini, diced
1 red bell pepper, diced
2 to 3 tablespoons apple cider vinegar (as needed)
Sea salt to taste

Garnish
¼ cup chopped fresh cilantro
Sour Cream (page 98)
Sliced avocado

Melt the coconut oil in a large pot set over medium-high heat. Lightly sauté the onions until they are translucent, 3 to 4 minutes. Stir in the cumin and oregano and mix the herbs well with the onions. Slightly increase the heat, then add the turkey and incorporate it into the onion mixture. When the turkey meat is nearly cooked through, add the chili powder, cinnamon, cacao, bay leaves, and the soaked beans. Stir the mixture well, then add the tomato purée, tomato paste, and stock or water. Simmer the chili, covered, for 30 minutes. Remember to stir it often to prevent any sticking. Then add in the celery, zucchini, and bell pepper, and simmer for an additional 15 to 20 minutes.

At this point the chili should be nice and thick. Season it with a splash of apple cider vinegar and salt. Serve it garnished with fresh cilantro, sour cream, and avocado slices.

CHICKEN AND WILD RICE SOUP

C Cleanse

Serves: 2

Prep time: overnight plus 10 minutes on serving day

Cooking time: 25 minutes

This soup is immune-boosting and delicious. Soups warm the heart and our bones when we need strengthening and to shake off a chill. Wrap your hands around a steaming bowl of this nourishing soup and feel the cold melt away.

1 quart Chicken Stock (page 224)
½ cup wild rice, soaked overnight
1 strip kelp, soaked for 20 minutes, then roughly chopped
1 medium carrot, finely diced
½ cup finely diced yellow onion
2 celery stalks, finely diced
Pinch of dried thyme
1 cup cooked pasture-raised shredded chicken meat
Sea salt to taste
½ teaspoon freshly ground black pepper
2 to 3 tablespoons miso (South River brand is good)

In a large pot set over medium-low heat, lightly simmer the chicken stock with the rice, kelp, carrot, onion, celery, and thyme for 20 minutes. Then add the chicken meat, season the soup with salt and pepper, and simmer an additional 5 minutes. Stir in the miso, and serve immediately.

SPICY BLACK BEAN SOUP

© Cleanse
V Vegan

Serves: 4 to 6

Prep time: overnight, if using dried beans instead of canned

Cooking time: 45 minutes

Warming and full of protein, this soup has a definite and delicious kick.

2 cups canned or dried and soaked black beans (see instructions)
2 tablespoons coconut oil
1 onion, chopped roughly
1 large carrot, chopped roughly
2 garlic cloves, minced
1 teaspoon dried oregano
1 teaspoon dried thyme
2 teaspoons ground cumin
1 bay leaf
½ teaspoon chipotle chili powder
Juice of 1 to 2 limes
2 tablespoons to ¼ cup (depending on desired taste) apple cider vinegar
Sea salt to taste
2 scallions, minced
Chopped fresh cilantro leaves

If using canned beans, proceed to the next paragraph, but if using dry beans soak the beans overnight in a bowl of water with a strip of kelp. After about 8 to 12 hours, strain and rinse the beans, and drain them well.

Melt the coconut oil in a large soup pot set over medium-high heat. Sauté the onion and carrot for about 3 to 4 minutes, stirring occasionally. Add the garlic and keep stirring frequently, until the mixture is fragrant. Stir in the oregano, thyme, cumin, bay leaf, chipotle chili powder, and black beans. Sauté for a few more minutes, continuing to stir often. Before the beans start to dry out, add enough water to completely cover them, and allow the mixture to come to a boil. Reduce the heat to medium, cover the pot, and simmer for another 30 minutes. Continue to stir the beans every so often. If the liquid gets very low and the beans are not yet tender, add a bit more water to the pot and continue to simmer. When the beans are soft, remove the pot from the heat and allow the beans to cool slightly.

Working in batches, purée the mixture in a blender with the lime juice until you have a thick and creamy soup.

Experiment with the flavor, adding a touch of apple cider vinegar to help balance out the flavors. Season the soup with salt and serve it garnished with scallions and cilantro.

BROCCOLI CHEDDAR SOUP

C Cleanse

G Gut

V Vegan

Serves: 2 to 4

Prep time: 5 minutes

Cooking time: 30 minutes

This is comfort food that's healthy and packed with antioxidants. Garlic and chicken are also wonderful for the immune system, and turmeric is anti-inflammatory and uniquely flavors this soup.

2 tablespoons coconut oil
1 leek, green top discarded, white section sliced into ½-inch-thick rounds
2 garlic cloves, minced
1 head broccoli, stem discarded, and cut into florets (should equal about 4 cups)
3 cups chicken or vegetable stock
1 bay leaf
¼ teaspoon ground turmeric
½ cup nutritional yeast
Sea salt and freshly ground black pepper to taste

Melt the coconut oil in a large soup pot set over medium-high heat. Sauté the leeks until they begin to soften, roughly 3 to 4 minutes. Add the garlic and cook it until it's fragrant. Stir in the broccoli and combine everything well. Sauté the mixture for an additional 2 minutes, then add the stock, bay leaf, and turmeric. Lower the heat, cover the pot, and let the soup simmer for 20 minutes.

Before serving, stir in the nutritional yeast and season with salt and pepper to taste. Serve warm.

SHAKES, ELIXIRS, DRINKS, AND TONICS

Shakes have been a staple at Clean since the beginning. They are an important part of our Cleanse and Gut programs and are an easy way to give your body water and easily digestible nutrients. We've also included warm medicinal elixir recipes, juices, and assorted drinks. From our Coconut Water and Lime Rickey to our Mango Slushie, and our Reishi Cappuccino to our Raspberry Lemon-Aide, there is a great-tasting and healthy beverage here for everyone.

ALMOND "MILK"

C Cleanse

G Gut

V Vegan

Makes: 3 to 4 cups

Prep time: overnight plus 10 minutes on serving day

Almond milk is easy and nutritious; why buy it when you can make your own from scratch in minutes? This is a great recipe for those who have sensitivities to gums or additives in store-bought nut milk.

1 cup raw almonds
3 cups water
Pinch of sea salt

Soak the almonds overnight (about 8 to 10 hours) in 4 cups of water. In the morning, drain the water and rinse the almonds well.

Place the almonds in a blender with the 3 cups of water and a tiny pinch of salt. Blend the mixture on a high setting for 45 seconds. Using a fine-mesh strainer or a cloth food bag, strain the pulp from the liquid, pressing with your hands or a rubber spatula to get as much liquid out of the pulp as possible.

Store the milk, refrigerated, in an airtight container for up to three days. The pulp can be dried, used fresh, or frozen, and used in a variety of other recipes.

Variations: Any nut or seed can be used here, but just be mindful of the soaking time. Fatty nuts like pecans, cashews, and macadamia nuts do not need to be soaked. Smaller seeds only need to soak for 2 to 3 hours. And for a thicker, cream-like consistency, reduce the water by 1 cup.

CHIA GEL

C Cleanse

G Gut

V Vegan

Makes: 1 pint

Prep time: 20 to 30 minutes

Soaking chia seeds in water helps break down phytic acid and increase digestion. The gel can be used to thicken smoothies, elixirs, soups, and desserts. This can become a staple in clean cooking and would be a great item to keep a constant supply of in the fridge.

3 tablespoons chia seeds
1¾ cups water

Simply mix the chia and water together in a small bowl or cup and allow the chia to soak up the liquid for 20 to 30 minutes. Store the gel in an airtight container in the fridge for up to one week.

GINGER JUICE

C Cleanse
G Gut
V Vegan

Makes: 1 pint
Prep time: 5 minutes

Here's a simple way to extend the life of your fresh ginger and easily incorporate it into both your sweet and savory meals. This potent juice can be used as a supplement and consumed whenever you feel chilly or a little under the weather, as it boosts circulation and gives your immune system a kick.

1 cup freshly sliced ginger
2 cups water

Place the ginger and water in a blender and blend on a high setting for 30 seconds, then pour the mixture through a fine-mesh strainer. Store the juice, refrigerated, in a container for up to two weeks.

SPRING DANDELION DETOX ELIXIR

C Cleanse

G Gut*

V Vegan†

Serves: 1

Prep time: overnight plus 15 minutes

This is a wonderful, medicinal, and cleansing drink to support the liver and clear out stagnant bile and winter buildup. It's traditionally consumed in the spring, but you can enjoy this anytime of the year.

1 tablespoon milk thistle seeds
2 tablespoons dried dandelion leaf
1 tablespoon dried nettle leaf
¼ cup shredded unsweetened coconut
1 tablespoon coconut oil
1 to 2 tablespoons coconut nectar
½ teaspoon vanilla extract

Soak the milk thistle seeds in 1 cup of water overnight, then strain and rinse them well.

Place the dandelion and nettle leaf in a jar and cover them with 1½ cups of boiling water. Secure the jar's lid and let the herbs infuse for 10 minutes.

Strain the herb infusion and pour it into a blender along with the soaked milk thistle and shredded coconut. Blend the mixture on a high setting for 45 seconds, then pour it through a fine-mesh strainer.

Return the strained milk to the blender and blend it with the coconut oil, a touch of coconut nectar or honey, and the vanilla.

*Omit sweetener; use stevia, xylitol, or Lakanto
†Using coconut nectar

MAKE JUICE, NOT WAR GREEN JUICE

Kris Carr, wellness activist, cancer thriver

Ⓒ Cleanse

Ⓥ Vegan

Makes: almost 4 cups (32 ounces)

Prep time: 15 minutes

It's my motto and my morning beverage.

2 large cucumbers (peeled, if not organic)
4 to 5 kale leaves
4 to 5 romaine leaves
4 celery stalks
1 to 2 big broccoli stems
1 to 2 pears
1-inch chunk ginger

Using a vegetable juicer, juice all the ingredients.

Variations: A few other optional greens to add are parsley, spinach, and dandelion.

RASPBERRY LEMON-AIDE

C Cleanse

G Gut

V Vegan

Serves: 2

Prep time: 5 minutes

This is a refreshing twist on a summertime classic. The MSM (methyl-sulfonyl-methane) powder helps relax muscles, which is great after a day in the garden or after a long workout, heightened by the natural electrolytes and potassium coconut water provides.

1 cup frozen raspberries
4 cups chilled coconut water
¼ cup lemon juice
4 to 6 drops liquid stevia
1 tablespoon MSM powder
Pinch of sea salt

Place all the ingredients in a blender and blend on a high setting until the mixture is well combined. Fill two glasses and enjoy!

Variations:

Any frozen fruit can replace the raspberries.

Use lime instead of lemon.

Add a few splashes of Ginger Juice (page 248).

HIBISCUS ROSE SPLASH

C Cleanse

G Gut*

V Vegan†

Serves: 4

Brewing time: 10 minutes to 8 hours

This is refreshing and not too sweet, and it has plenty of hydrating and nourishing benefits. It's a healthy drink that tastes like a treat!

2 tablespoons dried hibiscus flowers
1 tablespoon dried nettle leaf
1 teaspoon rose hips
4 cups chilled coconut water
3 cups chilled sparkling water
Juice of 1 lime
4 to 6 drops liquid stevia, coconut nectar, or honey
1 tray of ice

Place the dried herbs in a 1-quart mason jar. Top the herbs with 4 cups of boiling water, cover, and let the mixture infuse for a minimum of 10 minutes or up to 8 hours.

Strain the tea and pour 1⅓ cups of it into a large serving glass. Mix in 1 cup of the coconut water and ¾ cup of the sparkling water. Stir in a portion of the lime juice and sweetener, to taste, mix well, and add ice. Any extra tea can be stored in the fridge for up to a week and used as a base for other smoothies and drink recipes.

*Use stevia
†With stevia or coconut nectar

REISHI CAPPUCCINO

C Cleanse
G Gut*
V Vegan

Serves: 2
Prep time: 5 minutes

Reishi mushroom is a powerful immune-boosting mushroom that can be found in many parts of the world. It's highly prized in China for its health benefits and has been used for thousands of years.

2 cups unsweetened almond milk
1 teaspoon or the powder from 6 capsules reishi mushroom extract (in capsule form, look for "dual extraction" type)
2 tablespoons coconut oil
1 teaspoon ground cinnamon
½ teaspoon vanilla extract
Pinch of sea salt
1 to 2 tablespoons coconut palm sugar

In a saucepan, gently warm the almond milk, then place all the cappuccino ingredients in a blender and blend on a high setting until the mixture is frothy. Divide the mixture between two glasses and enjoy!

*Omit coconut palm sugar; use stevia, xylitol, or Lakanto

ADAM'S A.M. PRE-WORKOUT SHAKE

Adam Cobb, Health Head Lifter, founder FYCNYC

C Cleanse

G Gut

V Vegan

Prep time: 5 minutes

I recommend this shake to all my clients as a great pre-workout option. It has all the elements of a balanced nutritional shake with easily digestible protein. It will provide a quick burst of energy without making you feel bloated. Most important, this shake tastes amazing, and it gives you the momentum to start your movement for the day and live my phrase "eight days a week."

2 scoops plant protein powder (rice, pea, hemp)
1 cup unsweetened almond milk
¼ cup coconut water
Flesh of ¼ medium ripe avocado
1 tablespoon almond butter
Pinch of pink Himalayan salt
1 teaspoon maca powder
½ cup frozen blueberries
Dash of cinnamon
4 ice cubes

Place all ingredients in a blender and blend for 1 minute. I recommend you drink this shake 1 to 2 hours before any workout.

REJUVENATING EGGNOG

John Rosania, Clean VP of Product

G Gut

Vegetarian*

Serves: 1

Prep time: 5 minutes

This is a delicious warm eggnog-type drink. The eggs and collagen give absorbable protein while the coconut oil adds good saturated fat. Finish it off with some spices, and you get a sweet, sugar-free drink that deeply nourishes the body.

2 to 3 pasture-raised eggs
2 tablespoons coconut oil
1 to 2 tablespoons Great Lakes collagen hydrolysate
1 scoop of vanilla protein powder (optional)
1 teaspoon ground cinnamon
½ teaspoon ground nutmeg, or to taste
Pinch of cloves
Pinch of sea salt
Stevia to taste

Add all ingredients to blender. Slowly pour 2 to 2½ cups boiling water into the blender. Boiled water will cook the eggs. If you are making larger quantities, do not fill the blender too high, as it will spurt out. Blend on low and then increase speed for 15 to 20 seconds. Drink immediately or transfer to a thermos. It will keep for several hours.

Variations: Add 1 tablespoon of grass-fed butter to this drink if dairy works for you.

*Contains eggs

BLACKBERRY COCONUT MILK SHAKE

C Cleanse

G Gut*

V Vegan

Serves: 1

Prep time: 5 minutes

This is a winning combination. Blackberries are often overlooked when other berries are present, but they have the most varied sweet-tart flavor and pair perfectly with rich coconut and vanilla.

1 cup frozen blackberries
¾ cup chilled unsweetened coconut milk
1½ cups chilled coconut water
½ teaspoon vanilla extract
2 Medjool dates

Place all the ingredients in a blender and blend on a high setting for 30 seconds, then serve.

*Omit dates

The Doc on Shakes and Smoothies

Shakes are an important item in our wellness toolbox. Not only are they easy to make and great tasting, but you can also use them strategically to improve your health. Having a breakfast shake a few days a week is a simple way to provide your body with more water and easily absorbable nutrients and to reduce the work of the digestive system. When you do this, digestive energy is freed up to be utilized by other parts of the body for cleanup and repair.

TURMERIC ALMOND MILK

Carly de Castro, cofounder, Pressed Juicery

Ⓒ Cleanse*

Ⓖ Gut*

Ⓥ Vegan†

Makes: 2 cups

Nothing beats homemade almond milk. It's creamy like cow's milk but free of dairy and soy, and it has protein to boot. At Pressed Juicery, our signature almond "milk" is flavored with vanilla and dates, and many people have told us it tastes like melted vanilla ice cream. Over the years we've experimented with various ingredients and come up with a holiday spiced almond milk, and even chocolate almond milk that no child would turn down!

In this recipe, the star (besides almonds, of course) is turmeric, which has been used as a medicinal spice in ancient ayurvedic practices and continues to be popular today. Turmeric is anti-inflammatory and high in antioxidants, making it a choice supplement to boost the immune system. I've made this at home for my family and they love the earthy, sweet flavor of the turmeric combined with cardamom and honey. Another variation is to heat it up for a soothing "tea," which always does the trick for sore throats.

Note: as well as a blender you will need a nut milk bag or two pieces of cheesecloth to form a double layer for straining the milk.

1 cup raw almonds, soaked overnight, then rinsed and drained
2 cups water
1½ teaspoons ground turmeric
½ teaspoon ground cardamom
1 tablespoon raw honey
Freshly grated ginger to taste
1 cinnamon stick

Place the almonds in a blender with the water. Blend them on the lowest setting and gradually increase the speed for about 2 minutes. The water should be milky and white. Once the mixture is smooth, add the turmeric, cardamom, and honey, and gently blend again.

Place your nut milk bag (or cheesecloth) over an empty container, such as a jar. Pour the almond and spice mixture into the bag and strain it, using your hands to squeeze everything through. Make sure to get as much of the milk out as possible. Store the milk in a sealed container in the refrigerator for up to two days.

Serve it with freshly grated ginger on top and a cinnamon stick, if you'd like.

*Omit honey and use gut- or cleanse-approved sweetener
†Omit honey and use coconut nectar

MANGO SLUSHIE

C Cleanse

V Vegan

Serves: 1

Prep time: 5 minutes

Ginger, mango, and lime are always an amazing combination, and the kiwifruit just adds to the yumminess. Kombucha is readily found just about everywhere now, but this may also nudge you to make your own, if you're inspired to try it out.

1 cup frozen mango slices
2 kiwifruits, peeled, quartered, and frozen ahead of time
Juice of 1 lime
Ginger-flavored kombucha (we like GT's brand, and it's the easiest to find)
1 tablespoon coconut nectar or 2 to 4 drops stevia liquid

Place all the ingredients in a blender and blend on a high setting until the frozen fruit has broken down. Serve immediately.

JUST PEACHY

C Cleanse

V Vegan

Serves: 2

Prep time: 5 minutes

Creamy with an added coconut crunch on top, this is delectable and a wonderful sweet treat with coconut milk, which boosts metabolism and regulates blood sugar.

1 cup frozen peach slices
¼ cup raw pecans
2 cups unsweetened coconut milk
2 teaspoons ground pumpkin-pie spice (most health food stores have this in bulk, or you can use a mix of ground cinnamon, clove, nutmeg, and allspice)
1 teaspoon freshly grated ginger
Toasted or raw unsweetened coconut flakes (optional)

Place all the ingredients in a blender and blend on a high setting until the mixture is smooth and creamy. Top with a few sprinkles of toasted or raw coconut for an extra-crunchy treat.

MALTED MACA MILK SHAKE

C Cleanse

G Gut*

V Vegan

Serves: 1

Prep time: 5 minutes

Maca and mesquite are ancient South American powders that, between the two, are packed with fiber, B vitamins, iron, calcium, magnesium, and immune-strengthening properties. This shake tastes like a treat, but it's actually incredibly healthy. So drink up like Incan warriors used to!

1½ cups cold water
4 ice cubes
¼ cup raw cashews
2 teaspoons maca powder
1 tablespoon mesquite meal
½ teaspoon vanilla extract
1 to 2 tablespoons coconut nectar
Pinch of sea salt

Place all the ingredients in a blender and blend on a high setting for 30 seconds, then serve.

*Omit sweetener; use stevia, xylitol, or Lakanto

DREAMY BLUEBERRY SMOOTHIE

Ⓒ Cleanse

Ⓖ Gut*

Ⓥ Vegan

Serves: 1

Prep time: 5 minutes

Antioxidant- and protein-packed, this is a simple and low-sugar shake that will become a household staple the minute you try it.

1½ cups water or nut milk
½ cup frozen blueberries
1 soft Medjool date, pit removed
2 tablespoons unsalted almond butter, chunky or smooth
1 tablespoon Chia Gel (page 247)
1 tablespoon shredded unsweetened coconut

Place all the ingredients in a blender and blend on a high setting for 45 seconds, until the mixture is smooth and creamy, then serve.

*Omit dates; use stevia, xylitol, or Lakanto

HEALING CHOCOLATE ELIXIR

C Cleanse   **Serves:** 1

G Gut   **Prep time:** 30 minutes

We are surrounded by an abundant medicine cabinet here on earth. Almost every plant has some healing qualities, and when we know how to use them, our lives (and palates) become richer and our bodies benefit. Even chocolate has medicinal qualities; without the sugar and dairy, it's full of nutrients. Blended with healing herbal tea and some added powders and seeds, this is an incredible drink that will carry you through every season.

1 cup hot herbal tea, such as nettle, pau d'arco, or horsetail, or hot water
1 tablespoon coconut oil
2 tablespoons raw cashews
2 heaping tablespoons cacao powder
1 to 2 teaspoons L-glutamine powder
1 tablespoon Great Lakes collagen hydrolysate gelatin (Great Lakes uses bones from grass-fed animals and is superior in quality.
2 tablespoons Chia Gel (page 247)
Pinch of sea salt
Stevia to taste, or 1 to 2 teaspoons birch xylitol

Blend all the ingredients in a blender until the mixture is smooth, about 45 seconds. Serve warm.

CLEAN HOT COCOA

C Cleanse

G Gut*

V Vegan

Makes: about 3 cups

Prep time: 15 minutes

Cooking time: 3 minutes

Rich, creamy, and entirely soul-satisfying, this is a warming comfort drink at its best, one that kids and grownups alike will love. It's a million times better than packaged, sugar-filled versions. Plus, it's nondairy and something you can whip up and enjoy all winter long.

1 cup raw Brazil nuts (raw cashews or macadamia nuts work too)
2 cups water
Up to ¼ cup coconut palm sugar
⅔ cup cacao powder
½ teaspoon vanilla extract
Pinch of sea salt

Place the Brazil nuts and the water in a blender and blend on a high setting for 45 seconds. Strain the mixture, then pour it into a saucepan. Slowly heat it, then whisk in the coconut sugar, cacao powder, vanilla, and salt. Simmer the cocoa for about 3 minutes, continuously whisking to avoid scorching. Serve immediately.

*Omit coconut palm sugar for a strong coffee-like drink; use stevia instead

CRANBERRY CIDER SPRITZER

C Cleanse

V Vegan

Serves: 6

Prep time: 20 minutes

This is a festive holiday spritzer. Feel free to add libations to it for adult gatherings, but serve it as is to kids when there's a party or special occasion.

1 cup fresh or frozen cranberries
2 tablespoons coconut palm sugar
½ teaspoon vanilla extract
1 cinnamon stick
3 cups water
4 cups (32 ounces) apple cider
1 small bottle (8 ounces) club soda (or sparkling mineral water)

Place the cranberries, coconut sugar, vanilla, cinnamon, and water into a pot and simmer them until the cranberries burst, about 15 minutes. Remove the cinnamon stick, then transfer the mixture to a blender and blend on a high setting for 30 seconds. Pour it through a fine-mesh sieve.

To serve, mix 1 cup of the apple cider with a splash of club soda and ½ cup of the cranberry concentrate.

Any leftover concentrate can be refrigerated for up to one week in a container or frozen for future use.

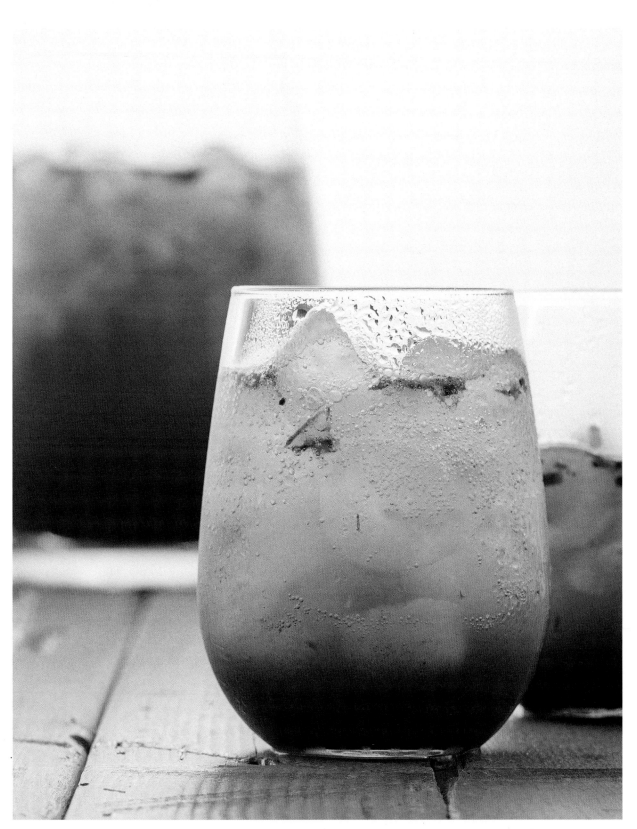

Cranberry Cider Spritzer, page 264

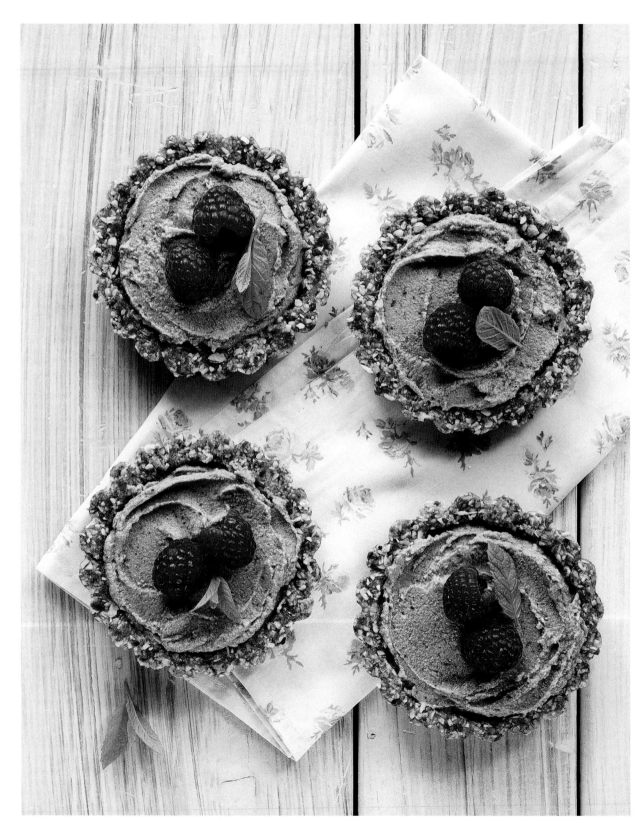

Mini Raspberry and Coconut Cream Tarts, page 274

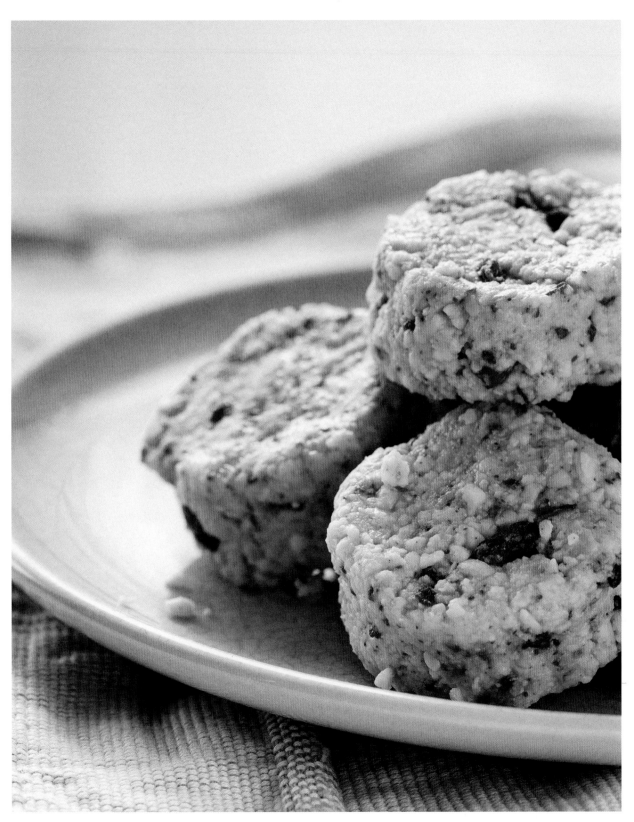

Cashew No-Bake Cookies, page 275

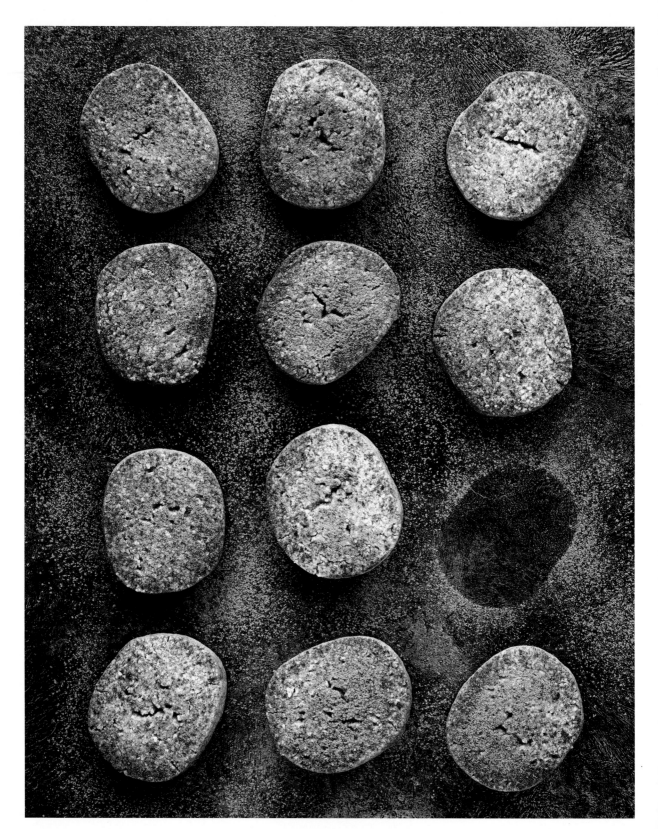

Almond Spice Cookies, page 285

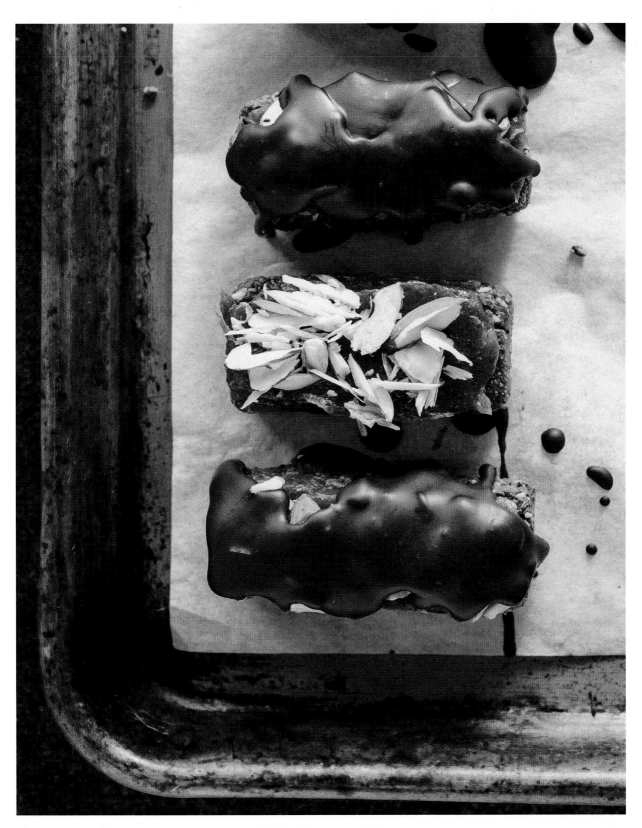

Snicker Bars, page 278

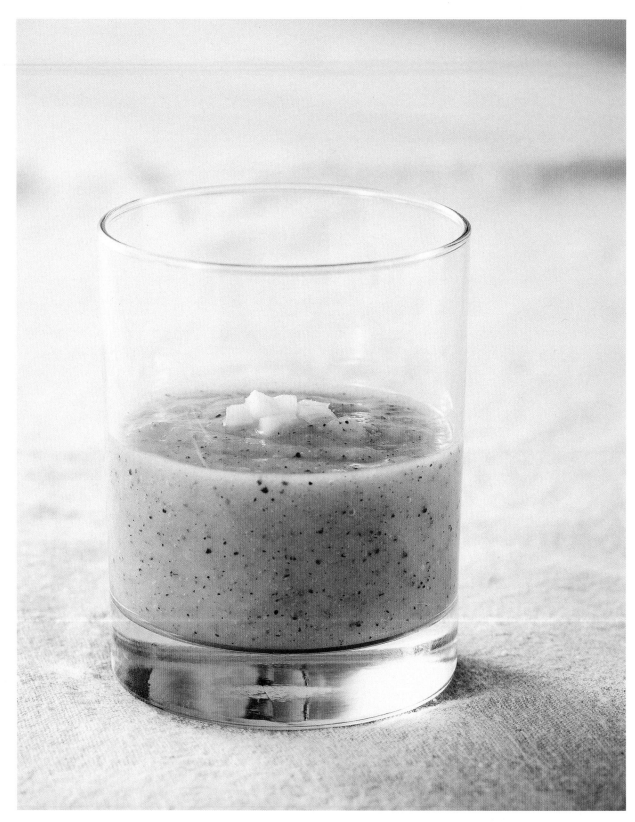

Mango Slushie, page 258

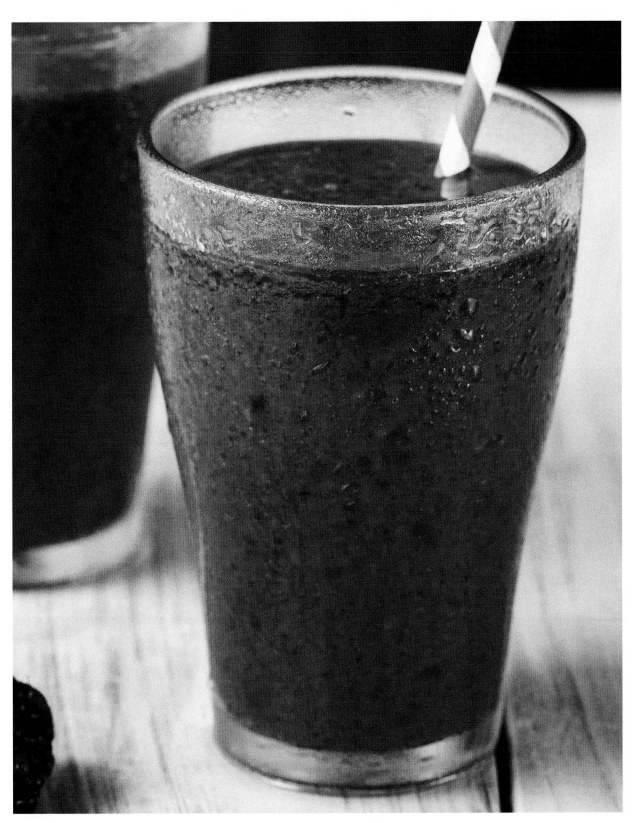

Blackberry Coconut Milk Shake, page 256

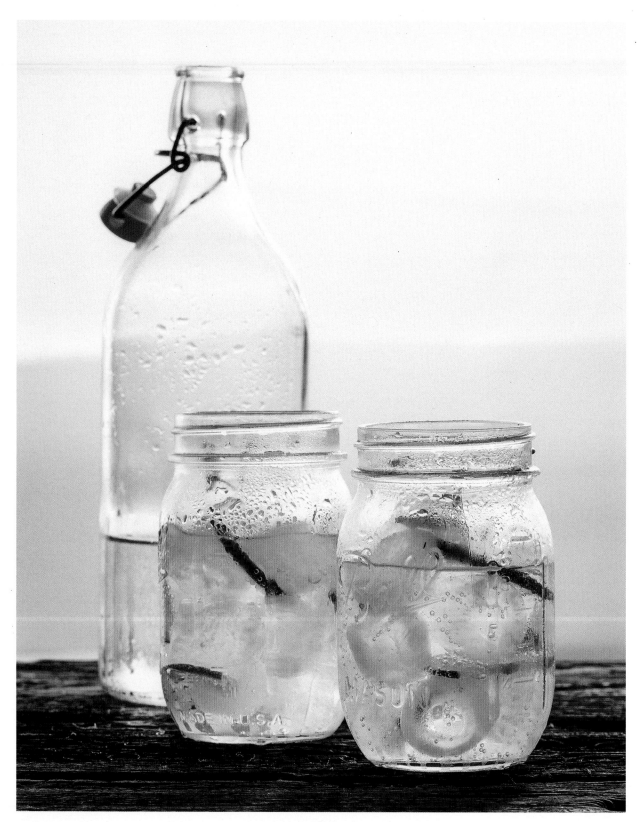

Coconut Water and Lime Rickey, page 265

COCONUT WATER AND LIME RICKEY

C Cleanse

G Gut

V Vegan

Serves: 2

Prep time: 5 minutes

A traditional highball drink that's very low in sugar, it's also incredibly popular at soda fountains *sans* alcohol. The lime and bitters are a great pairing with the naturally sweet coconut water.

1 cup chilled coconut water
2 tablespoons freshly squeezed lime juice
2 to 4 drops liquid stevia
3 drops bitters (optional)
½ cup club soda

In a jar, stir or shake together the coconut water, lime juice, stevia, and optional bitters. Divide the mixture between two glasses, then fill each glass with ¼ cup or more club soda and serve.

DESSERTS

The sweet taste is essential to life. We're programmed from birth to associate the sweet taste with satiety and survival, and this deep connection never fully vanishes. We seem to reach for sugary snacks and desserts at every occasion, in times of joy, in times of sadness, and in times of boredom. With our deep love of sweetness, it's a losing battle to reclaim our health by forbidding all sweet treats. The key is to let go of the ones that are loaded with gluten, dairy, processed sugar, and chemicals, and to substitute them for the amazing recipes we have included here. Once you try the Clean version of our Summer Fruit Crêpes with Vanilla Cream or the Peach Pie, there's no going back.

BLACKBERRY COBBLER

Ⓒ Cleanse

Ⓥ Vegan*

Serves: 4 to 6

Prep time: 20 minutes

Cooking time: 30 minutes

This is a paleo-inspired, grain-free version of a delicious dessert, snack, breakfast, or even dinner(!) that's sure to please everyone, and it's easy to make in a pinch. You'll never be stuck without a cobbler again, no matter how clean you're eating. Watch people ask you for this recipe over and over the more you share it.

4 apples, peeled, cored, and cut into large chunks
1 teaspoon ground cinnamon
¼ teaspoon stevia powder or a few drops of stevia liquid (optional)
1 cup fresh or frozen blackberries
2 teaspoons coconut oil

For the Topping
1 cup raw almonds
1 cup raw Brazil nuts
¼ cup shredded unsweetened coconut
1 tablespoon mesquite meal (optional but recommended)
2 dashes cinnamon
2 tablespoons coconut nectar or honey
1 tablespoon coconut oil, melted
2 teaspoons vanilla extract

Preheat the oven to 350°F.

In a large bowl, gently toss the chopped apples with the cinnamon and stevia (if using). Carefully, so they don't get too smashed, stir in the blackberries.

Oil an 8 × 8-inch square cake pan or a 9 × 4-inch rectangular loaf pan with the coconut oil. (As long as it's deep and the crumble doesn't spill over the top, any variety of pan will work.) Spread the apple and blackberry mixture in the pan, then make the topping.

In a food processor, pulse the almonds and Brazil nuts together until they are crumbly. Add the coconut, optional mesquite, cinnamon, coconut nectar or honey, coconut oil, and vanilla, and pulse a few more times until everything is combined but still chunky.

Sprinkle the topping evenly over the apple and blackberry mixture. Bake the cobbler for 30 minutes, checking and baking a bit longer if you want softer and mushier apples. The top should be brown and crispy.

Note: Be careful with stevia. If you decide to use it, you don't need much. It's super sweet and the apples and berries are already bursting with sweet flavor.

*Using coconut nectar

ROASTED PEARS WITH DATE CARAMEL SAUCE

C Cleanse

V Vegan

Serves: 4

Prep time: 20 minutes

Cooking time: 20 to 30 minutes

This is entirely elegant and dinner-party worthy. The lucuma powder is the secret ingredient, a low-glycemic sweetener that has a unique maple taste and is high in beta-carotene, iron, zinc, and calcium.

10 dates, soaked in warm water until soft (roughly 20 minutes), then strained and the liquid reserved
1 tablespoon Ginger Juice (page 248)
Juice of 1 lemon
Pinch of sea salt
¼ cup lucuma powder
1 to 2 tablespoons coconut nectar or maple syrup
4 crisp pears (any variety), cut into quarters and cored
¼ cup shredded unsweetened coconut
Freshly grated nutmeg to taste

Preheat the oven to 350°F.

In a blender, purée the strained dates with the ginger juice, lemon juice, salt, and lucuma powder. Add the coconut nectar, then blend the mixture again until it is smooth and runny. Use some of the reserved date soaking liquid to reach a desired consistency, if needed.

Set the pears in an oiled baking dish. Drizzle them with the sauce, then bake them until they are tender, roughly 20 to 30 minutes. Remove them from the oven, and let them cool slightly.

Spoon a ¼ cup or so of the sauce leftover in the baking dish onto four serving plates. Set the pears in the sauce, and sprinkle them with the coconut and grate a bit of nutmeg over each plate.

CLEAN ENERGY BARS

C Cleanse

V Vegan

Makes: 9 bars

Prep time: 15 minutes

While there are a few energy bars out there that are "clean," why not make your own? They're super easy and you'll know exactly what ingredients are in them, plus you'll save a lot of extra wrappers and packaging from being tossed in the trash. These are great clean fuel for all of your adventures.

¼ cup raw pumpkin seeds
¼ cup raw sunflower seeds
½ cup raw pistachios
1½ cups unsalted almond butter
½ cup coconut nectar
4 Medjool dates, cut into small chunks
2 tablespoons chia seeds
¼ cup raw hemp seeds
½ teaspoon ground cinnamon
2 tablespoons mesquite meal
1 teaspoon vanilla extract

If you wish, heat the oven to 350°F and dry roast the pumpkin seeds, sunflower seeds, and pistachios until they are golden brown, about 10 minutes, or you can keep them all raw.

In a large bowl, combine all the ingredients until the mixture is well incorporated. Line a 9 × 11-inch baking dish with parchment paper, then press the mixture into the dish, compacting it to form a solid layer about ½-inch thick. Score the surface into 2 × 2-inch bars, then place the dish into the fridge for the bars to set. After about 30 minutes, remove them from the fridge and cut them into squares. Leftovers can be stored for up to a month in the fridge or portioned and kept in the freezer.

APPLE CRISP (AKA MIRACLE CRISP)

Gabrielle Bernstein, New York Times *bestselling author and speaker*

Ⓒ Cleanse   **Cooking time:** 20 minutes

Ⓥ Vegan

As a woman who doesn't partake in sugar, yeast, gluten, or dairy, I find it hard to eat most desserts. This amazing recipe always curbs my sweet tooth and is a perfect apple pie replacement during the holiday season.

Note: I created this recipe with my friend Jamie Graber, the owner of Gingersnap's Organic.

5 medium red apples, thinly sliced
Ground cinnamon to taste
1 cup almond flour
3 tablespoons coconut oil
½ cup crushed walnuts
Pinch of ground nutmeg

Layer the apples in a baking dish, and generously sprinkle them with the cinnamon.

In a small bowl, combine the almond flour, coconut oil, walnuts, and nutmeg. Then sprinkle the mixture over the apples. Bake the crisp for 20 minutes (stick a fork in to make sure the apples are soft). Serve warm.

If there are any leftovers, try putting a few scoops of the crisp in a bowl with almond milk and eating it for breakfast or as a cold treat.

SUMMER FRUIT CRÊPES WITH VANILLA CREAM

Vegetarian*

Serves: 2 to 4

Prep time: 30 minutes

A bit of preparation goes into this, but the results are well worth it. Add some chocolate, if you wish, and use any fruit that's in season. Apples sautéed in cinnamon are delicious in the fall!

4 to 5 cups sliced fresh fruit, such as peaches, berries, apricots, and/or mango
2 tablespoons julienned fresh mint leaves
Coconut oil for the skillet

For the Crêpes
2 pasture-raised eggs
2 tablespoons coconut oil, melted
1 cup unsweetened almond milk (more, if you prefer a thinner crêpe)
1¼ cups all-purpose gluten-free flour mix (Bob's Red Mill is a good brand)
1½ tablespoons coconut palm sugar
1 teaspoon ground cardamom

For the Vanilla Cream
½ cup raw cashews, soaked in 2 cups of water for 30 minutes, then strained
1 teaspoon vanilla extract
1 to 2 tablespoons coconut nectar
¾ to 1 cup water

First, make the vanilla cream. Place all the ingredients for the cream in a blender and blend on a high setting, adding enough water to create a smooth and creamy consistency thin enough to drizzle. Pour the cream into a jar, and set aside.

Next, make the crêpes. In a large bowl, whisk the eggs, then stir in the melted coconut oil and almond milk. In another bowl, combine the flour mix, coconut palm sugar, and cardamom, then mix the dry ingredients into the wet ingredients. If the batter is too thick, add more almond milk 1 tablespoon at a time until the final consistency is thick but runny.

Oil well a 5- to 6-inch skillet and heat it until it's very hot. Pour into the pan about ¼ cup of the crêpe batter and cook the crêpe for about 1 to 2 minutes before flipping it and cooking for another 30 to 45 seconds. Set the crêpe aside, repeating these steps until all the batter is used up.

Lay the cooked crêpes on a cutting board and fill the center of each with some of the fresh fruit and chopped mint. Roll the crêpes, arrange them on serving plates, and drizzle them with the vanilla cream.

*Contains eggs

AVOCADO CHOCOLATE PUDDING

Stacy Keibler, entrepreneur, SK Philosophy

C Cleanse

G Gut

V Vegan

Serves: 1 to 2

Prep time: 5 minutes

Refrigeration time: 30 minutes

This dish is the perfect portion size for nights when you are having chocolate or sweet cravings but don't want to overindulge. I know I have a serious sweet tooth, so I always whip up a bit when I'm feeling the need for a sweet but satisfying treat! Free of preservatives, sugar, dairy, and wheat, this avocado pudding is the most nutritious option, perfect for children's school lunches, adults, and all chocolate addicts!

This pudding is simple and inexpensive, taking only about 5 minutes of your time. Make a big batch for the whole week, and store it in the fridge to keep fresh and ready to enjoy. Regardless of how much you decide to make, you don't have to feel guilty if you finish the whole bowl of avocado pudding, because it's not only addicting and delicious, it's completely healthy. Enjoy!

Flesh of 1 ripe avocado
¼ cup cacao powder
¼ cup almond milk
1 teaspoon vanilla extract
1 teaspoon coconut oil
1 tablespoon coconut butter
2 droppers chocolate liquid stevia
2 teaspoons xylitol

Place all the ingredients in a blender and blend on a high setting until the mixture is a pudding-like consistency, which shouldn't be more than 1 minute. Taste and adjust for sweetness. If it doesn't seem sweet enough, add 1 more dropper of chocolate liquid stevia. Then scoop the pudding into a bowl and place it in the fridge for 30 minutes.

Garnish the pudding with any desired toppings before serving, such as shredded coconut, ground cinnamon, fresh berries, nuts, granola, cacao nibs, or a dollop of almond butter!

MINI RASPBERRY AND COCONUT CREAM TARTS

C Cleanse

V Vegan

Makes: 4 mini tarts

Prep time: 30 minutes

Elegant, sweet, and delectable, these are true treats that fit every occasion. Definitely adjust the filling for what ingredients are local and in season where you live, and you'll have an endlessly surprising dessert.

You will need four mini tart pans for this recipe, each about 3 inches in diameter.

For the Crusts
1 cup whole raw pecans
¾ cup grated unsweetened coconut
4 teaspoons coconut oil, melted
8 soft Medjool dates
½ teaspoon vanilla extract
Pinch of sea salt

For the Filling
1 cup unsweetened coconut milk
1 cup coconut butter, softened in a double boiler
2½ tablespoons coconut palm sugar
1 cup frozen raspberries

For the Topping
1 pint fresh raspberries
Ground cinnamon for dusting

First, make the crusts. In a food processor, combine all the ingredients for the crust until the mixture is crumbly but moist enough to form a ball in your hand. Divide the mixture into four portions and press each portion into the four tart pans. Place the pans in the fridge to set while you prepare the filling.

Place all the ingredients for the filling in a blender and blend on a high setting until smooth, then pour the filling into the set tart shells. Top each with some fresh berries and a sprinkle of cinnamon. Place them back into the fridge to set further before serving.

Note: Because of the coconut, the crust may want to stick to the tin after it has cooled. If so, use a knife to crack the seal, then tip the pan gently (tapping the bottom) to remove the tart.

CASHEW NO-BAKE COOKIES

C Cleanse   **Makes:** about 20 1-ounce cookies

V Vegan   **Prep time:** 15 to 20 minutes

These are wonderful energy powerhouses, a cross between a treat and a protein bar. These are quick and easy since there's no cooking required. Great fun for kids to help make.

4 cups raw cashews
¼ cup soft dates (pitted)
1 teaspoon vanilla bean powder
3 tablespoons coconut oil, melted
4 drops lemon extract
¼ cup plus 2 tablespoons coconut butter (manna, not oil)
Pinch of sea salt
2 to 4 drops liquid stevia or 2 tablespoons coconut nectar

In a food processor, combine all the ingredients until the mixture forms a ball. Test its consistency by squeezing a pinch of the cashew mixture. It should hold together.

Using a spoon, scoop approximately 20 equal portions of the dough and form each into cookie shapes in your hand. Place the cookies onto a parchment-lined baking sheet, then chill in the fridge or freezer until they harden.

PEACH PIE

Farrell Feighan, Clean team blogger

C Cleanse

V Vegan

Makes: 1 9-inch pie

Prep time: 1 hour

Cooking time: 45 minutes

As soon as summer starts to turn to fall, I experience an immediate urge to bake pie. This peach pie is the perfect blend of sweet and savory and is best served with whipped coconut cream or all-natural ice cream. Enjoy it with friends!

For the Crust
2 cups brown rice flour
½ cup coconut oil, plus about 1 to 2 tablespoons melted for brushing the crust before baking
6 to 10 tablespoons water

For the Filling
5 cups sliced fresh peaches
2 tablespoons lemon juice
½ cup brown rice flour
½ cup coconut palm sugar
1 teaspoon ground cinnamon
¼ teaspoon ground nutmeg
¼ teaspoon sea salt

First, make the crust. In a large bowl, combine the brown rice flour and coconut oil. Use two butter knives to cut the flour and oil together until the mixture resembles coarse crumbs. Stir in the water, 1 tablespoon at a time, until the mixture forms a ball. Wrap the dough in plastic and refrigerate it for 1 hour.

Preheat the oven to 450°F.

Take the dough out of the fridge and divide into two parts. Roll the two parts of dough flat into roughly 9-inch circles. Line the bottom and sides of a 9-inch pie plate with one of the pie crusts and brush it with coconut oil so the crust does not get soggy while baking.

Place the sliced peaches in a large bowl, and sprinkle them with the lemon juice. Stir the peaches gently.

In a separate bowl, combine the flour, sugar, cinnamon, nutmeg, and salt. Pour the dry ingredients over the peaches, and mix them gently.

Fill the pie crust with the peach mixture, then cover it with the second pie crust. Fold the edges of the crusts under and press the edges together to seal them with the tines of a fork. Brush the top of the pie with coconut oil, then with a sharp knife cut several slits in the top crust to vent steam while the pie cooks.

Bake the pie for 10 minutes, then reduce the heat to 350°F and bake for an additional 35 minutes, until the crust is brown and the juice begins to bubble through the vents. About halfway through baking, cover the edges of the crust with strips of aluminum foil, to keep them from burning.

Cool the pie before serving. It is enjoyed best warm, not hot.

Peach Pie Afternoon by the Clean Team

We were steadily working away one afternoon in our Santa Monica office. Slowly we began to notice an exquisite smell wafting up from the kitchen. Pulled from our computers, we ran down the steps to see what was being prepared. Our team member, Farrell, on a whim, had had the urge to make a Peach Pie. A few minutes before, she had pulled it from the oven and the pie was now cooling on the counter. We each had a piece and fell over in food ecstasy. This pie was incredible. Our idea of what a clean dessert could be was changed forever. We knew we had to include it here. Now whenever we feel the urge for something sweet at the office, we look to Farrell hoping the whim will strike her again.

SNICKER BARS

C Cleanse
V Vegan*

Makes: 12 bars
Prep time: 1 hour

People are jumping on the make-your-own candy bandwagon and it's such a cool trend. We're happy to give what we think is one of the healthiest homemade candy bars out there. These are addictively good, but don't worry, they're lower glycemic and packed with healthy fat and protein, both of which keep blood sugar levels stable and metabolism fired up.

For the Base
2 cups plus 2 tablespoons raw almonds
2 tablespoons almond flour
1 tablespoon mesquite meal
⅛ teaspoon sea salt
¼ cup coconut nectar or honey (if not on cleanse)

For the Filling
1 cup packed dates (about a dozen), pits removed
2 tablespoons water
Just under ¼ teaspoon sea salt
½ teaspoon vanilla extract
1 tablespoon coconut oil, melted
¼ cup chopped raw almonds

For the Chocolate Topping
1 pound baking chocolate, 70 percent cacao or higher, cut into smaller chunks
1 teaspoon vanilla extract
½ cup finely ground coconut palm sugar
Pinch of sea salt

Preheat the oven to 350°F.

First, make the base dough. Spread the almonds on a baking sheet and toast them in the oven for 10 to 12 minutes, stirring occasionally, until they are lightly browned. Remove them from the oven and let them cool. Set aside 2 tablespoons of the almonds for a garnish, and roughly chop them.

Place the remaining 2 cups of toasted almonds in a food processor, and chop them finely. Add the almond flour, mesquite meal, salt, and honey or coconut nectar, and process further, using a spatula as needed to scrape down the sides, until the mixture begins to form a ball.

Shape the dough into 12 even-size cookies, just under 1 inch wide. Place them on a parchment-lined baking sheet and keep them in the fridge or freezer for 15 minutes to harden.

*Using coconut nectar

After the cookie bases have hardened, make the filling. Place all the ingredients for the filling into a blender and blend on a high setting until the mixture forms a smooth paste. Use a spoon or transfer the mixture to a pastry bag to spread a layer on top of each cookie. Place these in the fridge to set for 15 minutes. For the chocolate topping, place the chunks of baking chocolate in a double boiler and heat them slowly until they are fully melted. Stir in the vanilla, coconut palm sugar, and salt. Use a whisk, blender, or food processor to combine all the ingredients well.

Line a baking sheet with parchment paper and set a cooling rack on top of the baking sheet. Place the cookies on the cooling rack. Use a ladle to drizzle just enough chocolate topping to cover each entire cookie-and-filling mound. Once each is fully covered, top each with the reserved chopped almonds. Again, place them in the fridge to set, storing them there until ready to eat, about 30 minutes.

Save any extra chocolate topping in a jar or pour it into molds for a delicious candy-like treat.

HONEY PECAN BALLS

V Vegan

Makes: 12 balls

Prep time: 15 minutes

These are sweet little morsels of decadent goodness. Protein-rich from both the nuts and the honey, they use a sweetener that actually has enzymes to add to your store and help digestion. Healthy fats from the coconut butter help keep blood sugar levels stable and metabolism fired up. These are energy bars that taste like dessert.

2 cups raw pecans
½ cup coconut butter
2 tablespoons honey or coconut nectar
1 teaspoon freshly ground nutmeg
½ teaspoon vanilla extract
Pinch of sea salt

Place all the ingredients in a food processor and combine them until the mixture forms a ball. In your hands or with a melon scoop, form the dough into 1-inch balls. Place them in the fridge to set and store any extras also in the fridge for several weeks.

Chef Frank on Honey

Honey is a wonderful natural sweetener that contains enzymes and proteins. It strengthens the immune system, is antibacterial and antiviral, and has been known to help seasonal allergies, stabilize blood pressure, and balance blood sugar. It's also an anti-inflammatory, antioxidant-rich food that is one of the oldest sources of energy and sweetness known to man (and animals). When purchasing honey, look for varieties that are local and raw, unpasteurized or unheated, as they will be the most nutritious.

CLEAN CHOCOLATE

C Cleanse

G Gut*

V Vegan

Makes: about 2 pounds

Prep time: 30 minutes

Refrigeration time: 15 minutes

Yes! The rumors about the health benefits of chocolate are true. So make your own for the healthiest chocolate out there. You can vary it based on your sweet tooth (or lack of one) and any spices or additions, such as coconut or nuts, that you prefer. Add in herbs and tinctures to make your own medicinal treats.

1½ pounds cacao butter, roughly chopped into chunks
3 cups cacao powder (sifted before measuring)
½ cup mesquite meal
Pinch sea salt
1 teaspoon vanilla extract
¼ cup granulated coconut palm sugar

Place the cacao butter pieces into a double boiler or a small metal bowl set over a pot of hot water. Heat the butter slowly until it's fully melted. Remove it from the heat, transfer it to a large bowl, and whisk or blend in the cacao powder, mesquite meal, salt, vanilla, and coconut sugar.

Pour the chocolate into molds or ice cube trays, or spread it with a spatula onto a parchment-lined baking sheet. Place it in the fridge to set and keep it refrigerated.

*Omit coconut palm sugar; use stevia, xylitol, or Lakanto

FREEZER FUDGE

C Cleanse

V Vegan

Makes: about 1 pound

Prep time: 20 minutes

Refrigeration time: 2 hours or overnight

No one will ever know this doesn't contain sugar or dairy. Shhh, it's our clean little secret. Our freezer fudge is a great source of antioxidants, metabolism-boosting fats, and stimulating cacao.

1 tablespoon coconut oil
1 cup unsweetened coconut milk
12 ounces dark or baking chocolate, 70% or higher, chopped into smaller chunks
1 teaspoon ground cinnamon
2 teaspoons mesquite meal
½ teaspoon vanilla extract
¼ teaspoon sea salt
2 tablespoons coconut palm sugar
½ cup cacao powder for dusting

In a saucepan set over low heat, slowly warm the coconut oil and coconut milk.

In a large bowl, combine the chopped chocolate, cinnamon, mesquite meal, vanilla, and salt. When the coconut milk mixture is hot, pour it over the chocolate and stir until all the chocolate is completely melted and a thick consistency is achieved.

Transfer the mixture to a parchment-lined baking dish or baking sheet, doing your best to mold it into a ½-inch-thick log. Place the fudge in the freezer for a few hours or in the fridge overnight to harden.

When it's ready to serve, cut it into chunks and dust each chunk with cacao powder.

Chocolate Love by the Clean Team

Chocolate is one of our favorite desserts. It's also a great item to make with friends, family, and kids. Try making larger batches using clean ingredients so you have something to satisfy your sweet tooth free of sugar, dairy, and chemicals. Dried cacao or cocoa powder can also quickly be made into a comforting drink by adding a tablespoon or two to warm almond milk, a pinch of salt, and a dash of stevia or honey.

ROASTED CASHEW CURRANT BARK

C Cleanse

V Vegan

Serves: 4, as a snack

Prep time: 30 minutes

Refrigeration time: 20 minutes

This would make a wonderfully healthy and antioxidant-rich holiday treat for everyone on your list, especially if you make large batches. Wrap a handful of pieces in parchment or brown paper, and tie them up with a pretty ribbon and a sprig of evergreen or rosemary tucked inside. What better gift than the gift of health?

1 cup raw cashews
16 ounces Clean Chocolate (page 281)
½ cup dried currants
¼ cup shredded unsweetened coconut

Preheat the oven to 350°F.

Place the cashews on a baking sheet and toast them in the oven until they are golden brown, about 8 to 10 minutes, stirring and checking them occasionally so they don't burn. Remove them from the oven, let them cool, and chop them into smaller pieces.

When making the Clean Chocolate recipe, don't allow the 2 cups of it needed for this treat to set in the fridge but to instead remain soft. Place it in a bowl and stir in the cashews, currants, and coconut. Spread the mixture onto a parchment-lined baking sheet, and set it in the fridge or freezer to harden for 20 minutes. Once the chocolate is set, break up into smaller pieces and store them for months in the freezer.

CINNAMON-BAKED APPLES

C Cleanse

V Vegan

Serves: 2

Prep time: 15 minutes

Cooking time: 20 minutes

A very simple after-dinner treat; this is also just the thing on a cold morning. Whenever you make it, be prepared for your entire house to smell irresistibly delicious.

2 large crisp apples (we love using any local heirloom variety or a mix of them)
2 teaspoons ground cinnamon
3 to 4 tablespoons coconut palm sugar
½ teaspoon vanilla extract
¼ teaspoon ground clove

Preheat the oven to 375°F.

Peel and core the apples. Cut them in half, then into ⅛- to ¼-inch-thick slices. Place the slices in the center of a piece of parchment paper that is about 18 inches long. Top the slices with the cinnamon, coconut palm sugar, and vanilla. Gently toss the mixture, then bring the two ends of the parchment together and roll them toward the apples. Crumple up the ends to make an apple-filled pouch.

Place the pouch on a baking sheet and bake for 15 to 20 minutes. Remove from the oven, unwrap the pouch, and serve the apples in a bowl as is, or with a scoop of your favorite ice cream, whipped cream, or gelato.

ALMOND SPICE COOKIES

C Cleanse

G Gut*

V Vegan

Makes: 12 cookies

Prep time: 10 minutes plus 30 minutes to 24 hours
refrigeration time

Cooking time: 10 minutes

This is a great cookie recipe to make any time of year, and something kids will love to help with (and of course probably want to lick the spoon and bowl). The dough is as tasty as the cookies, so feel free to use it as you would uncooked cookie dough (aka eating straight from the bowl) or as a post-workout snack that's easy to travel with in a plastic container.

2½ cups almond flour
2 tablespoons coconut flour
½ cup arrowroot powder
1 teaspoon baking soda
¼ teaspoon sea salt
1 teaspoon ground cinnamon, plus more for sprinkling
¼ cup plus 1 tablespoon coconut oil, melted
½ cup coconut nectar
1 teaspoon almond extract

In a large bowl, combine the flours, baking soda, salt, and cinnamon. Stir in the melted coconut oil, coconut nectar, and almond extract. Mix just until everything is combined.

Wrap the dough in plastic wrap, tightening the sides and shaping it to form a long, even cylinder. Place it in the fridge to solidify, for a minimum of 30 minutes or up to one day.

When you're ready to bake the cookies, preheat the oven to 350°F.

Remove the dough from the plastic wrap and slice it into ¼-inch rounds. Place the cookies on a parchment-lined baking dish, and sprinkle each cookie with cinnamon. Bake them for 5 minutes, then flip each cookie and bake them for an additional 4 to 5 minutes, until they feel set.

*Omit coconut nectar; use stevia, xylitrol, or Lakanto

COCONUT ALMOND TAPIOCA PUDDING

Maribeth Evezich, dietitian and blogger

Ⓒ Cleanse

Ⓖ Gut

Ⓥ Vegan

Serves: 4

My mother would make tapioca pudding for special occasions, such as my father's birthday. I have "cleaned up" this childhood favorite, making it vegan and sugar-free. Be conservative with your sweetener, as the coconut milk, especially when condensed through cooking, provides ample sweetness. If it doesn't seem sweet enough at the end, consider adding a pinch of sea salt which balances the flavors rather than adding extra sweetener. I favor the large pearl tapioca for the toothy texture it creates, but the small pearl variety will also work. Just don't use "minute" tapioca.

3 tablespoons ground pearls or tapioca flour
⅓ cup large or small pearl tapioca
2 cups unsweetened almond milk
1 cup unsweetened coconut milk
¼ teaspoon sea salt
½ teaspoon almond or vanilla extract
Stevia to taste

In a spice grinder or blender, process the 3 tablespoons of tapioca pearls until they are a powder consistency (or use tapioca flour). In a bowl, combine the ground tapioca with the whole pearl tapioca and 1 cup of the almond milk. Stir the mixture thoroughly and let the tapioca soak for 2 hours, refrigerated. (If you are using large pearl tapioca, it can soak overnight.)

Combine the remaining cup of almond milk, the coconut milk, and the salt in a 2-quart saucepan. Add the soaked tapioca and almond milk mixture, whisking or stirring until it is well combined. Stirring constantly, bring the mixture to a boil over medium heat, about 12 to 15 minutes. Lower the heat and, continuing to stir often, let the mixture simmer for another 15 to 20 minutes. When the tapioca is translucent, turn the heat back up to medium, add the almond or vanilla extract and stevia, and continue to cook until the mixture thickens, stirring constantly. Adjust the sweetener and salt to taste.

Serve the pudding warm or cooled. If you wish to refrigerate it before serving, let it cool and place a piece of parchment paper directly on the surface of the pudding to prevent a skin forming.

BLACKBERRY POMEGRANATE MOUSSE

Ⓒ Cleanse

Ⓖ Gut

Makes: 3 cups

Prep time: 20 minutes

Refrigeration time: 2 to 3 hours to "set"

Gelatin made from grass-fed cows is incredibly healing for the gut. We love the Great Lakes brand. This is a wonderfully gut-building dessert and a great healthy treat that kids love. You could just as easily serve this gorgeous dessert at a dinner party and you'll receive rave reviews from adults too!

1 13.5-ounce can unsweetened coconut milk
1 tablespoon Great Lakes gelatin
½ cup cold water
½ pint fresh or frozen and thawed blackberries
½ teaspoon vanilla extract
2 tablespoons pomegranate concentrate
¼ cup pomegranate seeds

Heat half of the coconut milk (6.75 ounces) in a saucepan set over medium heat.

While the coconut milk is warming up, dissolve the gelatin in cold water in a medium bowl. Then stir the heated coconut milk into the gelatin water. Once it's mixed, stir in the remaining (unheated) half of the coconut milk.

Pour the mixture into a blender along with the blackberries, vanilla, and pomegranate concentrate. Purée the mixture, fold in the pomegranate seeds, then pour it into either silicon molds or ramekins. Place them in the fridge for several hours to set. You can also sprinkle the pomegranate seeds on top when you're ready to serve.

OUR PROGRAMS

Clean Cleanse | cleanprogram.com

The Clean Cleanse is a twenty-one-day program designed to support the body's natural ability to heal itself. It focuses on cleansing and detoxification through a mixture of dietary change and supplementation. The program was created to be easily incorporated into a busy schedule while providing all the practical tools necessary to support and rejuvenate the body. The effect is transformative. Typical benefits include improved skin, sleep, digestion, energy, and mental clarity with a reduction in bloating, constipation, headaches, and joint pain.

The program consists of a nutrient-dense shake for breakfast, a solid meal from the Cleanse diet for lunch, and a shake for dinner. Throughout the day you will also take a few key supplements. After your twenty-one-day program is complete, we lead you through a reintroduction process and continued education to help you stay clean beyond your cleanse.

Clean Gut Program | cleangut.com

All of today's most-diagnosed ailments can be traced back to an injured and irritated gut. The gut is an intricate and powerful system, naturally designed to protect and heal the body every moment of every day. And yet for far too many of us, this remarkable system is in disrepair, leading to all kinds of health problems—from extra pounds, aches and pains, allergies, mood swings, and lack of libido to heart disease, cancer, autoimmune disorders, insomnia, and depression.

The Clean Gut program is a twenty-one-day program that gets to the root of health and disease by supporting digestive health and gut repair. The program follows a simple structure that starts with a shake in the morning, a lunch meal and an evening salad from the Clean Gut diet, and a powerful combination of gut-restorative supplements.

Refresh | cleanprogram.com

Everyone falls off track with their health from time to time. Falling off track isn't a big deal. It's normal, but it becomes a problem when we stay off track. What we need is a reminder from time to time, a reminder of simple health principles that work.

Refresh is a seven-day structured program you do between cleanses that focuses on supporting energy levels, good digestion, and mental clarity. The program consists of a shake for breakfast and dinner with some targeted supplements. In the afternoon, you will have a lunch meal from the Refresh diet and a Refresh Boost. The Refresh Boost is a powerful combination of B vitamins formulated to help with stress and reduce after-meal sluggishness. After seven days on the program, your body will be primed to continue making healthier food and lifestyle choices.

21-DAY CLEAN CLEANSE MEAL PLAN

	Breakfast	Lunch	Dinner
MONDAY	Blackberry Coconut Milk Shake, p. 256	Thai Marinated Turkey Breast, p. 164	Mushroom Parsnip Stew (puréed), p. 231
TUESDAY	Reishi Cappuccino, p. 253	Mushroom Risotto, p. 220	Broccoli Cheddar Soup (puréed), p. 244
WEDNESDAY	Adam's A.M. Pre-Workout Shake, p. 254	Lemon Herb Chicken Burgers with Thousand Island Dressing, p. 156	Mango Slushie, p. 258
THURSDAY	Just Peachy, p. 259	Poached Cod with Soba Noodles and Ponzu Sauce, p. 146	Mushroom Parsnip Stew (puréed), p. 231
FRIDAY	Almond "Milk" with your choice of proteins, powders, and greens, p. 246	Roasted Cauliflower with Pistachio Dressing, p. 203	Gingered Carrot Purée (heated with coconut milk for a thick soup), p. 104
SATURDAY	Blackberry Coconut Milk Shake, p. 256	Savory Lentil Loaf, p. 218	Almond "Milk" with your choice of proteins, powders, and greens, p. 246
SUNDAY	Reishi Cappuccino, p. 253	Garlic-Crusted Chicken, p. 162	Blackberry Coconut Milk Shake, p. 256
MONDAY	Mango Slushie, p. 258	Zucchini-Wrapped Whitefish with Chive Oil, p. 144	Broccoli Cheddar Soup (puréed), p. 244
TUESDAY	Dreamy Blueberry Smoothie, p. 261	Stuffed Mushrooms and Asian Lettuce Wraps, pp. 111 and 112	Almond "Milk" with your choice of proteins, powders, and greens, p. 246
WEDNESDAY	Blackberry Coconut Milk Shake, p. 256	Salmon Stir-Fry, p. 150	Cucumber Avocado Soup (chilled or warmed), p. 235
THURSDAY	Just Peachy, p. 259	Sesame Noodles (add extra protein like chicken if you wish), p. 193	Mushroom Parsnip Stew (puréed), p. 231
FRIDAY	Almond "Milk" with your choice of proteins, powders, and greens, p. 246	Wild Rice with Middle Eastern Flavors (omit tomatoes), p. 210	Malted Maca Milk Shake, p. 260
SATURDAY	Healing Chocolate Elixir, p. 262	Crispy Roasted Chicken (serve with mixed greens dressed with balsamic vinegar), p. 169	Carrot, Cumin, and Cauliflower Soup (puréed), p. 232
SUNDAY	Mango Slushie, p. 258	Roasted Cauliflower with Pistachio Dressing, p. 203	Roasted Cauliflower with Pistachio Dressing (puréed into a soup), p. 203
MONDAY	Dreamy Blueberry Smoothie, p. 261	Pan-Roasted Halibut, p. 137	Blackberry Coconut Milk Shake, p. 256
TUESDAY	Malted Maca Milk Shake, p. 260	Roasted Cabbage with Chipotle and Caraway Sour Cream, p. 214	Almond "Milk" with your choice of proteins, powders, and greens, p. 246
WEDNESDAY	Blackberry Coconut Milk Shake, p. 256	Mustard-Baked Chicken, p. 159	Reishi Cappucino, p. 253
THURSDAY	Just Peachy, p. 259	Greek Quinoa with Hearts of Palm, p. 202	Healing Chocolate Elixir, p. 262
FRIDAY	Malted Maca Milk Shake, p. 260	Slow-Cooked Chicken with Fennel and Wild Mushrooms, p. 161	Onion Soup (puréed), p. 229
SATURDAY	Reishi Cappuccino, p. 253	Roasted Vegetables with Silky Hummus, p. 213	Malted Maca Milk Shake, p. 260
SUNDAY	Almond "Milk" with your choice of proteins, powders, and greens, p. 246	Harissa-Coated Haddock, p. 151	Mushroom Parsnip Soup (puréed), p. 231

21-DAY CLEAN GUT MEAL PLAN

	Breakfast	Lunch	Dinner
MONDAY	Malted Maca Milk Shake, p. 260	Vegetable Frittata, p. 56	Romaine and Sea Vegetable Salad, p. 64
TUESDAY	Adam's A.M. Pre-Workout Shake, p. 254	Sunken Eggs, p. 53	Chicken Paillard with Butternut Squash, p. 66
WEDNESDAY	Clean Hot Cocoa, p. 263	Coconut Zucchini Noodles and Spiced Meatballs, p. 184	Bitter Greens and Herb Salad, p. 70
THURSDAY	Blackberry Coconut Milk Shake, p. 256	Portobello Steaks with Mashed Celery Root, p. 221	Sesame Bok Choy Salad, p. 71
FRIDAY	Dreamy Blueberry Smoothie, p. 261	Chicken with Kale and Olives, p. 170	Spirulina Sprout Salad, p. 75
SATURDAY	Healing Chocolate Elixir, p. 262	Baked Turnip Casserole, p. 217	Smoked Salmon and Fennel Salad, p. 81
SUNDAY	Reishi Cappuccino, p. 253	Lemon and Thyme Baked Sea Bass, p. 138	Chinese Chicken Salad, p. 83
MONDAY	Malted Maca Milk Shake, p. 260	Vegetable Napoleon, p. 212	Romaine and Sea Vegetable Salad, p. 64
TUESDAY	Adam's A.M. Pre-Workout Shake, p. 254	Charred Lemon-Broiled Sole, p. 135	Chicken Paillard with Butternut Squash, p. 66
WEDNESDAY	Clean Hot Cocoa, p. 263	Garlic-Crusted Chicken, p. 162	Bitter Greens and Herb Salad, p. 70
THURSDAY	Blackberry Coconut Milk Shake, p. 256	Zucchini Manicotti, p. 197	Sesame Bok Choy Salad, p. 71
FRIDAY	Dreamy Blueberry Smoothie, p. 261	Lamb and Wild Mushroom Stuffed Eggplant, p. 176	Spirulina Sprout Salad, p. 75
SATURDAY	Healing Chocolate Elixir, p. 262	Egg Salad, p. 76	Smoked Salmon and Fennel Salad, p. 81
SUNDAY	Reishi Cappuccino, p. 253	Pan-Roasted Halibut, p. 137	Chinese Chicken Salad, p. 83
MONDAY	Malted Maca Milk Shake, p. 260	Baked Spaghetti Squash, p. 216	Romaine and Sea Vegetable Salad, p. 64
TUESDAY	Adam's A.M. Pre-Workout Shake, p. 254	Roasted Lamb Loin, p. 183	Chicken Paillard with Butternut Squash, p. 66
WEDNESDAY	Clean Hot Cocoa, p. 263	Lemon and Thyme Baked Sea Bass, p. 138	Bitter Greens and Herb Salad, p. 70
THURSDAY	Blackberry Coconut Milk Shake, p. 256	Mushroom Parsnip Stew, p. 231	Sesame Bok Choy Salad, p. 71
FRIDAY	Dreamy Blueberry Smoothie, p. 261	Chicken Osso Bucco, p. 166	Spirulina Sprout Salad, p. 75
SATURDAY	Healing Chocolate Elixir, p. 262	Herbed Buffalo Burgers, p. 187	Smoked Salmon and Fennel Salad, p. 81
SUNDAY	Reishi Cappuccino, p. 253	Chicken with Kale and Olives, p. 170	Chinese Chicken Salad, p. 83

7-DAY CLEAN REFRESH MEAL PLAN

	Breakfast	Lunch	Dinner
MONDAY	Malted Maca Milk Shake, p. 260	Farmers' Market Salad, p. 79	Mushroom Parsnip Stew (puréed), p. 231
TUESDAY	Adam's A.M. Pre-Workout Shake, p. 254	Shredded Chicken (over mixed greens), p. 168	Malted Maca Milk Shake, p. 260
WEDNESDAY	Clean Hot Cocoa, p. 263	Egg Salad, p. 76	Carrot, Cumin, and Cauliflower Soup (puréed), p. 232
THURSDAY	Blackberry Coconut Milk Shake, p. 256	Gingered Beef Ramen, p. 185	Almond "Milk" (with your choice of protein powered and greens), p. 246
FRIDAY	Dreamy Blueberry Smoothie, p. 261	Smoked Salmon and Fennel Salad, p. 81	Blackberry Coconut Milk Shake, p. 256
SATURDAY	Healing Chocolate Elixir, p. 262	Garlicky Greens, p. 114; and Snappy Crackers, p. 127; with optional leftover Silky Hummus, p. 213	Onion Soup (puréed), p. 229
SUNDAY	Reishi Cappuccino, p. 253	Sunken Eggs, p. 53	Chicken and Wild Rice Soup, p. 242

CONTRIBUTORS

The community recipes in this book were created by guest contributors from diverse backgrounds. We hope their delicious creations inspire you to explore the world of clean eating and to make it your own.

Susana Belen   *Hearty Winter Soup (p. 230)*

Susana is the founder of We Care Spa, a holistic detoxification spa in Desert Hot Springs, California. WCS has been leading the movement of juice fasting and colonics to detox the body, the mind, and the spirit for over twenty-five years. Wecarespa.com.

Gabrielle Bernstein   *Apple Crisp (aka Miracle Crisp) (p. 271)*

Gabrielle is the *New York Times* bestselling author of *May Cause Miracles*. She appears regularly as an expert on NBC's *Today* show, has been featured on Oprah's *Super Soul Sunday* as a next-generation thought leader, and was named "a new role model" by the *New York Times*. She is also the author of the books *Add More ~ing to Your Life, Spirit Junkie,* and *Miracles Now*. Gabrielle is the founder of Herfuture.com, a social networking site for women to inspire, empower, and connect.

Orlando Bloom   *Salmon Scramble with Cauliflower and Dill Purée (p. 52)*

Orlando is an actor and UNICEF Goodwill Ambassador.

Alison Burger   *Cashew Almond Nut Butter (p. 130)*

Alison is a lifelong health and fitness enthusiast and a California native. Her financial consulting career eventually took a backseat to her passion for wellness. She is now instructing fitness classes in Los Angeles. She shares her health journey, fitness tips, and Clean recipes at Alisonburger.com.

Kris Carr   *Make Juice, Not War Green Juice (p. 250)*

Kris is a *New York Times* and number-one Amazon bestselling author, wellness activist, and cancer thriver. Her books include *Crazy Sexy Diet, Crazy Sexy Kitchen,* and *Crazy Sexy Cancer Tips*. Visit her website at Kriscarr.com.

Adam Cobb   *Adam's A.M. Pre-Workout Shake (p. 254)*

Coach Adam is the founder of FYCNYC, a health and wellness lifestyle brand. He is a coach, motivational speaker, and certified nutritional consultant who has spent the last ten years carving out his own unique perspective on health and wellness. Check out his method at Fycnyc.com.

Peggy and Megan Curry   *Spinach Patties (p. 192)*

Curry Girls Kitchen was created by mother-daughter duo Peggy and Megan. Peggy is also the cofounder of GrowingGreat, a nationwide community-based nonprofit nutrition education organization. Visit Peggy and Megan at Currygirlskitchen.com.

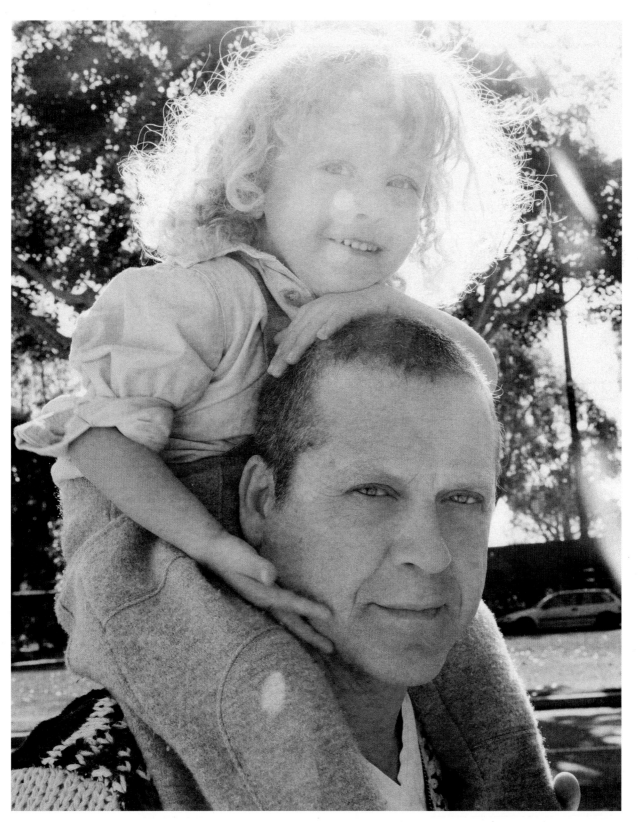

Market, Kitchen, Table: A day of clean eating with the Junger family

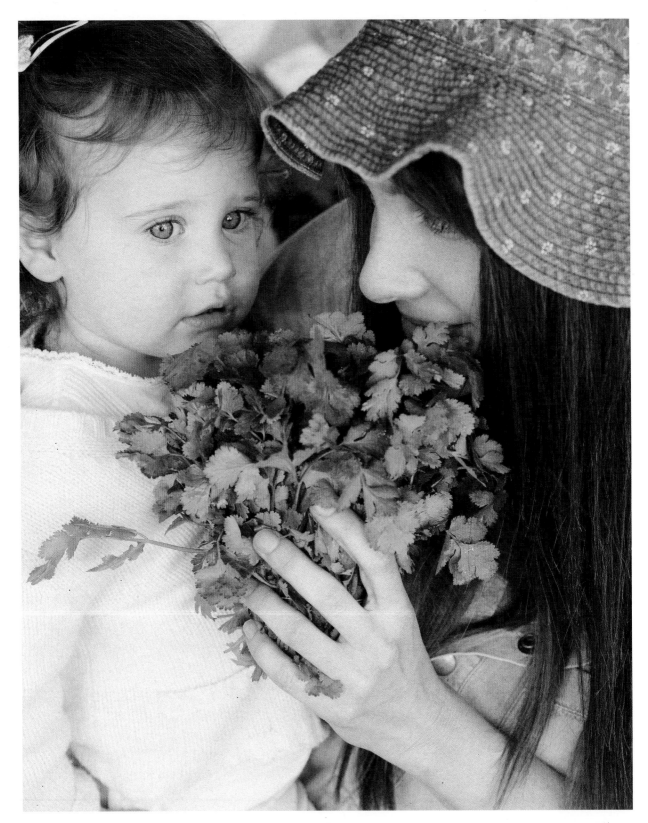

Market

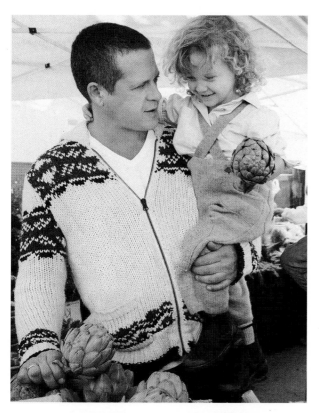

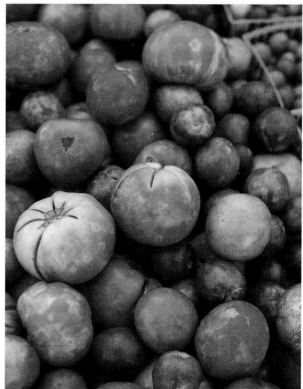

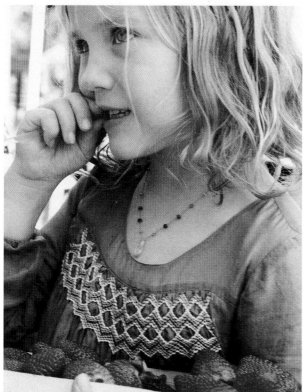

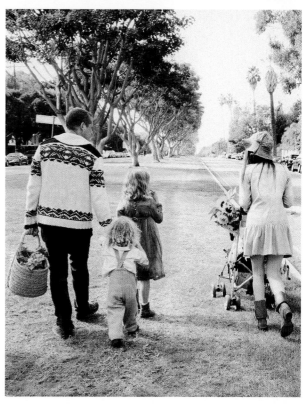

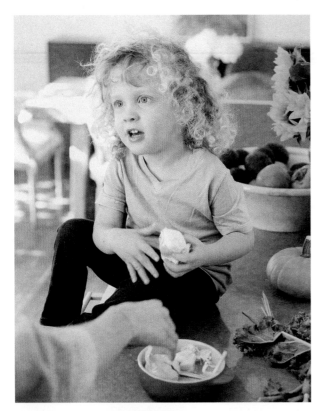
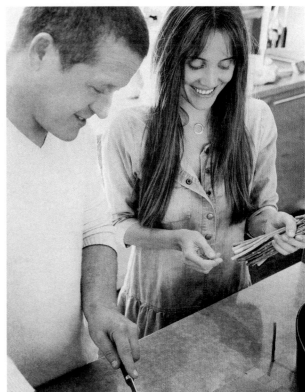
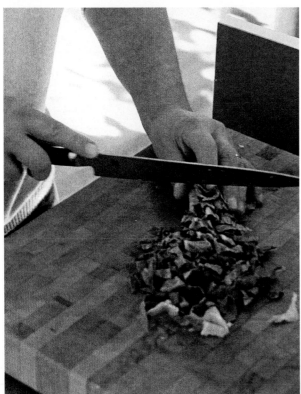
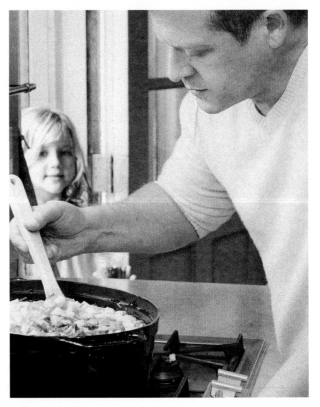

Kitchen

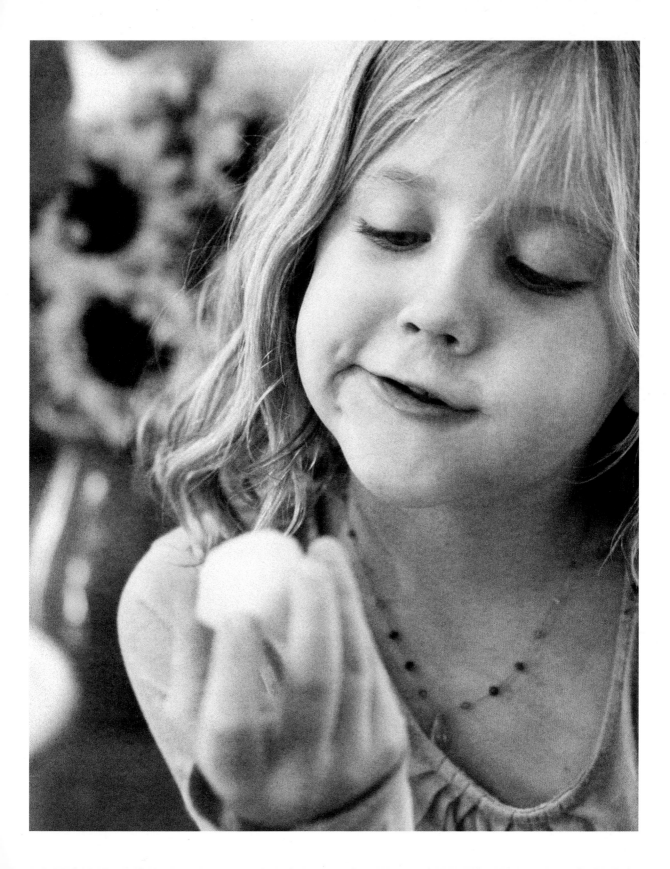

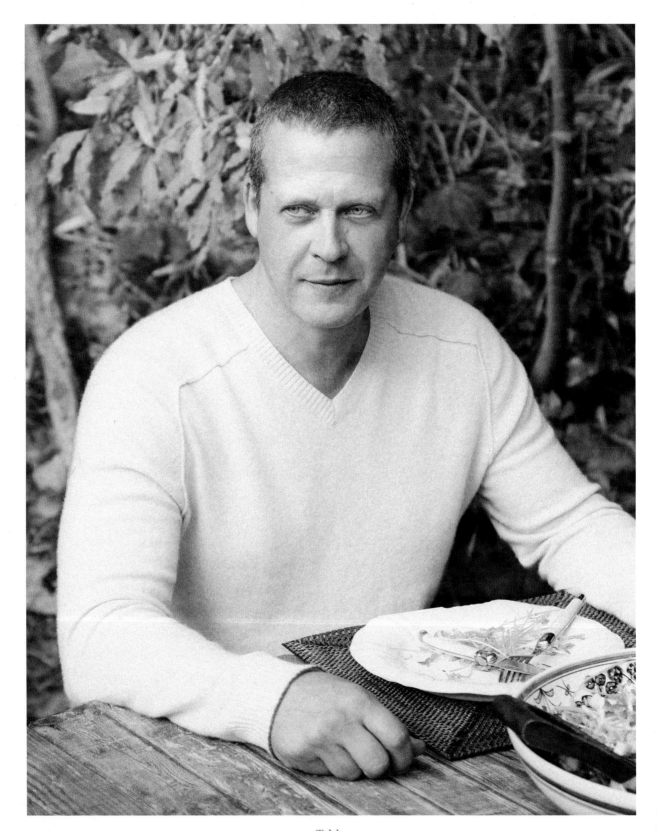

Table

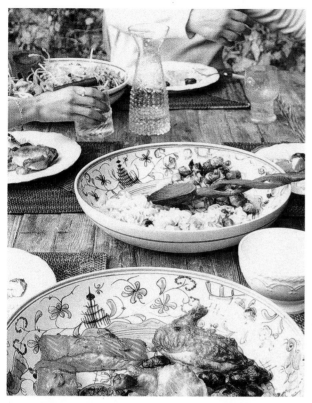
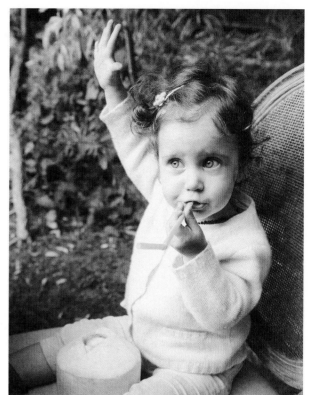
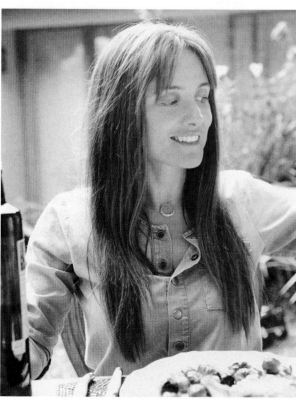
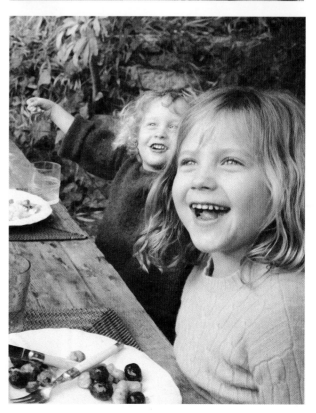

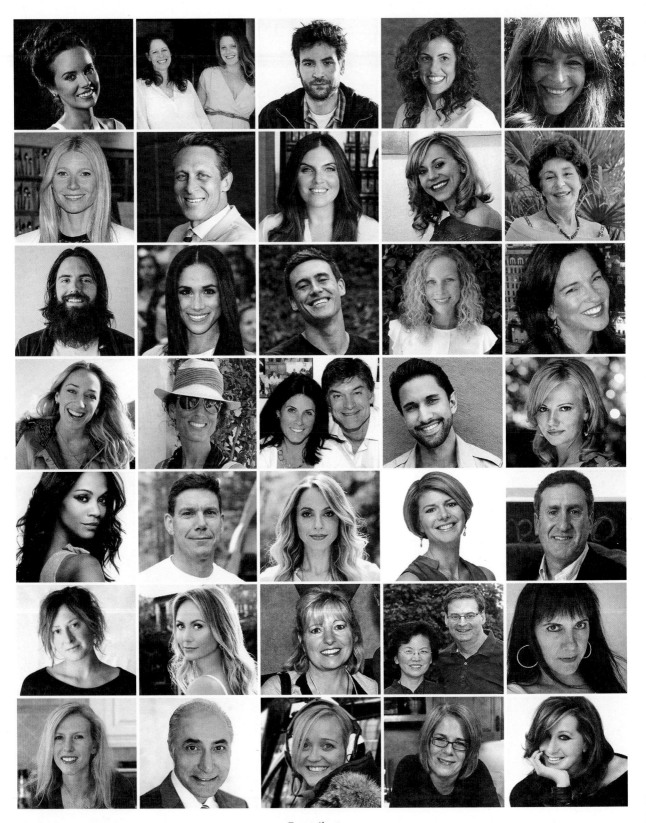

Contributors

Carly de Castro *Turmeric Almond Milk (p. 257)*
Carly co-founded Pressed Juicery in 2010 with Hayden Slater and Hedi Gores. There are currently eighteen locations throughout Southern and Northern California in addition to national delivery. Their first book, *JUICE: Recipes for Juicing, Cleansing and Living Well,* will be released in the summer of 2014 by Ten Speed Press.

Cameron Diaz *Everything Kale Salad (p. 69)*
Cameron is a lover of life, professional laugher, eater, and make-believer.

Maribeth Evezich *Coconut Almond Tapioca Pudding (p. 286)*
Maribeth has a passion for exploring and sharing the world of whole foods cooking. Following experiences cooking in the Oregon and California wine countries, Maribeth received her master's in nutrition from Bastyr University. A Seattle native, Maribeth currently lives in New York City. Check out her blog at Wholefoodsexplorer.com.

Lina Fedirko *Blueberry Quinoa Cereal (p. 44)*
Lina is a native Ukrainian professional living in New York City and working on issues related to urban adaptation in response to climate change.

Farrell Feighan *Peach Pie (p. 276)*
Farrell is a community support member on the Clean team. She is also the co-creator of Sisterdisco.com, a lifestyle blog that combines spiritual, health, and wellness topics with individual style, creativity, music, and art.

Janet Goldman Weinberg *Roasted Cauliflower and Chicken Sausage Casserole (p. 172)*
Janet is a personal chef currently residing in Highland Park, Illinois. She received a degree in culinary arts from Kendall College of Chicago. Her true passion is culinary nutrition: inspiring others to discover better health through eating a variety of local, seasonal, and sustainable foods.

Howie Greene *Vincent Arpino's Clean Brooklyn Sicilian Pizza Pie (p. 206)*
Howie's worked with both a president and a godfather, but he is most at home in his beloved New York City. Born and raised in Brooklyn, Howie is a real estate agent, college professor, and manager of The JB's, featuring former members of James Brown's bands. Howie started his career working as an intern for then-president Reagan and also managed James Brown for several years. He discovered the Clean program in

October 2012 and it changed his life. He's since finished the Clean Gut program and has lost fifty-one pounds and eight inches off his waist. His type 2 diabetes, high blood pressure, and high cholesterol are all gone. Missing his beloved Brooklyn Sicilian pizza, he devised his own clean style.

Michelle Hartgrove   *Zesty Roasted Chicken Salad (p. 84)*
Whether cooking a seasonal dish at home in beautiful Fuschl am See, a small village on a lake surrounded by mountains in Austria, or jet-setting across the globe as a talent manager for Red Bull, Michelle always knows that living clean gives her the fuel she needs to make her dreams a reality.

Mark Hyman, M.D.   *Cod with Roasted Chili Peppers and Cayenne (p. 140)*
Mark was co-medical director of Canyon Ranch for ten years and is now the chairman of the Institute for Functional Medicine and founder and medical director of the UltraWellness Center. He is the author of six *New York Times* bestsellers, including *The Blood Sugar Solution Cookbook, The Blood Sugar Solution, UltraMetabolism, The UltraMind Solution,* and *The UltraSimple Diet,* and a coauthor of *UltraPrevention.* Visit Dr. Hyman at Drhyman.com.

Paul Jaminet, Ph.D., and Shou-Ching Jaminet, Ph.D.   *Cambridge Fried Rice (p. 181)*
Paul is a former astrophysicist and entrepreneur turned health writer. He is editor-in-chief of the *Journal of Evolution and Health* and founder of the Perfect Health Retreat. Shou-Ching is a molecular biologist and cancer researcher at Harvard Medical School and Beth Israel Deaconess Medical Center in Boston. Together, they wrote *Perfect Health Diet: Regain Health and Lose Weight by Eating the Way You Were Meant to Eat* (Scribner, 2012). Their blog can be found at Perfecthealthdiet.com.

Donna Karan   *Forever-Green Soup and Salad (p. 80)*
Donna is a designer and founder of the Urban Zen Initiative.

Mary Karlin   *Chile Rellenos Stuffed with Mushrooms, Sweet Potatoes, and Chipotle Cashew Crema (p. 204)*
Mary is a passionate cook, a cooking teacher both online and at prominent culinary venues, and the author of three books: *Wood-Fired Cooking, Artisan Cheese Making at Home,* and *Mastering Fermentation.* Learn more at Marykarlin.com.

Stacy Keibler *Avocado Chocolate Pudding* (*p. 273*)

Stacy is a health advocate whose lifelong passion for all things health and fitness has allowed her to be on the path of educating herself and others about food and its direct connection to health, well-being, and life. She currently manages the website SKphilosophy.com, on which she shares her journey with the hopes that others will benefit from some of these insights.

Brent Kronk *Asian Lettuce Wraps* (*p. 112*)

In Columbus, Ohio, where Brent lives, there are plentiful fresh, organic produce and other ingredients at local farms and markets, making it easy to cook healthily and support the local community. She is an artist and works in marketing communications when she's not outside biking or feeding her birds.

Wanda LeBlanc-Rushmer *Mulligatawny Soup* (*p. 234*)

Wanda is an adoption social worker with a passion for working with children and families. She loves travel and adventure and has focused on health and wellness for many years. In her forties she developed digestive issues and reports that being clean has made a significant difference in her life.

Todd Lepine, M.D. *Clean and Green Guacamole* (*p. 123*)

Todd is a Dartmouth Medical School graduate and is board-certified in internal medicine. He has advanced expertise in integrative functional medicine. He has worked as a staff physician at Canyon Ranch Health Spa and now practices in western Massachusetts. His website is Drlepine.com.

Sarah Marchand *Sardines on Endives* (*p. 109*)

A native New Yorker, Sarah is a busy mother of twins who loves to cook. As a chronic sufferer of digestive problems, she has used clean eating strategies for years to help her and her family live a better, healthier life.

Meghan Markle *Spicy Cashew Dip* (*p. 93*)

Meghan is an actress and foodie.

Sarma Melngailis *Heirloom Tomato, Fennel, and Avocado Pressed Salad* (*p. 74*)

Sarma is a cofounder of Pure Food and Wine restaurant in New York City as well as the founder of One Lucky Duck, an e-commerce boutique selling One Lucky Duck snacks and more, and two New York juice bar locations. She is also the coauthor of *Raw Food Real World* and author of *Living Raw Food*.

Amy Myers, M.D.   *Coconut Curry (p. 160)*
Amy is the medical director of Austin UltraHealth and an expert in functional medicine and nutrition. People from around the world have recovered from chronic and debilitating health issues by following her program, The Myers Way. Her website is AmyMyersMD.com.

Jenny Nelson   *Banana Bread (p. 50)*
Having been on the Clean team since 2009, Jenny's been able to share her passions for eating locally and seasonally, for herbalism, and for women's health issues with thousands of people. She's a Clean wellness coach, an editorial and lifestyle photographer, and an outdoor junkie. She loves living on the ocean in Portland, Maine.

Lisa and Mehmet Oz   *Roasted Cauliflower with a Middle Eastern Twist (p. 99)*
Lisa is a producer, writer, bestselling author, and host of *The Lisa Oz Show*. Mehmet is an author, cardiothoracic surgeon, and Emmy Award–winning host of *The Dr. Oz Show*.

Gwyneth Paltrow   *Coconut Poached Salmon (p. 136)*
Gwyneth is a mother, health advocate, actor, and the founder of Goop.com.

Dhru Purohit   *Papa D's Fresh Fall Salad (p. 72)*
Dhru is a wellness sherpa and CEO of Clean.

Belinda Rachman, Esq.   *Best Dip / Sauce / Salad Dressing Ever (p. 125)*
Belinda is a family law attorney in Carlsbad, New Mexico, who lost forty pounds on the Clean program. She does nothing but peaceful divorce mediation with honest Southern California couples.

Josh Radnor   *Chunky Avocado Salad (p. 77)*
Josh is an American film director, actor, producer, and screenwriter.

Farshid Sam Rahbar, M.D., and Annie McRae, N.C.   *SeeReal Bars (p. 131)*
Farshid is a leading integrative gastroenterologist in Los Angeles, California. He is the founder and medical director of Los Angeles Integrative Gastroenterology and Nutrition, where he incorporates anti-aging and functional medicine for an integrative-holistic approach to digestive care. See Laintegrativegi.com.

Annie has been practicing clinical nutrition for fifteen years, specializing in the digestive system. She brings her nutrition expertise to California through personal consultations in collaboration with Los Angeles Integrative Gastroenterology and Nutrition. Visit her site at Nutrition4good.com.

John Rosania *Rejuvenating Eggnog (p. 255)*
John is an actor, writer, and the VP of Product at Clean. You can find his writing at Johnrosania.com

Zoe Saldana *Lentils Seasoned in Dominican Sofrito (p. 194)*
Zoe is a Dominican-American actress.

Lara Whitley *Teriyaki Sauce (p. 89)*
As a mom, artist, and foodie, Lara loves making things from scratch. She cooks up meals for her family and friends (and sometimes even gets them to join her in the wild chopping and stirring) at 8,000 feet in Colorado.

Key to contributor photos

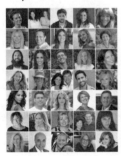

Alison Burger, Peggy and Megan Curry, Josh Radnor, Janet Goldman Weinberg, Brent Kronk

Gwyneth Paltrow, Mark Hyman, Carly de Castro, Lina Fedirko, Susana Belen

John Rosania, Meghan Markle, Adam Cobb, Farrell Feighan, Maribeth Evezich

Kris Carr, Lara Whitley, Lisa and Mehmet Oz, Dhru Purohit, Sarma Melngailis

Zoe Saldana, Todd Lepine, Gabrielle Bernstein, Amy Myers, Howie Greene
Jenny Nelson, Stacy Keibler, Wanda LeBlanc-Rushmer, Paul and Shou-Ching Jaminet, Belinda Rachman

Sarah Marchand, Farshid Sam Rahbar, Michelle Hartgrove, Mary Karlin, Donna Karan

NUTRIENT ANALYSES OF RECIPES

Nutrient analysis of recipes provides a good approximation of the calories and nutrients contained in the food. These can only be an approximation because of the nutrient variability common in natural foods and the variability in how people measure foods. Nevertheless, the recipe analyses provided can assist you in making the best food choices for you.

Nutrient analyses of recipes were conducted using the following conventions:

- When a recipe contains a choice of food ingredients, analysis is provided using the first ingredient unless otherwise indicated.

- When the ingredient amount varies, analysis uses the smallest amount unless otherwise indicated.

- Coarse sea salt is used whenever sea salt is listed.

- The following measures are used:

- A pinch is equivalent to $\frac{1}{16}$ teaspoon

- A dash is equivalent to $\frac{1}{12}$ teaspoon

- "Few" is analyzed as equaling to 2

- A drizzle is equal to 1 teaspoon

- Serving sizes used, when not otherwise indicated, are those used by the FDA for food product labeling. These are called Reference Amounts Customarily Consumed (RACC).

Breakfast Ideas

BANANA BREAD, p. 50

Makes 12 slices. Approximate Nutrient Analysis per slice (based on using pecans): 270 calories, 16 g fat, 6 g saturated fat, 30 mg cholesterol, 250 mg sodium, 30 g carbohydrate, 4 g fiber, 15 g sugar, 5 g protein

BLUEBERRY PANCAKES, p. 46

Makes 4 servings. Approximate Nutrient Analysis per serving (includes 3 tablespoons coconut oil for frying): 680 calories, 33 g fat, 22 g saturated fat, 95 mg cholesterol, 650 mg sodium, 89 g carbohydrate, 6 g fiber, 20 g sugar, 11 g protein

BLUEBERRY QUINOA CEREAL, p. 44

Makes 4 servings. Approximate Nutrient Analysis per serving (not including coconut yogurt or sweetener): 320 calories, 18 g fat, 14 g saturated fat, 0 mg cholesterol, 50 mg sodium, 35 g carbohydrate, 4 g fiber, 4 g sugar, 8 g protein

BUCKWHEAT GRANOLA, p. 42

Makes ½ gallon. Approximate Nutrient Analysis per ½ cup serving: 230 calories, 12 g fat, 2.5 g saturated fat, 0 mg cholesterol, 130 mg sodium, 26 g carbohydrate, 5 g fiber, 11 g sugar, 6 g protein

CASHEW YOGURT, p. 45

Makes 1 pint. Approximate Nutrient Analysis per ½ cup serving (not including suggested yogurt toppings): 300 calories, 24 g fat, 4 g saturated fat, 0 mg cholesterol, 10 mg sodium, 16 g carbohydrate, 2 g fiber, 3 g sugar, 10 g protein

CHAI-SPICED CHIA PORRIDGE, p. 51

Makes 2 servings. Approximate Nutrient Analysis per serving (based on sesame seeds, 2 tablespoons of coconut nectar, and including blueberries): 790 calories, 55 g fat, 12 g saturated fat, 0 mg cholesterol, 80 mg sodium, 59 g carbohydrate, 17 g fiber, 31 g sugar, 25 g protein

EGG-STUFFED SWEET POTATO WITH SPINACH PURÉE, p. 59

Makes 2 servings. Approximate Nutrient Analysis per serving (not including salt to taste): 880 calories, 64 g fat, 11 g saturated fat, 370 mg cholesterol, 550 mg sodium, 63 g carbohydrate, 11 g fiber, 12 g sugar, 18 g protein

FRENCH TOAST WITH VANILLA CREAM, p. 48

Makes 2 servings. Approximate Nutrient Analysis per serving: 1100 calories, 72 g fat, 57 g saturated fat, 370 mg cholesterol, 750 mg sodium, 98 g carbohydrate, 4 g fiber, 53 g sugar, 20 g protein

LACY POTATO CAKES, p. 58

Makes 8 pancakes. Approximate Nutrient Analysis per cake: 120 calories, 4 g fat, 3 g saturated fat, 25 mg cholesterol, 450 mg sodium, 18 g carbohydrate, 2 g fiber, 1 g sugar, 2 g protein

QUINOA AND SUGAR PUMPKIN PORRIDGE, p. 43

Makes 2 servings. Approximate Nutrient Analysis per serving (not including garnishes): 470 calories, 27 g fat, 22 g saturated fat, 0 mg cholesterol, 250 mg sodium, 54 g carbohydrate, 8 g fiber, 17 g sugar, 10 g protein

ROASTED ASPARAGUS WITH POACHED EGGS, p. 54

Makes 2 servings. Approximate Nutrient Analysis per serving (based on 2 eggs per person and not including sprinkle of sea salt): 280 calories, 23 g fat, 5 g saturated fat, 370 mg cholesterol, 150 mg sodium, 5 g carbohydrate, 2 g fiber, 2 g sugar, 15 g protein

ROOT VEGETABLE HASH, p. 60

Makes 2 servings. Approximate Nutrient Analysis per serving (not including salt to taste): 460 calories, 28 g fat, 24 g saturated fat, 0 mg cholesterol, 180 mg sodium, 51 g carbohydrate, 14 g fiber, 22 g sugar, 5 g protein

SALMON SCRAMBLE WITH CAULIFLOWER AND DILL PURÉE, p. 52

Makes 1 serving. Approximate Nutrient Analysis per serving (not including salt to taste or apple cider vinegar, lemon juice, or olive oil for the avocado): 750 calories, 58 g fat, 30 g saturated fat, 465 mg cholesterol, 250 mg sodium, 9 g carbohydrate, 6 g fiber, 2 g sugar, 49 g protein

SCALLION PANCAKES, p. 57

Makes 8 to 16 pancakes. Approximate Nutrient Analysis per pancake (based on 8 pancakes and including 2 tablespoons coconut oil for cooking): 100 calories, 7 g fat, 4.5 g saturated fat, 140 mg cholesterol, 300 mg sodium, 3 g carbohydrate, 1 g fiber, 1 g sugar, 5 g protein

SCRAMBLED EGGS WITH SMOKED SALMON, p. 55

Makes 1 serving. Approximate Nutrient Analysis per serving: 650 calories, 55 g fat, 20 g saturated fat, 750 mg cholesterol, 1100 mg sodium, 3 g carbohydrate, 0 g fiber, 1 g sugar, 37 g protein

SUNKEN EGGS, p. 53

Makes 2 servings. Approximate Nutrient Analysis per serving (not including salt to taste or optional sautéed vegetables): 230 calories, 10 g fat, 3 g saturated fat, 370 mg cholesterol, 1800 mg sodium, 19 g carbohydrate, 6 g fiber, 6 g sugar, 19 g protein

VEGETABLE FRITTATA, p. 56

Makes 2 servings. Approximate Nutrient Analysis per serving: 530 calories, 41 g fat, 27 g saturated fat, 560 mg cholesterol, 1150 mg sodium, 23 g carbohydrate, 4 g fiber, 8 g sugar, 24 g protein

Salads, Sauces, and Dressings

AIOLI (GARLIC MAYONNAISE), p. 92

Makes 1 pint. Approximate Nutrient Analysis per tablespoon (using 1 teaspoon sea salt and 1½ cups oil): 90 calories, 10 g fat, 1.5 g saturated fat, 10 mg cholesterol, 60 mg sodium, 0 g carbohydrate, 0 g fiber, 0 g sugar, 0 g protein

ARUGULA AND PEAR SALAD WITH WALNUT VINAIGRETTE, p. 73

Makes 2 servings. Approximate Nutrient Analysis per serving: 220 calories, 13 g fat, 1.5 g saturated fat, 0 mg cholesterol, 500 mg sodium, 25 g carbohydrate, 9 g fiber, 12 g sugar, 4 g protein

ARUGULA AND PERSIMMON SALAD WITH PISTACHIO VINAIGRETTE, p. 68

Makes 2 servings. Approximate Nutrient Analysis per serving (uses 2 tablespoons dressing): 350 calories, 22 g fat, 3 g saturated fat, 0 mg cholesterol, 500 mg sodium, 40 g carbohydrate, 9 g fiber, 25 g sugar, 7 g protein

BASIL VINAIGRETTE, p. 86

Makes about ⅔ cup. Approximate Nutrient Analysis per 2 tablespoons: 150 calories, 16 g fat, 2 g saturated fat, 0 mg cholesterol, 230 mg sodium, 1 g carbohydrate, 0 g fiber, 0 g sugar, 1 g protein

BITTER GREENS AND HERB SALAD, p. 70

Makes 4 servings. Approximate Nutrient Analysis per serving: 240 calories, 15 g fat, 1.5 g saturated fat, 0 mg cholesterol, 170 mg sodium, 19 g carbohydrate, 8 g fiber, 4 g sugar, 10 g protein

CHICKEN PAILLARD WITH BUTTERNUT SQUASH AND MUSTARD VINAIGRETTE, p. 66

Makes 2 servings. Approximate Nutrient Analysis per serving (not including salt to taste or coconut oil for coating and cooking): 600 calories, 29 g fat, 4.5 g saturated fat, 110 mg cholesterol, 1550 mg sodium, 48 g carbohydrate, 12 g fiber, 7 g sugar, 42 g protein

CHINESE CHICKEN SALAD, p. 83

Makes 2 servings. Approximate Nutrient Analysis per serving (not including salt to taste): 880 calories, 60 g fat, 9 g saturated fat, 150 mg cholesterol, 800 mg sodium, 29 g carbohydrate, 5 g fiber, 15 g sugar, 58 g protein

CHUNKY AVOCADO SALAD, p. 77

Makes 2 servings. Approximate Nutrient Analysis per serving (not including optional spirulina): 660 calories, 59 g fat, 8 g saturated fat, 0 mg cholesterol, 750 mg sodium, 32 g carbohydrate, 18 g fiber, 6 g sugar, 12 g protein

THE CLEAN NIÇOISE, p. 78

Makes 2 servings. Approximate Nutrient Analysis per serving (includes 2 tablespoons dressing): 750 calories, 57 g fat, 10 g saturated fat, 435 mg cholesterol, 2080 mg sodium, 33 g carbohydrate, 7 g fiber, 6 g sugar, 30 g protein

EGG SALAD, p. 76

Makes 2 servings. Approximate Nutrient Analysis per serving: 360 calories, 28 g fat, 7 g saturated fat, 560 mg cholesterol, 1350 mg sodium, 6 g carbohydrate, 1 g fiber, 3 g sugar, 20 g protein

EVERYTHING KALE SALAD, p. 69

Makes 1 serving. Approximate Nutrient Analysis per serving (not including salt to taste): 800 calories, 49 g fat, 8 g saturated fat, 155 mg cholesterol, 570 mg sodium, 53 g carbohydrate, 14 g fiber, 3 g sugar, 47 g protein

THE FARMERS' MARKET SALAD, p. 79

Makes 2 servings. Approximate Nutrient Analysis per serving (not including dressing): 170 calories, 9 g fat, 1.5 g saturated fat, 0 mg cholesterol, 75 mg sodium, 17 g carbohydrate, 6 g fiber, 9 g sugar, 9 g protein

FOREVER-GREEN SOUP AND SALAD, p. 80

Makes 4 servings. Approximate Nutrient Analysis per serving: 470 calories, 40 g fat, 6 g saturated fat, 0 mg cholesterol, 900 mg sodium, 25 g carbohydrate, 6 g fiber, 10 g sugar, 9 g protein

GREEN GODDESS DRESSING, p. 87

Makes just over 1 pint. Approximate Nutrient Analysis per 2 tablespoons: 150 calories, 15 g fat, 2 g saturated fat, 0 mg cholesterol, 300 mg sodium, 4 g carbohydrate, 1 g fiber, 0 g sugar, 3 g protein

HEIRLOOM TOMATO, FENNEL, AND AVOCADO PRESSED SALAD, p. 74

Makes 6 servings. Approximate Nutrient Analysis per serving (not including salt to taste): 560 calories, 53 g fat, 7 g saturated fat, 0 mg cholesterol, 400 mg sodium, 21 g carbohydrate, 9 g fiber, 6 g sugar, 5 g protein

MAYONNAISE, p. 91

Makes 1 pint. Approximate Nutrient Analysis per tablespoon (using 1 teaspoon sea salt and 1½ cups oil): 90 calories, 10 g fat, 1.5 g saturated fat, 10 mg cholesterol, 60 mg sodium, 0 g carbohydrate, 0 g fiber, 0 g sugar, 0 g protein

MEXICAN BLACK BEAN SALAD, p. 82

Makes 2 servings. Approximate Nutrient Analysis per serving: 720 calories, 39 g fat, 6 g saturated fat, 0 mg cholesterol, 2400 mg sodium, 75 g carbohydrate, 28 g fiber, 7 g sugar, 24 g protein

PAPA D'S FRESH FALL SALAD, p. 72

Makes 4 to 6 servings. Approximate Nutrient Analysis per serving (based on 4 servings): 570 calories, 49 g fat, 16 g saturated fat, 0 mg cholesterol, 500 mg sodium, 31 g carbohydrate, 7 g fiber, 7 g sugar, 7 g protein

ROASTED BEET SALAD WITH MISO DRESSING, p. 65

Makes 2 servings. Approximate Nutrient Analysis per serving (not including salt to taste): 540 calories, 37 g fat, 5 g saturated fat, 0 mg cholesterol, 1200 mg sodium, 44 g carbohydrate, 14 g fiber, 22 g sugar, 17 g protein

ROASTED SWEET POTATO AND SPINACH SALAD, p. 85

Makes 4 servings. Approximate Nutrient Analysis per serving (not including optional goat or feta cheese): 520 calories, 27 g fat, 3 g saturated fat, 0 mg cholesterol, 800 mg sodium, 66 g carbohydrate, 11 g fiber, 26 g sugar, 9 g protein

ROMAINE AND SEA VEGETABLE SALAD WITH CREAMY DILL DRESSING, p. 64

Makes 2 servings. Approximate Nutrient Analysis per serving (includes 2 tablespoons dressing): 150 calories, 8 g fat, 0.5 g saturated fat, 0 mg cholesterol, 250 mg sodium, 18 g carbohydrate, 9 g fiber, 6 g sugar, 8 g protein

ROSEMARY MUSTARD MARINADE, p. 94

Makes 1 cup. Approximate Nutrient Analysis per tablespoon: 70 calories, 7 g fat, 1 g saturated fat, 0 mg cholesterol, 130 mg sodium, 1 g carbohydrate, 0 g fiber, 1 g sugar, 0 g protein

SESAME BOK CHOY SALAD, p. 71

Makes 2 servings. Approximate Nutrient Analysis per serving: 250 calories, 17 g fat, 2.5 g saturated fat, 0 mg cholesterol, 950 mg sodium, 19 g carbohydrate, 4 g fiber, 5 g sugar, 10 g protein

SMOKED SALMON AND FENNEL SALAD, p. 81

Makes 2 servings. Approximate Nutrient Analysis per serving: 230 calories, 16 g fat, 2.5 g saturated fat, 15 mg cholesterol, 850 mg sodium, 12g carbohydrate, 5 g fiber, 1 g sugar, 12 g protein

SPICY CASHEW DIP, p. 93

Makes about ⅔ cup. Approximate Nutrient Analysis per 2 tablespoons: 50 calories, 4 g fat, 1 g saturated fat, 0 mg cholesterol, 0 mg sodium, 4 g carbohydrate, 0 g fiber, 1 g sugar, 1 g protein

SPIRULINA SPROUT SALAD, p. 75

Makes 2 servings. Approximate Nutrient Analysis per serving: 520 calories, 47 g fat, 6 g saturated fat, 0 mg cholesterol, 1140 mg sodium, 16 g carbohydrate, 6 g fiber, 3 g sugar, 13 g protein

TERIYAKI SAUCE, p. 89

Makes 1 cup. Approximate Nutrient Analysis per 1/4 cup: 120 calories, 0 g fat, 0 g saturated fat, 0 mg cholesterol, 1000 mg sodium, 23 g carbohydrate, 0 g fiber, 17 g sugar, 2 g protein

THAI DIPPING SAUCE, p. 88

Makes just over 1 pint. Approximate Nutrient Analysis per 2 tablespoons: 50 calories, 3.5 g fat, 0 g saturated fat, 0 mg cholesterol, 750 mg sodium, 3 g carbohydrate, 0 g fiber, 2 g sugar, 2 g protein

THOUSAND ISLAND DRESSING, p. 90

Makes just over 1 pint. Approximate Nutrient Analysis per 2 tablespoons: 70 calories, 6 g fat, 1 g saturated fat, 0 mg cholesterol, 280 mg sodium, 2 g carbohydrate, 1 g fiber, 1 g sugar, 1 g protein

ZESTY ROASTED CHICKEN SALAD, p. 84

Makes 4 servings. Approximate Nutrient Analysis per serving (includes 4 teaspoons lemon-flavored olive oil on the salad): 1270 calories, 81 g fat, 21 g saturated fat, 340 mg cholesterol, 660 mg sodium, 39 g carbohydrate, 8 g fiber, 4 g sugar, 93 g protein

Side, Starters, and Snacks

ALMOND POPPY SEED CRACKERS, p. 128

Makes about 2 dozen. Approximate Nutrient Analysis per cracker: 70 calories, 4.5 g fat, 0 g saturated fat, 0 mg cholesterol, 150 mg sodium, 6 g carbohydrate, 2 g fiber, 0 g sugar, 2 g protein

APPLE ONION CHUTNEY, p. 125

Makes about 1 cup. Approximate Nutrient Analysis per ¼ cup (not including salt to taste): 100 calories, 0 g fat, 0 g saturated fat, 0 mg cholesterol, 15 mg sodium, 26 g carbohydrate, 2 g fiber, 22 g sugar, 1 g protein

ASIAN-INSPIRED CHICKPEAS, p. 98

Makes 4 to 6 servings. Approximate Nutrient Analysis per serving (based on 4 servings): 360 calories, 12 g fat, 1.5 g saturated fat, 0 mg cholesterol, 720 mg sodium, 49 g carbohydrate, 13 g fiber, 9 g sugar, 17 g protein

ASIAN LETTUCE WRAPS, p. 112

Makes 4 servings. Approximate Nutrient Analysis per serving: 370 calories, 18 g fat, 4 g saturated fat, 75 mg cholesterol, 400 mg sodium, 31 g carbohydrate, 5 g fiber, 19 g sugar, 20 g protein

ASPARAGUS, SORREL, AND CHESTNUT PURÉE, p. 103

Makes 2 to 4 servings. Approximate Nutrient Analysis per serving (based on 4 servings and not including salt from water or salt to taste): 200 calories, 14 g fat, 1 g saturated fat, 0 mg cholesterol, 480 mg sodium, 19 g carbohydrate, 4 g fiber, 4 g sugar, 6 g protein

BEST DIP / SAUCE / SALAD DRESSING EVER, p. 125

Makes 2 cups. Approximate Nutrient Analysis per tablespoon: 110 calories, 11 g fat, 1 g saturated fat, 0 mg cholesterol, 85 mg sodium, 2 g carbohydrate, 1 g fiber, 0 g sugar, 1 g protein

BLACK OLIVE TAPENADE, p. 120

Makes about 1½ cups. Approximate Nutrient Approximate Nutrient Analysis per 2 tablespoons: 100 calories, 10 g fat, 1.5 g saturated fat, 0 mg cholesterol, 360 sodium, 3 g carbohydrate, 0 g fiber, 0 g sugar, 0 g protein

BRAZIL NUT PÂTÉ, p. 110

Makes 1 pint. Approximate Nutrient Analysis per 2 tablespoons (¼ cup olive oil only): 150 calories, 15 g fat, 3 g saturated fat, 0 mg cholesterol, 85 mg sodium, 4 g carbohydrate, 2 g fiber, 1 g sugar, 3 g protein

BUTTERNUT SQUASH RAGOUT, p. 115

Makes 2 to 4 servings. Approximate Nutrient Analysis per serving (based on 2 servings): 380 calories, 23 g fat, 20 g saturated fat, 5 mg cholesterol, 2550 mg sodium, 42 g carbohydrate, 9 g fiber, 11 g sugar, 6 g protein

CASHEW ALMOND NUT BUTTER, p. 130

Makes about 40 tablespoons. Approximate Nutrient Analysis per tablespoon (not including bee pollen): 100 calories, 9 g fat, 2 g saturated fat, 0 mg cholesterol, 25 mg sodium, 4 g carbohydrate, 1 g fiber, 1 g sugar, 3 g protein

CASHEW CHEESE, p. 97

Makes 1 pint. Approximate Nutrient Analysis per 2 tablespoons: 130 calories, 10 g fat, 2 g saturated fat, 0 mg cholesterol, 150 mg sodium, 7 g carbohydrate, 1 g fiber, 1 g sugar, 4 g protein

CLEAN AND GREEN GUACAMOLE, p. 123

Makes ½ pint. Approximate Nutrient Analysis per 2 tablespoons (not including salt to taste): 25 calories, 2 g fat, 0 g saturated fat, 0 mg cholesterol, 0 mg sodium, 3 g carbohydrate, 1 g fiber, 1 g sugar, 1 g protein

CRISPY POTATO WEDGES WITH ROASTED RED PEPPER AND CASHEW MAYO, p. 107

Makes 4 servings. Approximate Nutrient Analysis per serving: 800 calories, 50 g fat, 8 g saturated fat, 0 mg cholesterol, 500 mg sodium, 77 g carbohydrate, 7 g fiber, 4 g sugar, 14 g protein

CRUNCHY MESQUITE MAPLE WALNUTS, p. 132

Makes about 1 pound. Approximate Nutrient Analysis per 2 tablespoons: 90 calories, 8 g fat, 1g saturated fat, 0 mg cholesterol, 30 mg sodium, 5 g carbohydrate, 1 g fiber, 3 g sugar, 2 g protein

GARLICKY GREENS, p. 114

Makes 2 servings. Approximate Nutrient Analysis per serving (not including salt to taste): 240 calories, 21 g fat, 2.5 g saturated fat, 0 mg cholesterol, 130 mg sodium, 12 g carbohydrate, 3 g fiber, 1 g sugar, 4 g protein

GINGERED CARROT PURÉE, p. 104

Makes 2 cups. Approximate Nutrient Analysis per ½ cup serving: 90 calories, 3.5 g fat, 3 g saturated fat, 0 mg cholesterol, 200 mg sodium, 12 g carbohydrate, 4 g fiber, 6 g sugar, 2 g protein

GRACY'S AVOCUMBER ROLLS, p. 102

Makes 2 servings. Approximate Nutrient Analysis per serving: 250 calories, 21 g fat, 3 g saturated fat, 0 mg cholesterol, 45 mg sodium, 16 g carbohydrate, 11 g fiber, 3 g sugar, 4 g protein

MARINATED CARROT RIBBONS, p. 101

Makes 2 servings. Approximate Nutrient Analysis per serving (not including salt to taste): 380 calories, 31 g fat, 3.5 g saturated fat, 0 mg cholesterol, 1050 mg sodium, 27 g carbohydrate, 8 g fiber, 12 g sugar, 5 g protein

MINTY RICE DOLMAS WITH GARLIC DIPPING SAUCE, p. 106

Makes 10 to 12 dolmas. Approximate Nutrient Analysis per dolma (based on 10 dolmas): 250 calories, 20 g fat, 3 g saturated fat, 0 mg cholesterol, 500 mg sodium, 15 g carbohydrate, 3 g fiber, 0 g sugar, 4 g protein

THE PERFECT HARD-BOILED EGG, p. 96

Approximate Nutrient Analysis per egg: 80 calories, 5 g fat, 1.5 g saturated fat, 185 mg cholesterol, 60 mg sodium, 1 g carbohydrate, 0 g fiber, 1 g sugar, 6 g protein

PICKLED RADISHES, p. 100

Makes 1 pint. Approximate Nutrient Analysis per ounce: 5 calories, 0 g fat, 0 g saturated fat, 0 mg cholesterol, 250 to 350 mg sodium, 2 g carbohydrate, 1 g fiber, 1 g sugar, 0 g protein

ROASTED BEET CARPACCIO, p. 121

Makes 2 to 3 servings. Approximate Nutrient Analysis per serving (based on 2 servings and not including salt to taste): 310 calories, 27 g fat, 4 g saturated fat, 0 mg cholesterol, 300 mg sodium, 16 g carbohydrate, 4 g fiber, 10 g sugar, 3 g protein

ROASTED CAULIFLOWER WITH A MIDDLE EASTERN TWIST, p. 99

Approximate Nutrient Analysis per recipe (not including salt to taste): 210 calories, 9 g fat, 1 g saturated fat, 0 mg cholesterol, 120 mg sodium, 32 g carbohydrate, 4 g fiber, 14 g sugar, 6 g protein

ROASTED PEARS AND PARSNIPS, p. 117

Makes 4 servings. Approximate Nutrient Analysis per serving: 220 calories, 2 g fat, 0.5 g saturated fat, 0 mg cholesterol, 500 mg sodium, 45 g carbohydrate, 8 g fiber, 11 g sugar, 4 g protein

ROSEMARY DROP BISCUITS, p. 129

Makes about 1 dozen. Approximate Nutrient Analysis per biscuit: 140 calories, 7 g fat, 5 g saturated fat, 0 mg cholesterol, 450 mg sodium, 19 g carbohydrate, 1 g fiber, 0 g sugar, 2 g protein

ROSEMARY GARLIC WHITE BEAN DIP, p. 122

Makes 1½ cups. Approximate Nutrient Analysis per 2 tablespoons (not including salt to taste): 70 calories, 4 g fat, 0.5 g saturated fat, 0 mg cholesterol, 50 mg sodium, 7 g carbohydrate, 1 g fiber, 0 g sugar, 2 g protein

SARDINES ON ENDIVES, p. 109

Makes 2 servings. Approximate Nutrient Analysis per serving (not including salt to taste): 220 calories, 16 g fat, 4.5 g saturated fat, 80 mg cholesterol, 400 mg sodium, 5 g carbohydrate, 4 g fiber, 1 g sugar, 14 g protein

SEEREAL BARS, p. 131

Makes about 24 bars. Approximate Nutrient Analysis per bar: 90 calories, 5 g fat, 2.5 g saturated fat, 0 mg cholesterol, 10 mg sodium, 8 g carbohydrate, 2 g fiber, 2 g sugar, 3 g protein

SLOW-ROASTED GARLIC, p. 113

Makes about ½ cup. Approximate Nutrient Analysis per 2 tablespoons (and based on a pinch salt per garlic bulb): 80 calories, 5 g fat, 0.5 g saturated fat, 0 mg cholesterol, 150 mg sodium, 8 g carbohydrate, 1 g fiber, 0 g sugar, 2 g protein

SLOW-ROASTED TOMATOES, p. 118

Makes 2 quarts. Approximate Nutrient Analysis per cup (incudes ¼ cup drizzled oil but not salt to taste): 100 calories, 7 g fat, 1 g saturated fat, 0 mg cholesterol, 10 mg sodium, 9 g carbohydrate, 3 g fiber, 6 g sugar, 2 g protein

SNAPPY CRACKERS, p. 127

Makes 2 to 3 dozen. Approximate Nutrient Analysis per cracker (based on 24 crackers): 130 calories, 11 g fat, 1 g saturated fat, 15 mg cholesterol, 100 mg sodium, 4 g carbohydrate, 2 g fiber, 1 g sugar, 5 g protein

SOUR CREAM, p. 98

Makes ¾ cup. Approximate Nutrient Analysis per 2 tablespoons: 150 calories, 15 g fat, 1 g saturated fat, 0 mg cholesterol, 150 mg sodium, 3 g carbohydrate, 1 g fiber, 1 g sugar, 3 g protein

SPINACH PECAN PESTO, p. 119

Makes about 2 cups. Approximate Nutrient Analysis per ¼ cup serving (not including salt to taste): 210 calories, 22 g fat, 2.5 g saturated fat, 0 mg cholesterol, 20 mg sodium, 4 g carbohydrate, 2 g fiber, 1 g sugar, 2 g protein

STUFFED MUSHROOMS, p. 111

Makes 4 servings. Approximate Nutrient Analysis per serving (includes 3 tablespoons of olive oil and a pinch of salt): 250 calories, 18 g fat, 2.5 g saturated fat, 0 mg cholesterol, 200 mg sodium, 19 g carbohydrate, 5 g fiber, 8 g sugar, 4 g protein

SWEET AND SPICY SQUASH AND APPLE PURÉE, p. 116

Makes 4 to 6 servings. Approximate Nutrient Analysis per serving (based on 4 servings): 400 calories, 21 g fat, 10 g saturated fat, 0 mg cholesterol, 200 mg sodium, 59 g carbohydrate, 15 g fiber, 25 g sugar, 5 g protein

TOMATO SALSA, p. 124

Makes about 1 quart. Approximate Nutrient Analysis per 2 tablespoons: 20 calories, 1.5 g fat, 0 g saturated fat, 0 mg cholesterol, 170 mg sodium, 1 g carbohydrate, 0 g fiber, 1 g sugar, 0 g protein

VEGETABLE PAKORAS, p. 108

Makes 4 servings. Approximate Nutrient Analysis per serving (not including salt to taste): 430 calories, 30 g fat, 24 g saturated fat, 0 mg cholesterol, 45 mg sodium, 35 g carbohydrate, 9 g fiber, 7 g sugar, 10 g protein

ZA'ATAR ROASTED CARROTS, p. 105

Makes 4 servings. Approximate Nutrient Analysis per serving: 170 calories, 9 g fat, 1 g saturated fat, 0 mg cholesterol, 1350 mg sodium, 23 g carbohydrate, 7 g fiber, 11 g sugar, 3 g protein

Fish

CHARRED LEMON-BROILED SOLE, p. 135

Makes 2 servings. Approximate Nutrient Analysis per serving (based on 2 tablespoons olive oil): 290 calories, 18 g fat, 3 g saturated fat, 100 mg cholesterol, 1050 mg sodium, 2 g carbohydrate, 0 g fiber, 2 g sugar, 29 g protein

COCONUT FISH SOUP, p. 143

Makes 2 servings. Approximate Nutrient Analysis per serving: 1070 calories, 76 g fat, 51 g saturated fat, 185 mg cholesterol, 980 mg sodium, 26 g carbohydrate, 4 g fiber, 9 g sugar, 76 g protein

COCONUT POACHED SALMON, p. 136

Makes 2 servings. Approximate Nutrient Analysis per serving (not including salt to taste nor dark leafy greens): 500 calories, 40 g fat, 25 g saturated fat, 65 mg cholesterol, 300 mg sodium, 11 g carbohydrate, 0 g fiber, 1 g sugar, 27 g protein

COD WITH ROASTED CHILE PEPPERS AND CAYENNE, p. 140

Makes 4 servings. Approximate Nutrient Analysis per serving (not including salt to taste): 190 calories, 6 g fat, 1 g saturated fat, 75 mg cholesterol, 320 mg sodium, 3 g carbohydrate, 1 g fiber, 0 g sugar, 31 g protein

DILLY SALMON SALAD, p. 139

Makes 2 servings. Approximate Nutrient Analysis per serving (includes 1 tablespoon mayonnaise but not salt to taste): 420 calories, 26 g fat, 6.5 g saturated fat, 95 mg cholesterol, 415 mg sodium, 10 g carbohydrate, 2 g fiber, 3 g sugar, 38 g protein

FISH STICKS WITH TARTAR SAUCE, p. 142

Makes 2 servings. Approximate Nutrient Analysis per serving (includes 2 tablespoons tartar sauce but not salt to taste): 990 calories, 80 g fat, 44 g saturated fat, 290 mg cholesterol, 1300 mg sodium, 27 g carbohydrate, 14 g fiber, 5 g sugar, 47 g protein

FISH TACOS, p. 148

Makes 4 servings. Approximate Nutrient Analysis per serving: 480 calories, 24 g fat, 3.5 g saturated fat, 45 mg cholesterol, 470 mg sodium, 42 g carbohydrate, 5 g fiber, 13 g sugar, 26 g protein

HARISSA-COATED HADDOCK, p. 151

Makes 2 servings. Approximate Nutrient Analysis per serving: 200 calories, 3.5 g fat, .5 g saturated fat, 120 mg cholesterol, 780 mg sodium, 3 g carbohydrate, 1 g fiber, 1 g sugar, 37 g protein

LEMON AND THYME BAKED SEA BASS WITH BRUSSELS SPROUT HASH, p. 138

Makes 2 servings. Approximate Nutrient Analysis per serving (not including salt to taste): 1460 calories, 81 g fat, 12 g saturated fat, 230 mg cholesterol, 2300 mg sodium, 47 g carbohydrate, 13 g fiber, 16 g sugar, 118 g protein

OVEN-BAKED FLOUNDER WITH GARLIC AND GREEN OLIVES, p. 134

Makes 2 servings. Approximate Nutrient Analysis per serving (not including salt to taste): 360 calories, 25 g fat, 4 g saturated fat, 100 mg cholesterol, 1750 mg sodium, 3 g carbohydrate, 2 g fiber, 1 g sugar, 29 g protein

OVEN-ROASTED COD, p. 152

Makes 4 servings. Approximate Nutrient Analysis per serving (not including salt to taste): 300 calories, 15 g fat, 1.5 g saturated fat, 75 mg cholesterol, 200 mg sodium, 8 g carbohydrate, 3 g fiber, 2 g sugar, 34 g protein

PAN-ROASTED HALIBUT WITH ARTICHOKE AND CELERY SALAD AND A LAVENDER VINAIGRETTE, p. 137

Makes 2 servings. Approximate Nutrient Analysis per serving (not including salt to taste): 760 calories, 62 g fat, 7 g saturated fat, 85 mg cholesterol, 950 mg sodium, 21 g carbohydrate, 7 g fiber, 1 g sugar, 38 g protein

POACHED COD WITH SOBA NOODLES AND PONZU SAUCE, p. 146

Makes 2 servings. Approximate Nutrient Analysis per serving (includes 2 tablespoons ponzu sauce): 690 calories, 21 g fat, 3.5 g saturated fat, 75 mg cholesterol, 1050 mg sodium, 90 g carbohydrate, 2 g fiber, 3 g sugar, 41 g protein

SALMON STIR-FRY, p. 150

Makes 2 servings. Approximate Nutrient Analysis per serving: 730 calories, 56 g fat, 8 g saturated fat, 95 mg cholesterol, 2200 mg sodium, 17 g carbohydrate, 5 g fiber, 4 g sugar, 44 g protein

SPICED SALMON WITH BLUEBERRY VINAIGRETTE, p. 149

Makes 2 servings. Approximate Nutrient Analysis per serving (includes 2 tablespoons blueberry vinaigrette): 310 calories, 15 g fat, 4.5 g saturated fat, 95 mg cholesterol, 570 mg sodium, 9 g carbohydrate, 3 g fiber, 3 g sugar, 35 g protein

TUNA NOODLE CASSEROLE, p. 153

Makes 4 to 6 servings. Approximate Nutrient Analysis per serving (based on 4 servings): 760 calories, 24 g fat, 8 g saturated fat, 30 mg cholesterol, 1950 mg sodium, 109 g carbohydrate, 6 g fiber, 9 g sugar, 31 g protein

ZUCCHINI-WRAPPED WHITEFISH WITH CHIVE OIL, p. 144

Makes 2 servings. Approximate Nutrient Analysis per serving (includes 2 tablespoons chive oil): 510 calories, 40 g fat, 6 g saturated fat, 135 mg cholesterol, 1120 mg sodium, 6 g carbohydrate, 2 g fiber, 4 g sugar, 32 g protein

Poultry

CHICKEN AND BROCCOLI PAD THAI, p. 158

Makes 2 servings. Approximate Nutrient Analysis per serving (based on 6-ounce chicken breast and 1 teaspoon drizzled avocado oil): 780 calories, 28 g fat, 15 g saturated fat, 145 mg cholesterol, 1650 mg sodium, 103 g carbohydrate, 4 g fiber, 12 g sugar, 37 g protein

CHICKEN OSSO BUCCO, p. 166

Makes 2 servings. Approximate Nutrient Analysis per serving (not including salt to taste): 1160 calories, 77 g fat, 19 g saturated fat, 370 mg cholesterol, 460 mg sodium, 28 g carbohydrate, 6 g fiber, 11 g sugar, 65 g protein

CHICKEN WITH KALE AND OLIVES, p. 170

Makes 1 serving. Approximate Nutrient Analysis per serving: 620 calories, 37 g fat, 17 g saturated fat, 95 mg cholesterol, 1530 mg sodium, 38 g carbohydrate, 8 g fiber, 3 g sugar, 41 g protein

CHICKEN WITH PRESERVED LEMONS AND FRAGRANT SPICES, p. 171

Makes 4 servings. Approximate Nutrient Analysis per serving (not including salt to taste): 950 calories, 71 g fat, 30 g saturated fat, 305 mg cholesterol, 2000 mg sodium, 20 g carbohydrate, 6 g fiber, 8 g sugar, 57 g protein

COCONUT CURRY, p. 160

Makes 4 servings. Approximate Nutrient Analysis per serving (not including brown rice): 450 calories, 33 g fat, 20 g saturated fat, 25 mg cholesterol, 550 mg sodium, 29 g carbohydrate, 7 g fiber, 6 g sugar, 14 g protein

CRISPY ROASTED CHICKEN, p. 169

Makes 4 to 6 servings. Approximate Nutrient Analysis per serving (based on 4 servings): 560 calories, 41 g fat, 16 g saturated fat, 170 mg cholesterol, 1500 mg sodium, 1 g carbohydrate, 0 g fiber, 0 g sugar, 43 g protein

CURRIED COCONUT CHICKEN WITH CUCUMBER MANGO SALAD, p. 167

Makes 2 servings. Approximate Nutrient Analysis per serving (not including salt to taste): 710 calories, 42 g fat, 25 g saturated fat, 125 mg cholesterol, 2320 mg sodium, 44 g carbohydrate, 9 g fiber, 29 g sugar, 46 g protein

DUCK BREAST WITH CRANBERRY PEAR CHUTNEY, p. 165

Makes 2 servings. Approximate Nutrient Analysis per serving (based on 6-ounce duck and ¼ cup chutney): 770 calories, 67 g fat, 23 g saturated fat, 130 mg cholesterol, 300 mg sodium, 22 g carbohydrate, 4 g fiber, 14 g sugar, 20 g protein

GARLIC-CRUSTED CHICKEN, p. 162

Makes 2 servings. Approximate Nutrient Analysis per serving (based on 2-ounce chicken breasts with skin): 960 calories, 84 g fat, 13 g saturated fat, 165 mg cholesterol, 1100 mg sodium, 19 g carbohydrate, 8 g fiber, 2 g sugar, 41 g protein

LEMON HERB CHICKEN BURGERS WITH THOUSAND ISLAND DRESSING, p. 156

Makes 4 servings. Approximate Nutrient Analysis per serving (not including salt to taste): 570 calories, 27 g fat, 13 g saturated fat, 75 mg cholesterol, 650 mg sodium, 54 g carbohydrate, 7 g fiber, 13 g sugar, 30 g protein

THE MOST PERFECT CHICKEN BREAST, p. 163

Makes 2 servings. Approximate Nutrient Analysis per serving: 420 calories, 30 g fat, 6 g saturated fat, 110 mg cholesterol, 1000 mg sodium, 0 g carbohydrate, 0 g fiber, 0 g sugar, 35 g protein

MUSTARD-BAKED CHICKEN, p. 159

Makes 2 servings. Approximate Nutrient Analysis per serving (not including salt to taste): 700 calories, 59 g fat, 13 g saturated fat, 185 mg cholesterol, 2150 mg sodium, 3 g carbohydrate, 1 g fiber, 0 g sugar, 33 g protein

ROASTED CAULIFLOWER AND CHICKEN SAUSAGE CASSEROLE, p. 172

Makes 4 servings. Approximate Nutrient Analysis per serving (not including salt to taste): 410 calories, 24 g fat, 2 g saturated fat, 40 mg cholesterol, 550 mg sodium, 32 g carbohydrate, 10 g fiber, 13 g sugar, 23 g protein

SHREDDED CHICKEN, p. 168

Makes 2 to 4 servings. Approximate Nutrient Analysis per serving (based on 2 servings): 240 calories, 4.5 g fat, 1 g saturated fat, 110 mg cholesterol, 3200 mg sodium, 10 g carbohydrate, 2 g fiber, 3 g sugar, 38 g protein

SLOW-COOKED CHICKEN, p. 174

Makes 2 servings. Approximate Nutrient Analysis per serving: 1310 calories, 90 g fat, 23 g saturated fat, 345 mg cholesterol, 4100 mg sodium, 33 g carbohydrate, 8 g fiber, 13 g sugar, 90 g protein

SLOW-COOKED CHICKEN WITH FENNEL AND WILD MUSHROOMS, p. 161

Makes 4 servings. Approximate Nutrient Analysis per serving (not including salt to taste): 700 calories, 42 g fat, 11 g saturated fat, 175 mg cholesterol, 800 mg sodium, 19 g carbohydrate, 5 g fiber, 7 g sugar, 47 g protein

THAI MARINATED TURKEY BREAST, p. 164

Makes 4 servings. Approximate Nutrient Analysis per serving (based on 1.5-pound turkey breast without skin): 360 calories, 15 g fat, 2 g saturated fat, 105 mg cholesterol, 1600 mg sodium, 8 g carbohydrate, 1 g fiber, 4 g sugar, 46 g protein

Meat

BRAISED LAMB SHANKS, p. 180

Makes 2 servings. Approximate Nutrient Analysis per serving (not including salt to taste): 900 calories, 50 g fat, 27 g saturated fat, 175 mg cholesterol, 1550 mg sodium, 35 g carbohydrate, 8 g fiber, 16 g sugar, 55 g protein

CAMBRIDGE FRIED RICE, p. 181

Makes 6 to 8 servings. Approximate Nutrient Analysis per serving (based on 6 servings and not including salt to taste): 480 calories, 27 g fat, 15 g saturated fat, 255 mg cholesterol, 330 mg sodium, 38 g carbohydrate, 3 g fiber, 3 g sugar, 23 g protein

COCONUT ZUCCHINI NOODLES AND SPICED MEATBALLS, p. 184

Makes 2 to 3 servings. Approximate Nutrient Analysis per serving (based on 2 servings and not including salt to taste): 1250 calories, 109 g fat, 71 g saturated fat, 165 mg cholesterol, 1420 mg sodium, 29 g carbohydrate, 6 g fiber, 8 g sugar, 50 g protein

GINGERED BEEF RAMEN, p. 185

Makes 4 servings. Approximate Nutrient Analysis per serving: 480 calories, 23 g fat, 5 g saturated fat, 60 mg cholesterol, 600 mg sodium, 47 g carbohydrate, 1 g fiber, 3 g sugar, 23 g protein

HERBED BUFFALO BURGERS, p. 187

Makes 4 servings. Approximate Nutrient Analysis per serving: 190 calories, 10 g fat, 3.5 g saturated fat, 110 mg cholesterol, 1450 mg sodium, 1 g carbohydrate, 0 g fiber, 0 g sugar, 25 g protein

LAMB AND WILD MUSHROOM STUFFED EGGPLANT, p. 176

Makes 4 to 6 servings. Approximate Nutrient Analysis per serving (based on 4 servings): 340 calories, 21 g fat, 7 g saturated fat, 40 mg cholesterol, 1550 mg sodium, 26 g carbohydrate, 11 g fiber, 10 g sugar, 15 g protein

MOROCCAN LAMB KEBABS, p. 178

Makes about 12 kebabs. Approximate Nutrient Analysis per kebab skewer (not including salt to taste): 310 calories, 22 g fat, 6 g saturated fat, 50 mg cholesterol, 350 mg sodium, 11 g carbohydrate, 3 g fiber, 6 g sugar, 17 g protein

POMEGRANATE-GLAZED LAMB CHOPS, p. 182

Makes 2 servings. Approximate Nutrient Analysis per serving: 470 calories, 19 g fat, 5 g saturated fat, 130 mg cholesterol, 1950 mg sodium, 32 g carbohydrate, 1 g fiber, 29 g sugar, 41 g protein

ROASTED LAMB LOIN WITH MINT PESTO, p. 183

Makes 2 servings. Approximate Nutrient Analysis per serving (includes ¼ cup mint pesto): 770 calories, 67 g fat, 11 g saturated fat, 80 mg cholesterol, 4000 mg sodium, 14 g carbohydrate, 6 g fiber, 2 g sugar, 32 g protein

SHEPHERD'S PIE, p. 188

Makes 4 servings. Approximate Nutrient Analysis per serving (not including salt to taste): 670 calories, 42 g fat, 24 g saturated fat, 85 mg cholesterol, 600 mg sodium, 52 g carbohydrate, 11 g fiber, 14 g sugar, 25 g protein

SPAGHETTI AND MEATBALLS WITH THIRTY-MINUTE MARINARA, p. 186

Makes 4 servings. Approximate Nutrient Analysis per serving: 810 calories, 32 g fat, 8 g saturated fat, 120 mg cholesterol, 1450 mg sodium, 89 g carbohydrate, 4 g fiber, 7 g sugar, 34 g protein

Vegetables

BAKED SPAGHETTI SQUASH WITH AUTUMN PESTO, p. 216

Makes 2 servings. Approximate Nutrient Analysis per serving (includes ¼ cup pesto): 360 calories, 21 g fat, 3.5 g saturated fat, 0 mg cholesterol, 260 mg sodium, 41 g carbohydrate, 10 g fiber, 15 g sugar, 11 g protein

BAKED TURNIP CASSEROLE WITH WALNUT SAGE CREAM, p. 217

Makes 4 servings. Approximate Nutrient Analysis per serving: 580 calories, 50 g fat, 8 g saturated fat, 0 mg cholesterol, 1050 mg sodium, 29 g carbohydrate, 8 g fiber, 9 g sugar, 12 g protein

CHILE RELLENOS STUFFED WITH MUSHROOMS, SWEET POTATOES, AND CHIPOTLE CASHEW CREMA, p. 204

Makes 8 chile rellenos. Approximate Nutrient Analysis per chile relleno (includes 1 tablespoon crema but not extra salt for potatoes): 320 calories, 15.5 g fat, 3.5 g saturated fat, 0 mg cholesterol, 325 mg sodium, 43 g carbohydrate, 8 g fiber, 10 g sugar, 9 g protein

CLEAN KITCHARI, p. 211

Makes 4 servings. Approximate Nutrient Analysis per serving: 590 calories, 18 g fat, 12 g saturated fat, 0 mg cholesterol, 950 mg sodium, 88 g carbohydrate, 16 g fiber, 7 g sugar, 25 g protein

CLEAN SUSHI, p. 198

Makes 4 servings. Approximate Nutrient Analysis per serving (not including prepared wasabi, wheat-free tamari for dipping, or salt to taste): 320 calories, 13 g fat, 2 g saturated fat, 0 mg cholesterol, 35 mg sodium, 47 g carbohydrate, 10 g fiber, 5 g sugar, 9 g protein

CONFETTI VEGETABLES WITH SPICY SAUCE, p. 209

Makes 2 servings. Approximate Nutrient Analysis per serving (includes ¼ cup spicy sauce): 430 calories, 25 g fat, 14 g saturated fat, 0 mg cholesterol, 250 mg sodium, 45 g carbohydrate, 15 g fiber, 19 g sugar, 16 g protein

GREEK QUINOA WITH HEARTS OF PALM, p. 202

Makes 2 servings. Approximate Nutrient Analysis per serving: 750 calories, 43 g fat, 6 g saturated fat, 0 mg cholesterol, 3100 mg sodium, 76 g carbohydrate, 13 g fiber, 5 g sugar, 19 g protein

LENTILS SEASONED IN DOMINICAN SOFRITO, p. 194

Makes 4 servings. Approximate Nutrient Analysis per serving (includes ¼ cup sofrito): 710 calories, 30 g fat, 4 g saturated fat, 0 mg cholesterol, 70 mg sodium, 81 g carbohydrate, 20 g fiber, 9 g sugar, 34 g protein

MEDITERRANEAN RICE NOODLES, p. 200

Makes 2 servings. Approximate Nutrient Analysis per serving (based on 8.8 ounces noodles and 1 teaspoon salt): 550 calories, 19 g fat, 3.5 g saturated fat, 0 mg cholesterol, 1050 mg sodium, 93 g carbohydrate, 5 g fiber, 6 g sugar, 10 g protein

MEXICAN TOSTADAS, p. 215

Makes 4 servings. Approximate Nutrient Analysis per serving: 960 calories, 71 g fat, 8 g saturated fat, 0 mg cholesterol, 1850 mg sodium, 71 g carbohydrate, 23 g fiber, 11 g sugar, 22 g protein

MINTED PEA AND ASPARAGUS RISOTTO, p. 222

Makes 2 servings. Approximate Nutrient Analysis per serving: 670 calories, 19 g fat, 15 g saturated fat, 0 mg cholesterol, 3350 mg sodium, 99 g carbohydrate, 11 g fiber, 10 g sugar, 11 g protein

MUSHROOM RISOTTO, p. 220

Makes 2 servings. Approximate Nutrient Analysis per serving (includes 1 tablespoon avocado oil to sauté mushrooms but not salt to taste): 740 calories, 30 g fat, 4 g saturated fat, 0 mg cholesterol, 950 mg sodium, 100 g carbohydrate, 10 g fiber, 11 g sugar, 13 g protein

PORTOBELLO STEAKS WITH MASHED CELERY ROOT, p. 221

Makes 2 servings. Approximate Nutrient Analysis per serving: 590 calories, 42 g fat, 16 g saturated fat, 0 mg cholesterol, 2700 mg sodium, 45 g carbohydrate, 12 g fiber, 13 g sugar, 10 g protein

QUINOA WITH CELERY AND APPLES, p. 195

Makes 2 servings. Approximate Nutrient Analysis per serving (not including salt to taste): 850 calories, 35 g fat, 4.5 g saturated fat, 0 mg cholesterol, 110 mg sodium, 117 g carbohydrate, 16 g fiber, 25 g sugar, 20 g protein

ROASTED CABBAGE WITH CHIPOTLE AND CARAWAY SOUR CREAM, p. 214

Makes 2 servings. Approximate Nutrient Analysis per serving (not including salt to taste): 690 calories, 61 g fat, 5 g saturated fat, 0 mg cholesterol, 550 mg sodium, 35 g carbohydrate, 14 g fiber, 3 g sugar, 15 g protein

ROASTED CAULIFLOWER AND PISTACHIO DRESSING, p. 203

Makes 2 servings. Approximate Nutrient Analysis (includes 2 tablespoons dressing but not salt to taste): 460 calories, 40 g fat, 5 g saturated fat, 0 mg cholesterol, 280 mg sodium, 24 g carbohydrate, 8 g fiber, 9 g sugar, 7 g protein

ROASTED VEGETABLES WITH SILKY HUMMUS, p. 213

Makes 4 servings. Approximate Nutrient Analysis per serving (based on a mix of root crops): 630 calories, 39 g fat, 5 g saturated fat, 0 mg cholesterol, 3000 mg sodium, 63 g carbohydrate, 9 g fiber, 12 g sugar, 14 g protein

SAVORY LENTIL LOAF, p. 218

Makes 4 servings. Approximate Nutrient Analysis per serving (not including salt to taste): 560 calories, 21 g fat, 2.5 g saturated fat, 0 mg cholesterol, 1400 mg sodium, 78 g carbohydrate, 16 g fiber, 4 g sugar, 19 g protein

SAVORY STUFFED VEGETABLES, p. 196

Makes 3 to 4 cups stuffing. Approximate Nutrient Analysis per ½ cup serving (stuffing only and not including salt to taste): 330 calories, 28 g fat, 3 g saturated fat, 0 mg cholesterol, 35 mg sodium, 15 g carbohydrate, 6 g fiber, 5 g sugar, 10 g protein

SESAME NOODLES, p. 193

Makes 2 servings. Approximate Nutrient Analysis per serving (based on 8.8 ounces noodles): 680 calories, 35 g fat, 6 g saturated fat, 0 mg cholesterol, 970 mg sodium, 88 g carbohydrate, 3 g fiber, 2 g sugar, 11 g protein

SOUTH-OF-THE-BORDER VEGETABLE MILLET, p. 201

Makes 2 servings. Approximate Nutrient Analysis per serving: 720 calories, 30 g fat, 14 g saturated fat, 0 mg cholesterol, 2800 mg sodium, 100 g carbohydrate, 19 g fiber, 14 g sugar, 17 g protein

SPINACH PATTIES, p. 192

Makes 4 servings. Approximate Nutrient Analysis per serving (not including salt to taste): 300 calories, 22 g fat, 10 g saturated fat, 60 mg cholesterol, 300 mg sodium, 18 g carbohydrate, 4 g fiber, 4 g sugar, 10 g protein

SUMMER SQUASH PUTTANESCA, p. 208

Makes 1 quart. Approximate Nutrient Analysis per cup serving (with anchovies): 400 calories, 25 g fat, 3.5 g saturated fat, 5 mg cholesterol, 1800 mg sodium, 36 g carbohydrate, 7 g fiber, 18 g sugar, 10 g protein

VEGETABLE NAPOLEON, p. 212

Makes 2 servings. Approximate Nutrient Analysis per serving (not including extra-virgin olive oil and salt to taste): 470 calories, 29 g fat, 4 g saturated fat, 0 mg cholesterol, 300 mg sodium, 50 g carbohydrate, 16 g fiber, 21 g sugar, 12 g protein

VINCENT ARPINO'S CLEAN BROOKLYN SICILIAN PIZZA PIE, p. 206

Makes approximately 2 servings. Approximate Nutrient Analysis per serving (crust and tomato paste only): 900 calories, 71 g fat, 11 g saturated fat, 185 mg cholesterol, 1750 mg sodium, 46 g carbohydrate, 21 g fiber, 11 g sugar, 30 g protein

WILD RICE WITH MIDDLE EASTERN FLAVORS, p. 210

Makes 2 servings. Approximate Nutrient Analysis per serving (not including salt to taste): 650 calories, 35 g fat, 5 g saturated fat, 0 mg cholesterol, 25 mg sodium, 73 g carbohydrate, 9 g fiber, 7 g sugar, 16 g protein

ZUCCHINI MANICOTTI, p. 197

Makes 2 servings. Approximate Nutrient Analysis per serving (not including salt to taste): 1600 calories, 126 g fat, 20 g saturated fat, 0 mg cholesterol, 1450 mg sodium, 90 g carbohydrate, 15 g fiber, 33 g sugar, 49 g protein

Soups and Stews

BROCCOLI CHEDDAR SOUP, p. 244

Makes 2 to 4 servings. Approximate Nutrient Analysis per serving (based on 2 servings and not including salt to taste): 270 calories, 15 g fat, 12 g saturated fat, 0 mg cholesterol, 900 mg sodium, 26 g carbohydrate, 9 g fiber, 6 g sugar, 14 g protein

CARROT, CUMIN, AND CAULIFLOWER SOUP, p. 232

Makes 4 servings. Approximate Nutrient Analysis per serving: 290 calories, 21 g fat, 15 g saturated fat, 0 mg cholesterol, 1000 mg sodium, 23 g carbohydrate, 9 g fiber, 10 g sugar, 7 g protein

CHICKEN AND WILD RICE SOUP, p. 242

Makes 2 servings. Approximate Nutrient Analysis per serving (not including salt to taste): 400 calories, 7 g fat, 1.5 g saturated fat, 60 mg cholesterol, 2400 mg sodium, 50 g carbohydrate, 6 g fiber, 8 g sugar, 33 g protein

CHICKEN STOCK, p. 224

Makes 1 gallon. Approximate Nutrient Analysis per cup: 0 calories, g fat, 0 g fat, 0 mg cholesterol, 50 mg sodium, 0 g carbohydrate, 0 g fiber, 0 g sugar, 0 g protein

CHILLED CUCUMBER AVOCADO SOUP, p. 235

Makes 2 servings. Approximate Nutrient Analysis per serving: 650 calories, 52 g fat, 8 g saturated fat, 0 mg cholesterol, 1850 mg sodium, 41 g carbohydrate, 14 g fiber, 9 g sugar, 17 g protein

EGG DROP SOUP, p. 236

Makes 2 to 4 servings. Approximate Nutrient Analysis per serving (based on 2 servings): 120 calories, 6 g fat, 2 g saturated fat, 185 mg cholesterol, 750 mg sodium, 7 g carbohydrate, 2 g fiber, 2 g sugar, 9 g protein

GAZPACHO, p. 239

Makes 2 servings. Approximate Nutrient Analysis per serving: 460 calories, 39 g fat, 5 g saturated fat, 0 mg cholesterol, 2750 mg sodium, 28 g carbohydrate, 11 g fiber, 12 g sugar, 6 g protein

HARVEST SOUP WITH PUMPKIN MISO, p. 240

Makes 6 servings. Approximate Nutrient Analysis per serving (not including salt to taste): 260 calories, 16 g fat, 2.5 g saturated fat, 0 mg cholesterol, 650 mg sodium, 22 g carbohydrate, 6 g fiber, 8 g sugar, 11 g protein

LEMONY LENTIL SOUP, p. 232

Makes 4 servings. Approximate Nutrient Analysis per serving (not including salt to taste): 450 calories, 9 g fat, 1 g saturated fat, 0 mg cholesterol, 750 mg sodium, 81 g carbohydrate, 16 g fiber, 16 g sugar, 15 g protein

MAW MAW'S GUMBO, p. 238

Makes 6 to 8 servings. Approximate Nutrient Analysis per serving (based on 6 servings): 430 calories, 11 g fat, 6 g saturated fat, 65 mg cholesterol, 450 mg sodium, 54 g carbohydrate, 11 g fiber, 7 g sugar, 29 g protein

MINESTRONE, p. 228

Makes about 1 gallon. Approximate Nutrient Analysis per cup (not including salt to taste): 60 calories, 2 g fat, 0 g saturated fat, 0 mg cholesterol, 110 mg sodium, 9 g carbohydrate, 3 g fiber, 3 g sugar, 3 g protein

MULLIGATAWNY SOUP, p. 234

Makes approximately 6 servings. Approximate Nutrient Analysis per serving: 210 calories, 4.5 g fat, 2.5 g saturated fat, 35 mg cholesterol, 1200 mg sodium, 27 g carbohydrate, 5 g fiber, 10 g sugar, 16 g protein

MUSHROOM PARSNIP STEW, p. 231

Makes 4 to 6 servings. Approximate Nutrient Analysis per serving (based on 6 servings): 200 calories, 7 g fat, 0.5 g saturated fat, 0 mg cholesterol, 1200 mg sodium, 28 g carbohydrate, 6 g fiber, 8 g sugar, 6 g protein

MUSHROOM STOCK, p. 227

Makes ½ gallon. Approximate Nutrient Analysis per cup: 20 calories, 1.5 g fat, 0 g saturated fat, 0 mg cholesterol, 10 mg sodium, 0.5 g carbohydrate, 0 g fiber, 0 g sugar, 0 g protein

ONION SOUP, p. 229

Makes 4 servings. Approximate Nutrient Analysis per serving (not including salt to taste): 240 calories, 8 g fat, 1 g saturated fat, 0 mg cholesterol, 1150 mg sodium, 33 g carbohydrate, 5 g fiber, 11 g sugar, 4 g protein

SPICY BLACK BEAN SOUP, p. 243

Makes 4 to 6 servings. Approximate Nutrient Analysis per serving (based on 4 servings and not including salt to taste): 160 calories, 7 g fat, 7 g saturated fat, 0 mg cholesterol, 550 mg sodium, 25 g carbohydrate, 8 g fiber, 4 g sugar, 6 g protein

TURKEY CHILI, p. 241

Makes 6 to 8 servings. Approximate Nutrient Analysis per serving (based on 6 servings and not including salt to taste or garnish): 390 calories, 16 g fat, 7 g saturated fat, 85 mg cholesterol, 1100 mg sodium, 36 g carbohydrate, 11 g fiber, 14 g sugar, 30 g protein

VEGETABLE STOCK, p. 226

Makes 3 to 4 quarts. Approximate Nutrient Analysis per cup: 15 calories, 1.5 g fat, 0 g saturated fat, 0 mg cholesterol, 10 mg sodium, 1 g carbohydrate, 0 g fiber, 1 g sugar, 0 g protein

WHITE BEAN AND KALE SOUP, p. 233

Makes 4 servings. Approximate Nutrient Analysis per serving: 410 calories, 8 g fat, 1 g saturated fat, 0 mg cholesterol, 1850 mg sodium, 63 g carbohydrate, 16 g fiber, 7 g sugar, 23 g protein

Shakes, Elixirs, Drinks, and Tonics

ADAM'S A.M. PRE-WORKOUT SHAKE, p. 254

Makes 1 serving. Approximate Nutrient Analysis per serving (not including protein powder): 270 calories, 17 g fat, 1.5 g saturated fat, 0 mg cholesterol, 620 mg sodium, 28 g carbohydrate, 9 g fiber, 14 g sugar, 6 g protein

ALMOND "MILK," p. 246

Makes 3 to 4 cups. Approximate Nutrient Analysis per cup: 175 calories, 17 g fat, 1 g saturated fat, 0 mg cholesterol, 60 mg sodium, 2 g carbohydrate, 0 g fiber, 2 g sugar, 7 g protein

BLACKBERRY COCONUT MILK SHAKE, p. 256

Makes 1 serving. Approximate Nutrient Analysis per serving: 530 calories, 38 g fat, 33 g saturated fat, 0 mg cholesterol, 400 mg sodium, 50 g carbohydrate, 12 g fiber, 32 g sugar, 8 g protein

CHIA GEL, p. 247

Makes 1 pint. Approximate Nutrient Analysis per 2 tablespoons: 10 calories, 0.5 g fat, 0 g saturated fat, 0 mg cholesterol, 0 mg sodium, 1 g carbohydrate, 1 g fiber, 0 g sugar, 0 g protein

CLEAN HOT COCOA, p. 263

Makes about 3 cups. Approximate Nutrient Analysis per cup: 410 calories, 33 g fat, 9 g saturated fat, 0 mg cholesterol, 140 mg sodium, 34 g carbohydrate, 7 g fiber, 27 g sugar, 10 g protein

COCONUT WATER AND LIME RICKEY, p. 253

Makes 2 servings. Approximate Nutrient Analysis per serving: 30 calories, 0 g fat, 0 g saturated fat, 0 mg cholesterol, 140 mg sodium, 6 g carbohydrate, 1 g fiber, 4 g sugar, 1 g protein

CRANBERRY CIDER SPRITZER, p. 264

Makes 6 servings. Approximate Nutrient Analysis per serving: 120 calories, 0 g fat, 0 g saturated fat, 0 mg cholesterol, 30 mg sodium, 30 g carbohydrate, 1 g fiber, 24 g sugar, 0 g protein

DREAMY BLUEBERRY SMOOTHIE, p. 261

Makes 1 serving. Approximate Nutrient Analysis per serving: 280 calories, 22 g fat, 4.5 g saturated fat, 0 mg cholesterol, 90 mg sodium, 19 g carbohydrate, 7 g fiber, 8 g sugar, 7 g protein

GINGER JUICE, p. 248

Makes 1 pint. Approximate Nutrient Analysis per cup: 20 calories, 0 g fat, 0 g saturated fat, 0 mg cholesterol, 10 mg sodium, 4 g carbohydrate, 0 g fiber, 0 g sugar, 0 g protein

HEALING CHOCOLATE ELIXIR, p. 262

Makes 1 serving. Approximate Nutrient Analysis per serving: 320 calories, 25 g fat, 15 g saturated fat, 0 mg cholesterol, 35 mg sodium, 22 g carbohydrate, 4 g fiber, 6 g sugar, 16 g protein

HIBISCUS ROSE SPLASH, p. 252

Makes 4 servings. Approximate Nutrient Analysis per serving: 50 calories, 0 g fat, 0 g saturated fat, 0 mg cholesterol, 260 mg sodium, 11 g carbohydrate, 3 g fiber, 7 g sugar, 2 g protein

JUST PEACHY, p. 259

Makes 2 servings. Approximate Nutrient Analysis per serving: 570 calories, 58 g fat, 44 g saturated fat, 0 mg cholesterol, 30 mg sodium, 17 g carbohydrate, 3 g fiber, 7 g sugar, 6 g protein

MAKE JUICE, NOT WAR GREEN JUICE, p. 250

Makes almost 4 cups. Approximate Nutrient Analysis per cup: 90 calories, 1 g fat, 0 g saturated fat, 0 mg cholesterol, 80 mg sodium, 21 g carbohydrate, 6 g fiber, 9 g sugar, 4 g protein

MALTED MACA MILK SHAKE, p. 260

Makes 1 serving. Approximate Nutrient Analysis per serving: 280 calories, 16 g fat, 3 g saturated fat, 0 mg cholesterol, 400 mg sodium, 35 g carbohydrate, 5 g fiber, 16 g sugar, 7 g protein

MANGO SLUSHIE, p. 258

Makes 1 serving. Approximate Nutrient Analysis per serving: 290 calories, 1 g fat, 0 g saturated fat, 0 mg cholesterol, 25 mg sodium, 73 g carbohydrate, 8 g fiber, 61 g sugar, 4 g protein

RASPBERRY LEMON-AIDE, p. 251

Makes 2 servings. Approximate Nutrient Analysis per serving: 120 calories, 1 g fat, 1 g saturated fat, 0 mg cholesterol, 700 mg sodium, 27 g carbohydrate, 8 g fiber, 16 g sugar, 4 g protein

REISHI CAPPUCCINO, p. 253

Makes 2 servings. Approximate Nutrient Analysis per serving: 210 calories, 16 g fat, 12 g saturated fat, 0 mg cholesterol, 340 mg sodium, 17 g carbohydrate, 2 g fiber, 15 g sugar, 1 g protein

REJUVENATING EGGNOG, p. 255

Makes 1 serving. Approximate Nutrient Analysis per serving (not including protein powder): 410 calories, 37 g fat, 27 g saturated fat, 370 mg cholesterol, 550 mg sodium, 3 g carbohydrate, 2 g fiber, 1 g sugar, 19 g protein

SPRING DANDELION DETOX ELIXIR, p. 249

Makes 1 serving. Approximate Nutrient Analysis per serving: 270 calories, 21 g fat, 18 g saturated fat, 0 mg cholesterol, 25 mg sodium, 20 g carbohydrate, 4 g fiber, 15 g sugar, 1 g protein

TURMERIC ALMOND MILK, p. 257

Makes 2 cups. Approximate Nutrient Analysis per cup: 425 calories, 36 g fat, 2.5 g saturated fat, 0 mg cholesterol, 10 mg sodium, 20 g carbohydrate, 2 g fiber, 11 g sugar, 15 g protein

Desserts

ALMOND SPICE COOKIES, p. 285

Makes 12 cookies. Approximate Nutrient Analysis per cookie: 240 calories, 18 g fat, 6 g saturated fat, 0 mg cholesterol, 135 mg sodium, 19 g carbohydrate, 3 g fiber, 10 g sugar, 5 g protein

APPLE CRISP (AKA MIRACLE CRISP), p. 271

Makes 5 servings. Approximate Nutrient Analysis per serving: 400 calories, 28 g fat, 8 g saturated fat, 0 mg cholesterol, 10 mg sodium, 37 g carbohydrate, 9 g fiber, 24 g sugar, 9 g protein

AVOCADO CHOCOLATE PUDDING, p. 273

Makes 1 to 2 servings. Approximate Nutrient Analysis per serving (based on 1 serving): 460 calories, 39 g fat, 17 g saturated fat, 0 mg cholesterol, 55 mg sodium, 32 g carbohydrate, 16 g fiber, 10 g sugar, 8 g protein

BLACKBERRY COBBLER, p. 268

Makes 4 to 6 servings. Approximate Nutrient Analysis per serving (based on 4 servings): 680 calories, 50 g fat, 15 g saturated fat, 0 mg cholesterol, 15 mg sodium, 56 g carbohydrate, 16 g fiber, 34 g sugar, 14 g protein

BLACKBERRY POMEGRANATE MOUSSE, p. 287

Makes 3 cups. Approximate Nutrient Analysis per ½ cup serving: 160 calories, 14 g fat, 12 g saturated fat, 0 mg cholesterol, 10 mg sodium, 9 g carbohydrate, 1 g fiber, 5 g sugar, 3 g protein

CASHEW NO-BAKE COOKIES, p. 275

Makes 20 cookies. Approximate Nutrient Analysis per cookie (including coconut nectar): 210 calories, 17 g fat, 6 g saturated fat, 0 mg cholesterol, 25 mg sodium, 12 g carbohydrate, 2 g fiber, 5 g sugar, 5 g protein

CINNAMON-BAKED APPLES, p. 284

Makes 2 servings. Approximate Nutrient Analysis per serving: 200 calories, 0 g fat, 0 g saturated fat, 0 mg cholesterol, 10 mg sodium, 53 g carbohydrate, 4 g fiber, 45 g sugar, 1 g protein

CLEAN CHOCOLATE, p. 281

Makes about 2 pounds. Approximate Nutrient Analysis per 1-ounce serving: 210 calories, 22 g fat, 13 g saturated fat, 0 mg cholesterol, 15 mg sodium, 8 g carbohydrate, 4 g fiber, 2 g sugar, 2 g protein

CLEAN ENERGY BARS, p. 270

Makes 9 bars. Approximate Nutrient Analysis per bar: 440 calories, 33 g fat, 3 g saturated fat, 0 mg cholesterol, 110 mg sodium, 29 g carbohydrate, 8 g fiber, 18 g sugar, 14 g protein

COCONUT ALMOND TAPIOCA PUDDING, p. 286

Makes 4 servings. Approximate Nutrient Analysis per serving: 210 calories, 13 g fat, 11 g saturated fat, 0 mg cholesterol, 200 mg sodium, 22 g carbohydrate, 1 g fiber, 4 g sugar, 2 g protein

FREEZER FUDGE, p. 282

Makes about 1 pound. Approximate Nutrient Analysis per 1-ounce serving: 150 calories, 13 g fat, 8 g saturated fat, 0 mg cholesterol, 30 mg sodium, 13 g carbohydrate, 2 g fiber, 8 g sugar, 2 g protein

HONEY PECAN BALLS, p. 280

Makes 12 balls. Approximate Nutrient Analysis per ball: 190 calories, 18 g fat, 6 g saturated fat, 0 mg cholesterol, 35 mg sodium, 6 g carbohydrate, 3 g fiber, 4 g sugar, 2 g protein

MINI RASPBERRY AND COCONUT CREAM TARTS, p. 274

Makes 4 mini tarts. Approximate Nutrient Analysis per mini tart: 980 calories, 85 g fat, 58 g saturated fat, 0 mg cholesterol, 130 mg sodium, 49 g carbohydrate, 24 g fiber, 28 g sugar, 10 g protein

PEACH PIE, p. 276

Makes 1 9-inch pie (8 servings). Approximate Nutrient Analysis per serving: 450 calories, 17 g fat, 14 g saturated fat, 0 mg cholesterol, 60 mg sodium, 71 g carbohydrate, 4 g fiber, 32 g sugar, 4 g protein

ROASTED CASHEW CURRANT BARK, p. 283

Makes 4 servings. Approximate Nutrient Analysis per serving: 1090 calories, 109 g fat, 59 g saturated fat, 0 mg cholesterol, 70 mg sodium, 45 g carbohydrate, 17 g fiber, 10 g sugar, 13 g protein

ROASTED PEARS WITH DATE CARAMEL SAUCE, p. 269

Makes 4 servings. Approximate Nutrient Analysis per serving: 290 calories, 4 g fat, 3 g saturated fat, 0 mg cholesterol, 100 mg sodium, 63 g carbohydrate, 9 g fiber, 37 g sugar, 2 g protein

SNICKER BARS, p. 278

Makes 12 bars. Approximate Nutrient Analysis per bar: 500 calories, 31 g fat, 11 g saturated fat, 0 mg cholesterol, 100 mg sodium, 50 g carbohydrate, 9 g fiber, 35 g sugar, 9 g protein

SUMMER FRUIT CRÊPES WITH VANILLA CREAM, p. 272

Makes 2 to 4 servings. Approximate Nutrient Analysis per serving (based on 2 servings): 990 calories, 48 g fat, 24 g saturated fat, 185 mg cholesterol, 180 mg sodium, 132 g carbohydrate, 15 g fiber, 61 g sugar, 23 g protein

ACKNOWLEDGMENTS

Thank you:

To my wife, Carla.

To my kids, Grace, Beilo and Seraphina.

To Chef Frank Giglio for all the care and love you put into these incredible recipes. And to Aline Fiuza and Angela Gaines for helping Frank in the kitchen.

To Jenny Nelson for your writing, edits, and recipe inspiration.

To Vanessa Stump for your beautiful recipe photographs and Chris Hatcher for being a fantastic crop-master.

To Michael Dahan for the great family photos.

To Timothy Gold for your craftsmanship.

To Jason Hashmi for your design inspiration.

To Kaya Purohit and Farrell Feighan for your help organizing our recipe shoot.

To Lisa Zuniga for your careful and thoughtful editing.

To Laura Lind for your elegant design.

To the Clean Team: Albert Bitton, Dhru Purohit, Kaya Purohit, Harshal Purohit, Hema Shah, John Rosania, Jessi Heinze, Bonnie Gerlaugh, John Hand, Robert Domingo, Debbie Young, Farrell Feighan, Patricia Cleary, Philip and Casey McCluskey, Kalen Jorden, and Shannon Sinkin for being such a force for wellness.

To the Clean community and all our guest recipe contributors.

To my editor, Gideon Weil, for his expert guidance.

A special thanks to Dhru Purohit and John Rosania for making it all happen.

And to all my patients and readers, thank you.

INDEX

Adam's A.M. Pre-Workout Shake, 254
Aioli (Garlic Mayonnaise), 92
almond butter health benefits, 14
almond flour health benefits, 13
almond milk: Adam's A.M. Pre-Workout
    Shake, 254; Coconut Almond Tapioca
    Pudding, 286; health benefits of, 15;
    Reishi Cappuccino, 253; Summer Fruit
    Crêpes with Vanilla Cream, 272; Turmeric
    Almond Milk, 257
Almond "Milk" shake, 246
Almond Poppy Seed Crackers, 128
almonds: Best Dip /Sauce / Salad Dressing
    Ever, 125; Cashew Almond Nut Butter,
    130; Oven-Roasted Cod, 152; Savory
    Stuffed Vegetables, 196; Snicker Bars, 278–
    79. See also nuts
Almond Spice Cookies, 285
apple cider vinegar, 17
apples: Apple Crisp (aka Miracle Crisp), 271;
    Apple Onion Chutney, 126; Bitter Greens
    and Herb Salad, 70; Cinnamon-Baked
    Apples, 284; Moroccan Lamb Kebabs, 178–
    79; Mulligatawny Soup, 234; Quinoa with
    Celery and Apples, 195
arugula: Arugula and Pear Salad with Walnut
    Vinaigrette, 73; Arugula and Persimmon
    Salad with Pistachio Vinaigrette, 68;
    Roasted Beet Carpaccio, 121
Artichoke and Celery Salad, 137
Asian-Inspired Chickpeas, 98
Asian Lettuce Wraps, 112
asparagus: Asparagus, Sorrel, and Chestnut
    Purée, 103; The Clean Niçoise, 78; Clean
    Sushi, 198–99; Minted Pea and Asparagus
    Risotto, 222; Roasted Asparagus with
    Poached Eggs, 54
Austin UltraHealth, 160
avocado oil health benefits, 13
avocados: Adam's A.M. Pre-Workout Shake,
    254; Avocado Chocolate Pudding, 273;
    Chilled Cucumber Avocado Soup, 235;
    Chunky Avocado Salad, 77; Clean and
    Green Guacamole, 123; Clean Sushi,
    198–99; Coconut Curry, 160; Everything
    Kale Salad, 69; Gazpacho, 239; Gracy's
    Avocumber Rolls, 102; Heirloom Tomato,
    Fennel, and Avocado Pressed Salad, 74;
    Mexican Black Bean Salad, 82; Mexican
    Tostadas, 215; Papa D's Fresh Fall Salad,
    72–73; South-of-the-Border Vegetable
    Millet, 201; Zesty Roasted Chicken
    Salad, 84

Baked Spaghetti Squash with Autumn
    Pesto, 216
Baked Turnip Casserole with Walnut Sage
    Cream, 217
balsamic vinegar health benefits, 15
Banana Bread, 50
basic cooking skills: chef thinking skills as
    part of, 38–39; dry roasting, 19; elixirs,
    20–21; infusions vs. decoctions, 20; soak-
    ing, 19, 247. See also clean kitchen
Basil Vinaigrette, 86
beans: description and recommended clean,
    12; Mexican Black Bean Salad, 82; Mexican
    Tostadas, 215; Minestrone, 228; Roasted
    Cauliflower with a Middle Eastern Twist,
    99; Rosemary Garlic White Bean Dip, 122;
    soaking, 19; Spicy Black Bean Soup, 243;
    Turkey Chili, 241; Vegetable Pakoras, 108;
    White Bean and Kale Soup, 233. See also
    legumes
beef: Gingered Beef Ramen, 185;
    Herbed Buffalo Burgers, 187; Spaghetti
    and Meatballs with Thirty-Minute
    Marinara, 186
beets: Farmers' Market Salad, 79; Harvest
    Soup with Pumpkin Miso, 240; Roasted
    Beet Carpaccio, 121; Roasted Beet Salad
    with Miso Dressing, 65; Roasted Vegetables
    with Silky Hummus, 213; Root Vegetable
    Hash, 60

Bernstein, Gabrielle, 271

Best Dip / Sauce / Salad Dressing Ever, 125

beverages: Adam's A.M. Pre-Workout Shake, 254; Almond "Milk," 246; Blackberry Coconut Milk Shake, 256; Chia Gel, 247; Clean Hot Cocoa, 263; Coconut Water and Lime Rickey, 265; Cranberry Cider Spritzer, 264; Dreamy Blueberry Smoothie, 261; elixirs, 20–21; Ginger Juice, 248; Healing Chocolate Elixir, 262; health benefits of shakes and smoothies, 256; Hibiscus Rose Splash, 252; Just Peachy, 259; Make Juice, Not War Green Juice, 250; Malted Maca Milk Shake, 260; Mango Slushie, 258; Raspberry Lemon-Aide, 251; Reishi Cappuccino, 253; Rejuvenating Eggnog, 255; Spring Dandelion Detox Elixir, 249; Turmeric Almond Milk, 257

bitter greens: Bitter Greens and Herb Salad, 70; how to prepare, 71

black beans: Mexican Black Bean Salad, 82; Spicy Black Bean Soup, 243; Turkey Chili, 241

blackberries: Blackberry Cobbler, 268; Blackberry Coconut Milk Shake, 256; Blackberry Pomegranate Mousse, 287

Black Olive Tapenade, 120

Blendtec, 17

Bloom, Orlando, 52

blueberries: Adam's A.M. Pre-Workout Shake, 254; Blueberry Pancakes, 46; Blueberry Quinoa Cereal, 44; Dreamy Blueberry Smoothie, 261; Spiced Salmon with Blueberry Vinaigrette, 149; wild, 67

bone broths, 225

Bragg Liquid Aminos, 16, 102, 125

Braised Lamb Shanks, 180

Brazil Nut Pâté, 110

breakfast ideas: Banana Bread, 50; Blueberry Pancakes, 46; Blueberry Quinoa Cereal, 44; Buckwheat Granola, 42; Cashew Yogurt, 45; Chai-Spiced Chia Porridge, 51; Egg-Stuffed Sweet Potatoes with Spinach Purée, 59; French Toast with Vanilla Cream, 48; Lacy Potato Cakes, 58; Quinoa and Sugar Pumpkin Porridge, 43; Roasted Asparagus with Poached Eggs, 54; Root Vegetable Hash, 60; Salmon Scramble with Cauliflower and Dill Purée, 52; Scallion Pancakes, 57; Scrambled Eggs with Smoked Salmon, 55; Sunken Eggs, 53; Vegetable Frittata, 56

broccoli: Broccoli Cheddar Soup, 244; Chicken and Broccoli Pad Thai, 158; Clean Sushi, 198–99; Coconut Zucchini Noodles and Spiced Meatballs, 184–85; Make Juice, Not War Green Juice, 250; Roasted Beet Salad with Miso Dressing, 65; Tuna Noodle Casserole, 153; Vegetable Frittata, 56; Vegetable Pakoras, 108

Buckwheat Granola, 42

Butternut Squash Ragout, 115

cacao powder: Avocado Chocolate Pudding, 273; Clean Chocolate, 281; Clean Hot Cocoa, 263; Freezer Fudge, 282; Healing Chocolate Elixer, 262; Snicker Bars, 278–79. See also chocolate

Cambridge Fried Rice, 181

carrots: Carrot, Cumin, and Cauliflower Soup, 232; Clean Kitchari, 211; Confetti Vegetables with Spicy Sauce, 209; Gingered Carrot Purée, 104; Harvest Soup with Pumpkin Miso, 240; Marinated Carrot Ribbons, 101; Roasted Vegetables with Silky Hummus, 213; Root Vegetable Hash, 60; Za'atar-Roasted Carrots, 105; Zesty Roasted Chicken Salad, 84

cashews: Cashew Almond Nut Butter, 130; Cashew Basil Dressing, 80; Cashew Cheese, 97; Cashew Mayo, 107; Cashew No-Bake Cookies, 275; Cashew Yogurt, 45; Chile Rellenos Stuffed with Mushrooms, Sweet Potatoes, and Chipotle Cashew Crema, 204–5; Chilled Cucumber Avocado Soup, 235; Chinese Chicken Salad, 83; Chipotle Cashew Crema, 204; Malted Maca Milk Shake, 260; Roasted Cashew Currant Bark, 283; Spicy Cashew Dip, 93; Summer Fruit Crêpes with Vanilla Cream, 272; Thousand Island Dressing, 90; Zucchini Manicotti, 197. See also nuts

cauliflower: Carrot, Cumin, and Cauliflower Soup, 232; Roasted Cauliflower and

Chicken Sausage Casserole, 172–73; Roasted Cauliflower with a Middle Eastern Twist, 99; Roasted Cauliflower with Pistachio Dressing, 203; Salmon Scramble with Cauliflower and Dill Purée, 52; Vegetable Pakoras, 108
Celtic sea salt, 14, 15
Centers for Disease Control and Prevention, 35
Chai-Spiced Chia Porridge, 51
chard: Garlicky Greens, 114; Harvest Soup with Pumpkin Miso, 240; Lemony Lentil Soup, 237; Sunken Eggs, 53
Charred Lemon-Broiled Sole, 135
chia seeds: Almond Poppy Seed Crackers, 128; Chai-Spiced Chia Porridge, 51; Chia Gel, 247; Clean Energy Bars, 270; Savory Lentil Loaf, 218–19; soaking, 247; Spaghetti and Meatballs with Thirty-Minute Marinara, 186; Spinach Patties, 192. *See also* seeds
Chicken and Broccoli Pad Thai, 158
Chicken with Kale and Olives, 170
Chicken Osso Bucco, 166
Chicken with Preserved Lemons and Fragrant Spices, 171
chicken. *See* poultry
Chicken Stock, 224
Chicken and Wild Rice Soup, 242
chickpea flour, 13
chickpeas: Asian-Inspired Chickpeas, 98; Hearty Winter Soup, 230
Chile Rellenos Stuffed with Mushrooms, Sweet Potatoes, and Chipotle Cashew Crema, 204–5
Chilled Cucumber Avocado Soup, 235
Chinese Chicken Salad, 83
Chipotle Cashew Crema, 204
chocolate: Clean Team tips on, 282; Freezer Fudge, 282. *See also* cacao powder
Chunky Avocado Salad, 77
Cinnamon-Baked Apples, 284
cinnamon health benefits, 14
Clean: The Revolutionary Program to Restore the Body's Natural Ability to Heal Itself (Junger), 7, 113
Clean Chocolate, 281

Clean Cleanse program: Cleanse, Gut, AND Vegan icons used in, 7; Cleanse icon indicating recipes suitable for, 7; Frank Giglio's testimonial on the, 44, 89; overview of the, 289; testimonials on the, 89, 125, 207, 234; 21-Day Clean Cleanse Meal Plan, 291. *See also* Refresh Clean program
clean eating: cooking more as part of, 28–29; description of, 3, 24–25; financial benefits of, 31–32; living more through, 35; mastering five health meals, 30. *See also* foods
clean eating community, 34
Clean Energy Bars, 270
clean foods: clean team favorites, 15–16; favorite salad toppings, 16–17; must-haves listed, 14–15; recommendations on listed, 11–14
Clean and Green Guacamole, 123
Clean Gut (Junger), 7
Clean Gut program: Frank Giglio's testimonial on the, 44; overview of the, 289; recipes appropriate for the, 7; testimonial on the, 207; 21-Day Clean Gut Meal Plan, 292
Clean Hot Cocoa, 263
Clean Kitchari, 211
clean kitchen: chef thinking skills to use in your, 38–39; childhood memories of eating goulash in her home's, 9–10; clean foods and recommendations, 11–17; as the heart and soul of your clean lifestyle, 10; kitchen tools recommended, 17–18; utensils under twenty dollars, 18. *See also* basic cooking skills
Cleanse icon, 7
cleansing program benefits, 1–2
Clean Sushi, 198–99
Cobb, Adam, 254
Coconut Almond Tapioca Pudding, 286
coconut butter health benefits, 14
Coconut Curry, 160
Coconut Fish Soup, 143
coconut flour health benefits, 13
coconut manna health benefits, 15
coconut milk health benefits, 15
coconut oil health benefits, 13, 14
Coconut Poached Salmon, 136
coconut water health benefits, 15

Coconut Water and Lime Rickey, 265
Coconut Zucchini Noodles and Spiced
    Meatballs, 184–85
cod: Cod with Roasted Chili Peppers and
    Cayenne, 140, 141; Oven-Roasted Cod,
    152; Poached Cod with Soba Noodles and
    Ponzu Sauce, 146–47; Zucchini-Wrapped
    Whitefish with Chive Oil, 144
communities: benefits of belonging to,
    33–34; creating a clean eating, 34
Confetti Vegetables with Spicy Sauce, 209
"cooking more" concept, 28–29
Cranberry Cider Spritzer, 264
Cranberry Pear Chutney, 165
Creamy Dill Dressing, 64
Crispy Potato Wedges with Roasted Red
    Pepper and Cashew Mayo, 107
Crispy Roasted Chicken, 169
Crunchy Maple Mesquite Walnuts, 132
cucumbers: Chilled Cucumber Avocado
    Soup, 235; Chunky Avocado Salad, 77;
    Curried Coconut Chicken with Cucumber
    Mango Salad, 167; Farmers' Market Salad,
    79; Gazpacho, 239; Gracy's Avocumber
    Rolls, 102; Make Juice, Not War Green
    Juice, 250; Savory Stuffed Vegetables, 196;
    Spirulina Sprout Salad, 75; Zesty Roasted
    Chicken Salad, 84
Curried Coconut Chicken with Cucumber
    Mango Salad, 167

dairy: description and recommended clean,
    12; Frank Giglio on lactose intolerance
    and, 86; health benefits of removing from
    diet, 6–7; the problem with eating, 6; reci-
    pes that include sources of, 6
de Castro, Carly, 257
decoctions, 20
desserts: Almond Spice Cookies, 285; Apple
    Crisp (aka Miracle Crisp), 271; Avocado
    Chocolate Pudding, 273; Blackberry
    Cobbler, 268; Blackberry Pomegranate
    Mousse, 287; Cashew No-Bake Cookies,
    275; Cinnamon-Baked Apples, 284; Clean
    Chocolate, 281; Clean Energy Bars, 270;
    Coconut Almond Tapioca Pudding, 286;
    Freezer Fudge, 282; Honey Pecan Balls,

280; Mini Raspberry and Coconut Cream
    Tarts, 274; Peach Pie, 276–77; Roasted
    Cashew Currant Bark, 283; Roasted Pears
    with Date Caramel Sauce, 269; Snicker
    Bars, 278–79; Summer Fruit Crêpes with
    Vanilla Cream, 272
Dilly Salmon Salad, 139
dips: Best Dip / Sauce / Salad Dressing Ever,
    125; Clean and Green Guacamole, 123;
    Garlic Dipping Sauce, 106; Rosemary
    Garlic White Bean Dip, 122; Spicy Cashew
    Dip, 93; Thai Dipping Sauce, 88; Tomato
    Salsa, 124. See also sauces
Dreamy Blueberry Smoothie, 261
dressings: Best Dip / Sauce / Salad Dressing
    Ever, 125; Caper Dressing, 74; Cashew
    Basil Dressing, 80; for Clean Sushi, 198;
    Creamy Dill Dressing, 64; Green Goddess
    Dressing, 87; Miso Dressing, 65; Pistachio
    Dressing, 203; Spirulina Dressing, 75;
    Thousand Island Dressing, 90, 156. See
    also salads; vinaigrettes
drinks. See beverages
Dr. Schulze's SuperFood, 17
dry roasting, 19
Duck Breast Cranberry Pear Chutney, 165

"eating healthy on a budget," 32
Egg Drop Soup, 236
eggplant: Lamb and Wild Mushroom Stuffed
    Eggplant, 176–77; Vegetable Napoleon,
    212–13
eggs: The Clean Niçoise, 78; description and
    recommended clean, 11; Egg Salad, 76;
    Egg-Stuffed Sweet Potatoes with Spinach
    Purée, 59; French Toast with Vanilla
    Cream, 48; The Perfect Hard-Boiled Egg,
    96; Roasted Asparagus with Poached Eggs,
    54; Salmon Scramble with Cauliflower
    and Dill Purée, 52; Scallion Pancakes, 57;
    Scrambled Eggs with Smoked Salmon, 55;
    Sunken Eggs, 53; Vegetable Frittata, 56
elixirs: description and recommended ingre-
    dients, 20–21; Healing Chocolate Elixir,
    262; Spring Dandelion Detox Elixir, 249
Everything Kale Salad, 69
Evezich, Maribeth, 286

farmers' markets, 79

Farmers' Market Salad, 79

fats. *See* oils and fats

Fedirko, Lina, 44

Feighan, Farrell, 276

fennel: Clean Kitchari, 211; Forever-Green Soup and Salad, 80; Heirloom Tomato, Fennel, and Avocado Pressed Salad, 74; Mustard-Baked Chicken, 159; Slow-Cooked Chicken with Fennel and Wild Mushrooms, 161; Smoked Salmon and Fennel Salad, 81

fermented foods, 100

fish: Charred Lemon-Broiled Sole, 135; The Clean Niçoise, 78; Coconut Fish Soup, 143; Coconut Poached Salmon, 136; Cod with Roasted Chili Peppers and Cayenne, 140, 141; description and recommended clean, 11; Dilly Salmon Salad, 139; Fish Tacos, 148; Harissa-Coated Haddock, 151; Lemon and Thyme Baked Sea Bass with Brussels Sprout Hash, 138–39; Maw Maw's Gumbo, 238; Oven-Baked Flounder with Garlic and Green Olives, 134; Oven-Roasted Cod, 152; Pan-Roasted Halibut with Artichoke and Celery Salad and Lavender Vinaigrette, 137; Poached Cod with Soba Noodles and Ponzu Sauce, 146–47; Salmon Scramble with Cauliflower and Dill Purée, 52; Salmon Stir-Fry, 150; Sardines on Endives, 109; Scrambled Eggs with Smoked Salmon, 55; Smoked Salmon and Fennel Salad, 81; Spiced Salmon with Blueberry Vinaigrette, 149; Tuna Noodle Casserole, 153; Zucchini-Wrapped Whitefish with Chive Oil, 144

Food & Water Watch, 135

food information: phytonutrients, 26, 27; PUFAs (polyunsaturated fatty acids), 26–27

foods: fermented, 100; information role played by, 26–27; using local and seasonal, 61; toxic triggers, 25; wild, 67. *See also* clean eating

Forever-Green Soup and Salad, 80

Freezer Fudge, 282

French Toast with Vanilla Cream, 48

garbanzo beans: Roasted Cauliflower with a Middle Eastern Twist, 99; Vegetable Pakoras, 108

garlic: Garlic-Crusted Chicken, 162; Garlic Dipping Sauce, 106; Garlicky Greens, 114; Slow-Roasted Garlic, 113

Gazpacho, 239

Giglio, Frank: on cod as the perfect meal, 141; on cooking with herbs and spices, 168, 187, 223; on dairy, 86; on farmers' markets, 79; on fermented foods, 100; on five skills for thinking like a chef, 38–39; on flavored oils and vinegars, 145; on Food & Water Watch, 135; on gluten-free flours, 47; on his lifelong interest in cooking, 37–38; on honey, 280; on local and seasonal foods, 61; on making extra food to keep as snacks, 132; on preparing bitter greens, 71; recipes contributed by, 3, 5, 7; on root vegetables, 214; on saturated fats, 49; testimonial on the Clean program by, 44; on wild foods, 67

Gingered Beef Ramen, 185

Gingered Carrot Purée, 104

ginger health benefits, 14

Ginger Juice, 248

gluten: description and sources of the, 6; health benefits of removing from diet, 6–7; the problem with eating, 6

gluten-free flours: description and recommended clean, 13; Frank Giglio on using, 47

gluten sensitivity, 6

Gracy's Avocumber Rolls, 102

grains: description and recommended clean, 12; soaking, 19

Greek Quinoa with Hearts of Palm, 202

green bell peppers (Lentils Seasoned in Dominican Sofrito), 194

Green Goddess Dressing, 87

green powders, 15

Gut icon, 7

halibut: Pan-Roasted Halibut with Artichoke and Celery Salad and Lavender Vinaigrette, 137; Zucchini-Wrapped Whitefish with Chive Oil, 144

Harissa-Coated Haddock, 151
Harvest Soup with Pumpkin Miso, 240
Healing Chocolate Elixir, 262
HealthCorps, 99, 295
Hearty Winter Soup, 230
Heirloom Tomato, Fennel, and Avocado Pressed Salad, 74
herbal tea, 20
Herbed Buffalo Burgers, 187
herbs and spices: description and recommended clean, 13–14; Frank Giglio on cooking with, 168, 187, 223; infusions vs. decoctions of herbs, 20; Spice Rub for Moroccan Lamb Kebabs, 178; yerba maté, 16
Hibiscus Rose Splash, 252
Himalayan salt, 14, 15
honey: health benefits of, 280; Honey Pecan Balls, 280
Hyman, Mark, 140, 141

icons: Cleanse, 7; Gut, 7; Vegan, 7
infusions, 20

Jaminet, Paul, 181
Jaminet, Shou-Ching, 181
Junger, Grace, 102
Just Peachy, 259

kale: Chicken with Kale and Olives, 170; Everything Kale Salad, 69; Garlicky Greens, 114; Make Juice, Not War Green Juice, 250; Papa D's Fresh Fall Salad, 72–73; Scrambled Eggs with Smoked Salmon, 55; Sunken Eggs, 53; Vegetable Frittata, 56; White Bean and Kale Soup, 233
Karan, Donna, 80
kombucha, 16
Kronk, Brent, 112

lactose intolerance, 86
Lacy Potato Cakes, 58
lamb: Braised Lamb Shanks, 180; Coconut Zucchini Noodles and Spiced Meatballs, 184–85; Lamb and Wild Mushroom Stuffed Eggplant, 176–77; Moroccan Lamb Kebabs, 178–79; Pomegranate-Glazed Lamb Chops, 182; Roasted Lamb Loin with Mint Pesto, 183; Shepherd's Pie, 188–89
legumes: health benefits of, 12; soaking, 19. *See also* beans
Lemon Herb Chicken Burgers with Thousand Island Dressing, 156–57
Lemon Herb vinaigrette, 78
lemon juice (freshly squeezed), 17
Lemon and Thyme Baked Sea Bass with Brussels Sprout Hash, 138–39
Lemony Lentil Soup, 237
lentils: Hearty Winter Soup, 230; Lemony Lentil Soup, 237; Lentils Seasoned in Dominican Sofrito, 194; Savory Lentil Loaf, 218–19
liquid chlorophyll, 15
Living Raw Food (Melngailis), 74
lucuma powder, 17

maca powder, 16
Maine salt, 14
Make Juice, Not War Green Juice, 250
Malted Maca Milk Shake, 260
mango: Curried Coconut Chicken with Cucumber Mango Salad, 167; Mango Sauce, 148; Mango Slushie, 258
Marinated Carrot Ribbons, 101
Markle, Meghan, 93
Mashed Celery Root, 221
Mashed Root Vegetables, 188
master five meals, 30
Maw Maw's Gumbo, 238
mayonnaises: Aioli (Garlic Mayonnaise), 92; Cashew Mayo, 107; for Dilly Salmon Salad, 139; Mayonnaise, 91. *See also* sauces
meat dishes: Braised Lamb Shanks, 180; Cambridge Fried Rice, 181; clean meat recommendations, 11; Coconut Zucchini Noodles and Spiced Meatballs, 184–85; Gingered Beef Ramen, 185; Herbed Buffalo Burgers, 187; Lamb and Wild Mushroom Stuffed Eggplant, 176–77; Moroccan Lamb Kebabs, 178–79; Pomegranate-Glazed Lamb Chops, 182; Roasted Lamb Loin with Mint Pesto, 183; Shepherd's Pie, 188–89; Spaghetti and Meatballs with Thirty-Minute Marinara, 186

Mediterranean Rice Noodles, 200
Melngailis, Sarma, 74
Mexican Black Bean Salad, 82
Mexican Tostadas, 215
Minestrone, 228
Mini Raspberry and Coconut Cream
    Tarts, 274
Minted Pea and Asparagus Risotto, 222
Mint Pesto, 183
Minty Rice Dolmas with Garlic Dipping
    Sauce, 106
miso: Chicken and Wild Rice Soup, 242; Egg
    Drop Soup, 236; Forever-Green Soup and
    Salad, 80; Green Goddess Dressing, 87;
    Harvest Soup with Pumpkin Miso, 240;
    Roasted Beet Salad with Miso Dressing, 65
Moroccan Lamb Kebabs, 178–79
The Most Perfect Chicken Breast, 163
Mulligatawny Soup, 234
mushrooms: Cambridge Fried Rice, 181;
    Chile Rellenos Stuffed with Mushrooms,
    Sweet Potatoes, and Chipotle Cashew
    Crema, 204–5; Lamb and Wild Mushroom
    Stuffed Eggplant, 176–77; Mushroom
    Parsnip Stew, 231; Mushroom Risotto,
    220; Mushroom Stock, 227; Portobello
    Steaks with Mashed Celery Root, 221;
    Reishi Cappuccino, 253; Savory Lentil
    Loaf, 218–19; Slow-Cooked Chicken with
    Fennel and Wild Mushrooms, 161; Stuffed
    Mushrooms, 111; Tuna Noodle Casserole,
    153; Vegetable Napoleon, 212–13; Zesty
    Roasted Chicken Salad, 84
mustard: Mustard-Baked Chicken, 159;
    Mustard Vinaigrette, 66; Rosemary
    Mustard Marinade, 94; whole-grain, 15
Myers, Amy, 160

Nelson, Jenny, 50
nutritional yeast, 16
nuts: Argula and Pear Salad with Walnut
    Vinaigrette, 73; banana bread, 50;
    Blackberry Cobbler, 268; Buckwheat
    Granola, 42; Brazil Nut Pâté, 110; Clean
    Hot Cocoa, 263; Crunchy Maple Mesquite
    Walnuts, 132; description and recom-
    mended clean, 13; dry roasting, 19; soak-
    ing, 19; Walnut Sage Cream, 217. See also
    almonds; cashews; pecans
nut and seed oils, 13

oils and fats: description and recommended
    clean, 13; flavored oils, 145; Frank Giglio
    on saturated fats, 49; PUFAs (polyunsatu-
    rated fatty acids), 26–27; recommended
    elixir fats, 21
olive oil health benefits, 13, 17
olives: Chicken with Kale and Olives, 170;
    Greek Quinoa with Hearts of Palm, 202;
    Oven-Baked Flounder with Garlic and
    Green Olives, 134
Onion Soup, 229
Oven-Baked Flounder with Garlic and Green
    Olives, 134
Oven-Roasted Cod, 152
Oz, Lisa, 99, 295
Oz, Mehmet, 99, 295

Pan-Roasted Halibut with Artichoke and
    Celery Salad and Lavender Vinaigrette, 137
Papa D's Fresh Fall Salad, 72–73
parsnips: Mushroom Parsnip Stew, 231;
    Roasted Pears and Parsnips, 117; Roasted
    Vegetables with Silky Hummus, 213; Root
    Vegetable Hash, 60; Shepherd's Pie, 188–89
Peach Pie, 276–77
pears: Arugula and Pear Salad with Walnut
    Vinaigrette, 73; Bitter Greens and Herb
    Salad, 70; Duck Breast Cranberry Pear
    Chutney, 165; Roasted Pears with Date
    Caramel Sauce, 269; Roasted Pears and
    Parsnips, 117
peas: Confetti Vegetables with Spicy Sauce,
    209; Minted Pea and Asparagus Risotto, 222
pecans: Cashew Almond Nut Butter, 130;
    Honey Pecan Balls, 280; Spinach and
    Pecan Pesto, 119; Sweet and Spicy Squash
    and Apple Purée, 116. See also nuts
The Perfect Hard-Boiled Egg, 96
Perfect Health Diet (Jaminet and
    Jaminet), 181
persimmons, Arugula and Persimmon Salad
    with Pistachio Vinaigrette, 68
phytonutrients, 26, 27

Pickled Radishes, 100

pine nuts: Asparagus, Sorrel, and Chestnut Purée, 103; Cashew Cheese, 97; Marinated Carrot Ribbons, 101; Sour Cream, 98

pistachios: Clean Energy Bars, 270; Pistachio Dressing, 203; Pistachio Vinaigrette, 68

Poached Cod with Soba Noodles and Ponzu Sauce, 146–47

polyunsaturated fats, 13

pomegranates: Blackberry Pomegranate Mousse, 287; Pomegranate-Glazed Lamb Chops, 182

Ponzu Sauce, 146

Portobello Steaks with Mashed Celery Root, 221

potatoes: The Clean Niçoise, 78; Crispy Potato Wedges with Roasted Red Pepper and Cashew Mayo, 107; Lacy Potato Cakes, 58. *See also* sweet potatoes

potato flour, 13

poultry: Asian Lettuce Wraps, 112; Chicken and Broccoli Pad Thai, 158; Chicken with Kale and Olives, 170; Chicken Osso Bucco, 166; Chicken Paillard with Butternut Squash and Mustard Vinaigrette, 66–67; Chicken with Preserved Lemons and Fragrant Spices, 171; Chicken and Wild Rice Soup, 242; Chinese Chicken Salad, 83; Coconut Curry, 160; Crispy Roasted Chicken, 169; Curried Coconut Chicken with Cucumber Mango Salad, 167; Duck Breast Cranberry Pear Chutney, 165; Everything Kale Salad, 69; Garlic-Crusted Chicken, 162; Lemon Herb Chicken Burgers with Thousand Island Dressing, 156–57; Maw Maw's Gumbo, 238; The Most Perfect Chicken Breast, 163; Mulligatawny Soup, 234; Mustard-Baked Chicken, 159; Roasted Cauliflower and Chicken Sausage Casserole, 172–73; Shredded Chicken, 168; Slow-Cooked Chicken, 174; Slow-Cooked Chicken with Fennel and Wild Mushrooms, 161; Thai Marinated Turkey Breast, 164; Turkey Chili, 241; Zesty Roasted Chicken Salad, 84

produce: farmers' markets for buying, 79; recommendations for, 11. *See also* vegetables

PUFAs (polyunsaturated fatty acids), 26–27

Pumpkin Miso, 240

pumpkin seeds: Baked Spaghetti Squash with Autumn Pesto, 216; Clean Energy Bars, 270; Everything Kale Salad, 69; Farmers' Market Salad, 79; soaking, 19

quinoa: Blueberry Quinoa Cereal, 44; Everything Kale Salad, 69; Greek Quinoa with Hearts of Palm, 202; Quinoa with Celery and Apples, 195; Quinoa and Sugar Pumpkin Porridge, 43; Zesty Roasted Chicken Salad, 84

radishes (Pickled Radishes), 100

raspberries: Mini Raspberry and Coconut Cream Tarts, 274; Raspberry Lemon-Aide, 251

red bell peppers: Crispy Potato Wedges with Roasted Red Pepper and Cashew Mayo, 107; Lentils Seasoned in Dominican Sofrito, 194; Savory Stuffed Vegetables, 196; Slow-Cooked Chicken with Fennel and Wild Mushrooms, 161; South-of-the-Border Vegetable Millet, 201; Zucchini Manicotti, 197

Refresh Clean program: overview of the, 290; 7-Day Refresh Meal Plan, 293. *See also* Clean Cleanse program

Reishi Cappuccino, 253

Rejuvenating Eggnog, 255

rice: Cambridge Fried Rice, 181; Chicken and Wild Rice Soup, 242; Maw Maw's Gumbo, 238; Mushroom Risotto, 220; Savory Lentil Loaf, 218–19; Sushi Rice, 198; Wild Rice with Middle Eastern Flavors, 210

rice flour, 13

Roasted Asparagus with Poached Eggs, 54

Roasted Beet Carpaccio, 121

Roasted Beet Salad with Miso Dressing, 65

Roasted Cabbage with Chipotle and Caraway Sour Cream, 214

Roasted Cashew Currant Bark, 283

Roasted Cauliflower and Chicken Sausage Casserole, 172–73
Roasted Cauliflower with a Middle Eastern Twist, 99
Roasted Cauliflower with Pistachio Dressing, 203
Roasted Lamb Loin with Mint Pesto, 183
Roasted Pears with Date Caramel Sauce, 269
Roasted Pears and Parsnips, 117
Roasted Sweet Potato and Spinach Salad, 85
Roasted Vegetables with Silky Hummus, 213
Romaine and Sea Vegetable Salad with Creamy Dill Dressing, 64
Root Vegetable Hash, 60
root vegetables: Frank Giglio on cooking with, 214; Mashed Root Vegetables, 188. *See also specific root vegetable*
Rosemary Drop Biscuits, 129
Rosemary Garlic White Bean Dip, 122
Rosemary Mustard Marinade, 94

salads: Arugula and Pear Salad with Walnut Vinaigrette, 73; Arugula and Persimmon Salad with Pistachio Vinaigrette, 68; Bitter Greens and Herb Salad, 70; Chicken Paillard with Butternut Squash and Mustard Vinaigrette, 66–67; Chinese Chicken Salad, 83; Chunky Avocado Salad, 77; The Clean Niçoise, 78; Egg Salad, 76; Everything Kale Salad, 69; Farmers' Market Salad, 79; Forever-Green Soup and Salad, 80; Heirloom Tomato, Fennel, and Avocado Pressed Salad, 74; list of favorite toppings for, 16–17; Mexican Black Bean Salad, 82; Papa D's Fresh Fall Salad, 72–73; Roasted Beet Salad with Miso Dressing, 65; Roasted Sweet Potato and Spinach Salad, 85; Romaine and Sea Vegetable Salad with Creamy Dill Dressing, 64; Sesame Bok Choy Salad, 71; Spirulina Sprout Salad, 75; Zesty Roasted Chicken Salad, 84. *See also* dressings
salmon: The Clean Niçoise, 78; Coconut Fish Soup, 143; Coconut Poached Salmon, 136; description and recommended clean, 11; Dilly Salmon Salad, 139; Salmon Scramble with Cauliflower and Dill Purée, 52; Salmon Stir-Fry, 150; Scrambled Eggs with Smoked Salmon, 55; Smoked Salmon and Fennel Salad, 81; Spiced Salmon with Blueberry Vinaigrette, 149
salt, 14, 15
Sardines on Endives, 109
saturated fats, 49
sauces: Aioli (Garlic Mayonnaise), 92; Best Dip / Sauce / Salad Dressing Ever, 125; Clean and Green Guacamole, 123; Confetti Vegetables with Spicy Sauce, 209; Mango Sauce, 148; Mayonnaise, 91; Ponzu Sauce, 146; Rosemary Mustard Marinade, 94; Teriyaki Sauce (Kronk recipe), 112; Teriyaki Sauce (Whitley recipe), 89; Thai Dipping Sauce, 88; Tzatziki Sauce, 178, 179. *See also* dips; mayonnaises
Savory Lentil Loaf, 218–19
Savory Stuffed Vegetables, 196
Scallion Pancakes, 57
Scrambled Eggs with Smoked Salmon, 55
sea bass: Fish Tacos, 148; Lemon and Thyme Baked Sea Bass with Brussels Sprout Hash, 138–39
sea salt, 16
seaweed, 17
seeds: description and recommended clean, 13; dry roasting, 19; pumpkin, 19, 69, 79, 216, 270; soaking, 19. *See also* chia seeds; sesame seeds; sunflower seeds
Seereal Bars, 131
Sesame Bok Choy Salad, 71
Sesame Noodles, 193
sesame seeds: Asian-Inspired Chickpeas, 98; Asian Lettuce Wraps, 112; Chinese Chicken Salad, 83; as favorite salad topping, 17; Garlic Dipping Sauce, 106; Gingered Beef Ramen, 185; Poached Cod with Soba Noodles and Ponzu Sauce, 146; Salmon Stir-Fry, 150; Seereal Bars, 131; Sesame Bok Choy Salad, 71; Sesame Noodles, 193; soaking, 19; Wild Rice with Middle Eastern Flavors, 210. *See also* seeds
7-Day Refresh Meal Plan, 293
shakes. *See* beverages

338

Shepherd's Pie, 188–89

Shredded Chicken, 168

shrimp (Cambridge Fried Rice), 181

sides, starters, and snacks: Almond Poppy Seed Crackers, 128; Apple Onion Chutney, 126; Asian-Inspired Chickpeas, 98; Asian Lettuce Wraps, 112; Asparagus, Sorrel, and Chestnut Purée, 103; Best Dip / Sauce / Salad Dressing Ever, 125; Black Olive Tapenade, 120; Brazil Nut Pâté, 110; Butternut Squash Ragout, 115; Cashew Almond Nut Butter, 130; Cashew Cheese, 97; Clean and Green Guacamole, 123; Crispy Potato Wedges with Roasted Red Pepper and Cashew Mayo, 107; Garlicky Greens, 114; Gingered Carrot Purée, 104; Gracy's Avocumber Rolls, 102; Marinated Carrot Ribbons, 101; Minty Rice Dolmas with Garlic Dipping Sauce, 106; The Perfect Hard-Boiled Egg, 96; Pickled Radishes, 100; Roasted Beet Carpaccio, 121; Roasted Cauliflower with a Middle Eastern Twist, 99; Roasted Pears and Parsnips, 117; Rosemary Drop Biscuits, 129; Rosemary Garlic White Bean Dip, 122; Sardines on Endives, 109; Seereal Bars, 131; Slow-Roasted Garlic, 113; Slow-Roasted Tomatoes, 118; Snappy Crackers, 127; Sour Cream, 98; Spinach and Pecan Pesto, 119; Stuffed Mushrooms, 111; Sweet and Spicy Squash and Apple Purée, 116; Tomato Salsa, 124; Vegetable Pakoras, 108; Za'atar-Roasted Carrots, 105

Slow-Cooked Chicken, 174

Slow-Cooked Chicken with Fennel and Wild Mushrooms, 161

Slow-Roasted Garlic, 113

Slow-Roasted Tomatoes, 118

Smoked Salmon and Fennel Salad, 81

smoothies. See beverages

snacks. See sides, starters, and snacks

Snappy Crackers, 127

Snicker Bars, 278–79

soaking: beans, 19; chia seeds, 247

sole: Charred Lemon-Broiled Sole, 135; Oven-Baked Flounder with Garlic and Green Olives, 134

soups and stews: bone broths, 225; Broccoli Cheddar Soup, 244; Carrot, Cumin, and Cauliflower Soup, 232; Chicken Stock, 224; Chicken and Wild Rice Soup, 242; Chilled Cucumber Avocado Soup, 235; Coconut Fish Soup, 143; Egg Drop Soup, 236; Gazpacho, 239; Harvest Soup with Pumpkin Miso, 240; Hearty Winter Soup, 230; Lemony Lentil Soup, 237; Maw Maw's Gumbo, 238; Minestrone, 228; Mulligatawny Soup, 234; Mushroom Parsnip Stew, 231; Mushroom Stock, 227; Onion Soup, 229; Spicy Black Bean Soup, 243; Turkey Chili, 241; Vegetable Stock, 226; White Bean and Kale Soup, 233

Sour Cream, 98

South-of-the-Border Vegetable Millet, 201

Spaghetti and Meatballs with Thirty-Minute Marinara, 186

Spiced Salmon with Blueberry Vinaigrette, 149

Spice Rub (Moroccan Lamb Kebabs), 178

spices. See herbs and spices

Spicy Black Bean Soup, 243

Spicy Cashew Dip, 93

spinach: Asparagus, Sorrel, and Chestnut Purée, 103; Baked Spaghetti Squash with Autumn Pesto, 216; Egg-Stuffed Sweet Potatoes with Spinach Purée, 59; Forever-Green Soup and Salad, 80; Garlicky Greens, 114; Roasted Beet Carpaccio, 121; Roasted Sweet Potato and Spinach Salad, 85; Spinach Patties, 192; Spinach and Pecan Pesto, 119; Sunken Eggs, 53; Vegetable Frittata, 56

spirulina: as favorite salad topping, 16; Spirulina Sprout Salad, 75

Spring Dandelion Detox Elixir, 249

squash: Baked Spaghetti Squash with Autumn Pesto, 216; Butternut Squash Ragout, 115; Chicken Paillard with Butternut Squash and Mustard Vinaigrette, 66–67; Confetti Vegetables with Spicy Sauce, 209; Mexican Tostadas, 215; Summer Squash Puttanesca, 208; Sweet and Spicy Squash and Apple Purée, 116; Vegetable Frittata, 56; Vegetable Napoleon, 212–13 starches, 12–13

starters. *See* sides, starters, and snacks

Stuffed Mushrooms, 111

Summer Fruit Crêpes with Vanilla Cream, 272

Summer Squash Puttanesca, 208

sunflower seeds: Buckwheat Granola, 42; Chunky Avocado Salad, 77; Clean Energy Bars, 270; Everything Kale Salad, 69; Forever-Green Soup and Salad, 80; Savory Stuffed Vegetables, 196; Seereal Bars, 131; Snappy Crackers, 127; soaking, 19. *See also* seeds

Sunken Eggs, 53

Sushi Rice, 198

sweeteners: description and recommended clean, 14; honey health benefits as a, 280; recommended elixir, 21

sweet potatoes: Chile Rellenos Stuffed with Mushrooms, Sweet Potatoes, and Chipotle Cashew Crema, 204–5; Coconut Curry, 160; Egg-Stuffed Sweet Potatoes with Spinach Purée, 59; Lemony Lentil Soup, 237; Maw Maw's Gumbo, 238; Papa D's Fresh Fall Salad, 72–73; recommendations on how to use, 12–13; Roasted Sweet Potato and Spinach Salad, 85. *See also* potatoes

Sweet and Spicy Squash and Apple Purée, 116

tamari: Asian-Inspired Chickpeas, 98; Best Dip / Sauce / Salad Dressing Ever, 125; Chinese Chicken Salad, 83; Egg Drop Soup, 236; Mushroom Parsnip Stew, 231; Ponzu Sauce, 146; Roasted Beet Salad with Miso Dressing, 65; Rosemary Mustard Marinade, 94; Sesame Bok Choy Salad, 71; Teriyaki Sauce, 89

Teriyaki Sauce (Kronk recipe), 112

Teriyaki Sauce (Whitley recipe), 89

Thai Dipping Sauce, 88

Thai Marinated Turkey Breast, 164

Thousand Island Dressing, 90, 156

Tomato Basil Vinaigrette, 212–13

tomatoes: Chunky Avocado Salad, 77; Farmers' Market Salad, 79; Gazpacho, 239; Heirloom Tomato, Fennel, and Avocado Pressed Salad, 74; Maw Maw's Gumbo, 238; Mediterranean Rice Noodles, 200; Mexican Black Bean Salad, 82; Mulligatawny Soup, 234; Savory Stuffed Vegetables, 196; Slow-Roasted Tomatoes, 118; Stuffed Mushrooms, 111; Summer Squash Puttanesca, 208; Thousand Island Dressing, 90; Tomato Salsa, 124

toxic triggers, 25

Tuna Noodle Casserole, 153

Turkey Chili, 241

turkey. *See* poultry

Turmeric Almond Milk, 257

turmeric health benefits, 14

turnips: Baked Turnip Casserole with Walnut Sage Cream, 217; Root Vegetable Hash, 60

21-Day Clean Cleanse Meal Plan, 291

21-Day Clean Gut Meal Plan, 292

Tzatziki Sauce, 178, 179

Ultra Wellness Center, 140

Urban Zen Initiative, 80

Vegan icon, 7

Vegetable Frittata, 56

Vegetable Pakoras, 108

vegetables: Baked Spaghetti Squash with Autumn Pesto, 216; Baked Turnip Casserole with Walnut Sage Cream, 217; Chile Rellenos Stuffed with Mushrooms, Sweet Potatoes, and Chipotle Cashew Crema, 204–5; Clean Kitchari, 211; Clean Sushi, 198–99; Confetti Vegetables with Spicy Sauce, 209; Greek Quinoa with Hearts of Palm, 202; Lentils Seasoned in Dominican Sofrito, 194; Mashed Root Vegetables, 188; Mediterranean Rice Noodles, 200; Mexican Tostadas, 215; Minted Pea and Asparagus Risotto, 222; Mushroom Risotto, 220; Portobello Steaks with Mashed Celery Root, 221; Quinoa with Celery and Apples, 195; Roasted Cabbage with Chipotle and Caraway Sour Cream, 214; Roasted Cauliflower with Pistachio Dressing, 203; Roasted Vegetables with Silky Hummus, 213; Savory Lentil Loaf, 218–19; Savory Stuffed Vegetables, 196; Sesame Noodles,

vegetables *(continued)*
193; South-of-the-Border Vegetable
Millet, 201; Spinach Patties, 192; Summer
Squash Puttanesca, 208; Vegetable
Napoleon, 212–13; Vincent Appino's
Clean Brooklyn Sicilian Pizza Pie, 206;
Wild Rice with Middle Eastern Flavors,
210; Zucchini Manicotti, 197. *See also*
produce
Vegetable Stock, 226
vinaigrettes: Basil Vinaigrette, 86; Blueberry
Vinaigrette, 149; Lavender Vinaigrette,
137; Lemon Herb vinaigrette, 78; Mustard
Vinaigrette, 66; Pistachio Vinaigrette, 68;
for Sesame Noodles, 193; Tomato Basil
Vinaigrette, 212–13; Walnut Vinaigrette,
73. *See also* dressings
Vincent Appino's Clean Brooklyn Sicilian
Pizza Pie, 206
vinegars: apple cider, 17; balsamic, 15; fla-
vored, 145
Vitamin Angels, 295, 296
Vitamix, 17

walnuts: Apple Crisp (aka Miracle Crisp),
217; Arugula and Pear Salad with
Walnut Vinaigrette, 73; Crunchy Maple
Mesquite Walnuts, 132; Roasted Sweet

Potato and Spinach Salad, 85; Walnut
Sage Cream, 217
We Care Spa, 2
Weinberg, Janet Goldman, 172
wheat-free tamari, 15
White Bean and Kale Soup, 233
white beans (Rosemary Garlic White Bean
Dip), 122
Whitley, Lara, 89
Whole Foods Market, 31
whole-grain mustard, 15
wild foods, 67
Wild Rice with Middle Eastern Flavors, 210

xylitol chewing gum, 16

yerba maté, 16

Za'atar-Roasted Carrots, 105
Zesty Roasted Chicken Salad, 84
zucchini: Coconut Zucchini Noodles and
Spiced Meatballs, 184–85; Forever-Green
Soup and Salad, 80; Mexican Tostadas,
215; Turkey Chili, 241; Vegetable Frittata,
56; Vegetable Napoleon, 212–13; Vegetable
Pakoras, 108; Zucchini Manicotti, 197;
Zucchini-Wrapped Whitefish with Chive
Oil, 144

SCAN THIS CODE
WITH YOUR SMARTPHONE TO BE LINKED TO THE BONUS MATERIALS FOR

CLEAN EATS

on the Elixir website,
where you can also find information about other
healthy living books and related materials.

YOU CAN ALSO TEXT
CLEANEATS to READIT (732348)

to be sent a link to the Elixir website.

Also Available from
Dr. Alejandro Junger

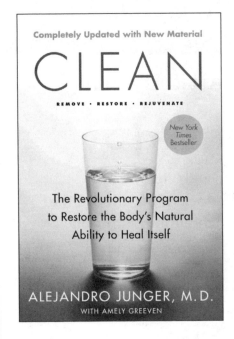

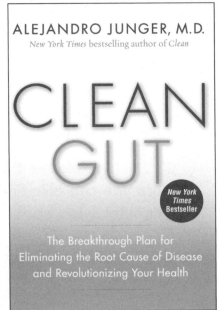

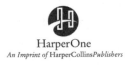

HarperOne
An Imprint of HarperCollinsPublishers